Pulmonary and Respiratory Diseases and Disorders

nova
Medicine & Health
New York

Pulmonary and Respiratory Diseases and Disorders

Interstitial Lung Disease: From Diagnosis to Treatment
Roberto G. Carbone, MD, FCCP,
Francesco Puppo, MD,
Keith Wille, MD, MSPH,
Pallav Shah, MD (Editors)
2022. ISBN: 978-1-68507-926-0 (Hardcover)
2022. ISBN: 979-8-88697-068-5 (eBook)

A Clinical Manual of Sarcoidosis
Vikas Pathak, MD,
Shambhu Aryal, MD (Editors)
2022. ISBN: 978-1-68507-681-8 (Hardcover)
2022. ISBN: 978-1-68507-782-2 (eBook)

Pulmonary Vascular Disorders
Francesco Puppo, MD,
Roberto G. Carbone, MD, FCCP,
Victor F. Tapson, MD, FCCP, FRCP (Editors)
2021. ISBN: 978-1-53619-458-6 (Hardcover)
2021. ISBN: 978-1-53619-553-8 (eBook)

Non-Invasive Mechanical Ventilation Complications: Essentials for Treatment and Prevention
Antonio M. Esquinas, M.D, Ph.D (Editor)
2021. ISBN: 978-1-53619-515-6 (Hardcover)
2021. ISBN: 978-1-53619-903-1 (eBook)

Practical Guide for Pulmonary Rehabilitation: The Essential Source for Pulmonary Rehabilitation Programs
Dr. Liana Pradan,
Florin Mihaltan,
Dr. Vishal Bansal (Editors)
2021. ISBN: 978-1-53619-045-8 (Hardcover)
2021. ISBN: 978-1-53619-125-7 (eBook)

More information about this series can be found at https://novapublishers.com/product-category/series/pulmonary-and-respiratory-diseases-and-disorders/

Jaber S. Alqahtani
Editor

Chronic Obstructive Pulmonary Disease

From Diagnosis to Treatment

nova
Medicine & Health
New York

DOI: 10.52305/SQCS9715.

NOTICE TO THE READER

Library of Congress Cataloging-in-Publication Data

ISBN: 979-8-88697-333-4

Published by Nova Science Publishers, Inc. † New York

Contents

Preface

Chronic obstructive pulmonary disease (often known as COPD) is a respiratory disease that affects more than 400 million people worldwide. In 2019, COPD was responsible for 3.23 million deaths globally. This makes COPD the third greatest cause of mortality worldwide. People with COPD frequently experience increasing levels of breathlessness as the disease advances. This can cause a significant financial burden due to the limitation of the workplace and home productivity, and costs of medical treatment. Therefore, delivering comprehensive management for people living with COPD is important to lessen such a burden. This book intends to provide comprehensive expert review chapters on the most significant aspects in the management of COPD from diagnosis to treatment through clear insights and explanations. It offers thorough evaluations that provide clinicians involved in COPD management at all levels with a brief, all-encompassing reference to symptoms, diagnosis, and treatment. This book covers four major areas in COPD management, including disease physiology and pathophysiology, diagnosis tools, disease burden, and management of stable and non-stable COPD.

Chapter 1 - Chronic Obstructive Pulmonary Disease (COPD) is one of the most common chronic diseases of the lungs; it is among the leading causes of death and health problems worldwide. The definition of the disease has been clearly presented in the current international guidelines, and early diagnosis and treatment of cases suffering from this disease help avert significant morbidities and ultimately mortality. Health expenditures allocated to this disease are ever-increasing worldwide, and this, in turn, leads countries to attach importance to awareness-raising efforts on its prevention and treatment. Annually, approximately 3 million people lose their lives due to COPD and the loss of Disability Adjusted Life Years (DALY) occurs in 29 million lives. In this section, the international definitions and epidemiological data of the disease will be discussed with current literature.

Chapter 2 - Chronic obstructive pulmonary disease (COPD) is a chronic, progressive and irreversible lung disorder. COPD is one of the leading causes of suffering and death in the world, affecting millions of people globally. It is not a curable disease, but it can be prevented with proper measures. Many factors contribute to the development or the worsening of COPD. The most commonly known risk factor is tobacco smoking, and long-term exposure has been shown to affect the lung parenchyma and the airways. In recent years it has been noted that a large number of patients develop COPD who have never smoked tobacco in their whole lives. Factors such as air pollution, genetics, age, gender, ethnicity, socioeconomic status, lung growth and exposure during childhood, and other diseases such as Asthma, tuberculosis, and Human Immunodeficiency Virus (HIV) infection also contribute to the development of COPD. It is essential for clinicians to know the factors that lead to COPD development to strategize ways to reduce the burden of the disease, lessen the suffering of patients, and understand and select the appropriate management plan. This chapter discusses all of these risk factors in detail.

Chapter 3 - Chronic obstructive pulmonary disease (COPD) is a group of diseases characterized by progressive irreversible airflow limitation. The major risk factor for developing COPD is smoking. The pathophysiology of COPD is not fully understood; however, the current hypothesis is that chronic exposure to tobacco or other noxious particles triggers the immune system leading to an extensive inflammation process. The inflammatory cell infiltration and the release of different cytokines result in pathological changes in airway epithelium, lung parenchyma, and blood vessel walls. These pathological changes result in increased mucus production, mucociliary dysfunction, airway narrowing, mucus plugging, airway fibrosis, and alveolar destruction. This leads to an increase in peripheral airway resistance and an increase in lung compliance, which affect ventilation/perfusion ratios and may lead to dynamic hyperinflation.

Chapter 4 - Chronic obstructive pulmonary disease (COPD) occurs alongside other chronic medical conditions called comorbidities. The most frequently occurring concomitant chronic diseases in individuals with COPD include cardiovascular disease, lung cancer, metabolic disorders, psychiatric disorders, skeletal muscle weakness, and osteoporosis. These comorbidities are associated with an increased risk of mortality, and they significantly contribute to morbidity and increased healthcare costs in individuals with COPD. The links between COPD and other chronic illnesses may be partially explained by shared risk factors, including smoking, physical inactivity, and advancing age; systemic inflammatory changes in COPD have also been linked to the development of comorbidities. Comorbidity prevalence does not necessarily correspond with lung disease severity, and the increased risk of various comorbidities is frequently independent of shared risk factors such as cigarette consumption. This chapter focuses on common comorbidities associated with COPD.

Chapter 5 - Mental health disabilities are among the most common comorbidities in patients with chronic obstructive pulmonary disease (COPD), with severe impacts on health, including functional disability, poor adherence to treatment, and increased risk of mortality. While international guidelines recommend identifying mental illnesses in COPD patients, assessing such comorbidities is not part of standard practice. Indeed, the current literature suggests that mental illness in COPD patients remains under-recognized, and thus many patients do not receive appropriate treatment. Several barriers have been proposed to the provision of treatment, including patients, physicians, and systems.

Early and accurate diagnosis of mental health facilitates the development of an appropriate treatment plan that meets patients' needs. Evidence regarding pharmacological interventions in patients with COPD remains limited. However, non-pharmacological interventions remain the first-line approach for managing mental health in patients. While there are also some promising findings on the effect of non-pharmacological interventions in alleviating mental health symptoms in patients with COPD, an integrated approach is recommended to improve clinical outcomes.

Chapter 6 - The importance of spirometry as a diagnostic tool in chronic obstructive pulmonary disease (COPD) has been addressed in the clinical practice guideline update from the American College of Physicians, American College of Chest Physicians, American Thoracic Society, and European Respiratory Society. The guideline update recommended that spirometry should be obtained to diagnose airflow obstruction in patients with respiratory symptoms and to screen for airflow obstruction in individuals without respiratory symptoms [1]. Therefore, it is essential that healthcare providers involved in managing COPD understand this physiological test, relevant measurements obtained from it, how to perform good quality tests and their value in diagnosing, monitoring, and assessing the severity of the disease. This chapter is intended to give an overview of all-important aspects related to spirometry.

Chapter 7 - Chronic obstructive pulmonary disease (COPD) is a complex disease with different clinical manifestations. Pulmonary diseases are usually assessed using physiological tests such as forced expiratory maneuver via spirometry. Indeed, spirometry is the most widely used physiological assessment for COPD. It is used in the diagnosis and monitoring of the disease progression or improvement. In clinical practice, the use of spirometry has some limitations, including being an effort-dependent test, and may not be tolerated in advanced disease stages or during exacerbations. Other physiological assessment modalities have been proposed to help in assessing airways diseases such as COPD. Unlike spirometry, body plethysmography is used in assessing lung volumes and airways resistance. Another method, oscillometry, soundwaves are used to obtain the impedance of the airways of which the resistance and reactance are obtained. In multiple and single breath washout tests, the exhaled gases fractions are used in determining lung volumes and ventilation heterogeneity. These modalities require minimal effort and may give more insights into the airways' conditions. In this chapter, the alternative physiological modalities (body plethysmography, oscillometry, and multiple/single breathe washout tests) will be explored and discussed to better understand their utility in clinical practice.

Chapter 8 - Chronic obstructive pulmonary disease (COPD) is a leading cause of morbidity and mortality worldwide. Raising awareness of COPD and early detection of the disease are recommended strategies to combat this important public health issue. COPD case-finding tools are promising useful alternatives to identify patients at-risk for COPD and refer to a confirmatory diagnosis and adequate early management favoring better clinical outcomes and prognosis. A simple, safe, feasible and accurate tool may be cost-effective to identify patients who require diagnostic spirometry. Questionnaires, peak expiratory flow (PEF) and a handheld micro-spirometer or a combination of them have emerged as COPD case-finding tools. Thus, the knowledge of these different approaches and their performances in different settings is essential for applications in clinical practice. However, there are some questions that are still unclear about the feasibility, effectiveness and long-term cost-effectiveness of COPD case-finding tools in health outcomes, in the primary care system and in different settings. In this chapter the authors will explore, in light of science, these alternative approaches and their evidence, challenges and future perspectives.

Chapter 9 - Tobacco smoking is the most common etiological factor in the development and progression of chronic obstructive pulmonary disease (COPD). Although most smokers with COPD are aware of the harmful effects of smoking, they continue to smoke, and those who quit smoking have a high risk of relapse. Smokers with COPD have a long and intense history of smoking and are highly attached to nicotine's rewarding effects. However, there are effective aids to assist smokers with COPD to quit, including pharmacotherapies and behavioral support. Indeed, smoking cessation was found to be the most effective intervention for slowing disease progression and improving lung function among smokers with COPD. Therefore, this chapter addresses smoking cessation in the management of stable COPD from different perspectives, including assessment, treatment, and prevention.

Chapter 10 - Pneumococcal vaccines have demonstrated substantial advancements in the treatment and prevention of invasive pneumococcal diseases. Both 13-valent pneumococcal conjugate vaccine and pneumococcal polysaccharide vaccine promote active immunization against the serotypes of pneumococcal bacteria. Inactivated influenza vaccines and live attenuated influenza vaccines are produced to protect against three different seasonal influenza viruses. The composition of both influenza vaccines is updated annually. Studies on the vaccine efficacy and effectiveness in COPD have revealed varied results. Since the beginning of the SARS-CoV-2 pandemic, different technologies were used for the development of SARS-CoV-2 vaccines that included weakened and inactive viruses, viral vectors, nucleic acids, and proteins. The efficacy and effectiveness of the various types of SARS-CoV-2 vaccines against infection are still under investigation which might largely depend on age, vaccine types, variants of the virus, and geographic region. The effectiveness and safety concerns for the related COPD vaccinations were discussed in this chapter.

Chapter 11 - Pulmonary rehabilitation (PR) is a multidisciplinary, patient-focused supplementary program for the treatment of patients with chronic obstructive pulmonary disease (COPD). This program is most suitable for patients with COPD because it involves thorough exercise training to strengthen their lungs and improve their breathing. A 4–12-week PR program with 2–3 supervised visits is effective in controlling dyspnea, tolerating exercise, improving mental health, achieving better Health-related quality of life (HRQOL), facilitating greater independence, reducing hospitalizations, and its consequent economic burden. Supplementation of the two major rehabilitation components—exercise and education—provides an added advantage by improving mental support.

Chapter 12 - Chronic Obstructive Pulmonary Disease is a condition of global proportions. This series of persistent respiratory illness may be common and treatable. However, the disease's progression, prevalence, and suddenness are significant points of concern as it ranks the fourth leading cause of death worldwide. Malnutrition of different forms persists and co-exists in COPD patients, further exacerbating the symptoms and leading to higher mortality. With the excessive production of Cytokines and a malnutrition-stricken body, consequences may include reduced exercise capacity, longer hospitalization, weaker body functions, and higher risk of mortality rate. Management of malnutrition included dietary advice and nutritional supplementation should be incorporated in COPD patients' management, aiming to stabilize body composition and improve functional status. Dietary advice allows for the intake of energy-dense or protein-rich foods that augments physical and weight development. Proper oral nutritional supplementation addresses malnutrition and improves the overall state of the body as it fills the gap in vitamins, amino acids, and the life necessary in maintaining the body.

Chapter 13 - Chronic obstructive pulmonary disease (COPD) is a serious chronic pulmonary illness that has a considerable impact on quality of life, health care utilization, comorbidity, and mortality. Limitation of the expiratory airflow is the fundamental pathophysiological feature of COPD, which limits the respiratory system's ability to breathe appropriately. Various societies have created disease severity classifications in order to predict and manage COPD patients. Lung function, patient-reported symptoms and the frequency of exacerbations are all factors in current classification scheme. Global Initiative for Chronic Obstructive Lung Disease (GOLD) classifies airflow limitation according to predicted values of the forced expiratory volume (FEV_1 %) into four stages, ranging from mild (GOLD1) to very severe (GOLD4). Despite the severity of COPD category, COPD patients are considered stable when their symptoms are well-managed and lung deterioration is minimal. This chapter will discuss the recent approaches to oxygen therapy and ventilatory support for stable COPD patients.

Chapter 14 - Chronic obstructive pulmonary disease (COPD) patients face a severe challenge regarding their quality of life. Pharmacotherapy, rehabilitation, and smoking cessation form important pillars of controlling the disease. But at times, despite these efforts, the patients are not optimized to lead a comfortable, independent life. Interventions, in the form of bronchoscopic and surgical procedures to change the course of the disease, come into the picture at this point. Bronchoscopic interventions include various methods to reduce the lung volume like valves, coils, and vapor ablation. Surgical procedures range from a bullectomy to the ultimate step of lung transplantation. While surgical procedures have inherent perioperative morbidity and mortality risks, bronchoscopic procedures also carry the risks of infection, pneumothoraces, and procedural failures. The cost of these interventions is another vital dimension of the decision-making process of management. Thereby, choosing the appropriate intervention for a patient and for a budding interventionalist, choosing the appropriate patient for intervention, are key to successful management. This chapter attempts to provide evidence-based answers to basic questions like what the options for intervention are, when one should intervene and what are the challenges before and after such an intervention in a patient with stable COPD.

Chapter 15 - Chronic obstructive pulmonary disease (COPD) is a common cause of morbidity and mortality worldwide, and its burden is expected to increase over the next decade. Proper management of COPD symptoms is vital for preventing disease progression and improving outcomes, particularly minimizing the risk of COPD exacerbation. Although non-pharmacologic management approaches are valuable and should be employed alongside pharmacologic management, this chapter focuses mainly on managing symptoms and dyspnea in patients with stable COPD using pharmacotherapy based on the best available evidence. Besides reviewing the current evidence of the value of using a pharmacologic approach (including bronchodilators and inhaled corticosteroids, either alone or in combination) to reduce the frequency and severity of COPD exacerbation and improve overall quality of life, this chapter discusses the potential of using a pharmacologic approach to improve the survival rate of patients with stable COPD.

Chapter 16 - Palliative and end-of-life care focuses on preventing and alleviating suffering through early identification, assessment and treatment of all physical, psychosocial and spiritual issues that affect the patient and their families. Chronic obstructive pulmonary disease (COPD) is characterized as a chronic and progressive disorder that, in its advanced stages, can be associated with significant physical, psychological and social damage. Patients with advanced COPD should receive palliative care to improve their quality of life and that of their families. A problem that makes care difficult is based on establishing a prognosis, making it necessary for the team to educate patients about palliative care, in addition to understanding and respecting their preferences. The end-of-life period for COPD patients is characterized by a progressive decline in health status, increasing symptoms, and greater dependence on family and caregivers to perform daily activities, such as personal hygiene and self-care. The role of palliative and end-of-life care must have an approach that focuses on managing symptoms, maintaining quality of life, and good communication between physician and patient, and family.

Chapter 17 - The treatment of chronic diseases needs patient's engagement to be successful, therefore, clinicians involved in the treatment of patients with chronic obstructive pulmonary disease must reserve time in medical appointments to teach self-management interventions and give patients trustworthy information about their disease. The ultimate goal of self-management strategies in COPD is to give the patients the knowledge and skills to cooperate with their health provider to improve disease control, improve quality of life and prevent exacerbations.

The self-management interventions include: education, the development of a COPD action plan, strategies for symptoms control, teaching adequate inhaler techniques, stimulating a healthy lifestyle and long term oxygen therapy use when required. The evidence that supports self-management strategies is controversial but it seems to improve health related quality of life and lower the risk of respiratory related hospital admissions. More evidence regarding the benefit of the specific interventions is required.

Chapter 18 - Aerosol delivery by pressurized metered-dose inhalers (pMDIs) and nebulizers attached by an adapter or spacer into a high flow nasal cannula (HFNC) system add great benefits in the management of obstructive lung disease patients. The inhaled medication, given during HFNC, offers better and quicker clinical effects than unassisted breathing. Unfortunately, there is no specific recommendation or guidelines to guide healthcare providers in their decisions while delivering aerosols through HFNC which puts the patients at risk of receiving either a sub-therapeutic or toxic dose of their inhaled medications. This increases the urgency for the development of recommendations or guidelines by a trusted board or society for aerosol delivery to such critically ill patients.

Chapter 19 - No single definition of acute (Chronic obstructive pulmonary disease) COPD exacerbation has been universally accepted. However, it can reasonably be defined as an acute change in a patient s initial shortness of breath, or sputum, that exceeds normal daily variability and needs a change in medication. The impact of exacerbations is significant and it may take several weeks for the patient s symptoms and lung function to return to baseline values. The most common causes of exacerbation are tracheobronchial tree infection and air pollution, but the cause of about a third of severe exacerbations cannot be determined. While managing the exacerbation of COPD with history, physical examination, laboratory, and imaging, alternative diagnoses that may be confused with the acute situation should also be kept in mind. Exacerbations significantly reduce the quality of life, deplete financial resources and accelerate a progressive decline in pulmonary function, causing frequent hospitalizations, relapses, and readmissions, contributing to death during or shortly after hospitalization. For this reason, patients should be made aware of exposure and should care about symptoms different from their current symptoms. It can also be controlled in the progression of the disease with the need for medical treatment support.

Chapter 20 - Chronic obstructive pulmonary disease (COPD) is widely prevalent in patients aged beyond the fourth decade across the globe. It has significant morbidity and impact on quality of life. Acute exacerbation of COPD (AECOPD) has even significant mortality if not detected and treated on time. It is characterized by the acute deterioration of the cough and shortness of breath, often requiring increasing medication and even emergency department visits and hospitalization. Multiple factors can predispose a COPD patient to AECOPD. Many cardiorespiratory conditions also co-exist and even mimic AECOPD when present as an isolated condition. These conditions need to be considered as differentials of AECOPD and managed accordingly. The present chapter briefly enumerates the differentials of AECOPD and puts forward a bedside algorithmic approach to reaching a differential diagnosis.

Chapter 21 - Although Chronic Obstructive Pulmonary Disease (COPD) is mainly a chronic disease, during its natural disease course, a significant number of patients suffer from COPD exacerbations, with consequences in terms of lower quality of life and higher morbidity and mortality rates in frequent exacerbators and particularly in severe exacerbations.

The most prevalent triggers for COPD exacerbations are airway infections (viruses and bacteria) and air pollution. Some risk factors like bronchiectasis, eosinophilia and frequent prior exacerbations are important predictors for exacerbations.

The pathophysiological hallmark of COPD exacerbation is increased airway inflammation, consequent expiratory flow limitation, reduced lung recoil pressure, and small airway obstruction. Thus, the ventilation (especially the expiratory time) is compromised, preventing end-expiratory lung volume from achieving natural relaxation volume at the end of a tidal expiration, leading to lung overinflation.

This chapter intends to give insight into relevant aspects of COPD exacerbations in terms of its pathophysiology to expand our understanding of the disease further and hopefully improve our clinical and therapeutic approach.

Chapter 22 - Chronic obstructive pulmonary disease (COPD) is the most common chronic lung disease in the world. Exacerbations of COPD determine disease-related morbidity, mortality, resource burden, and healthcare expenditures. Acute exacerbation care requirements extend from impulsive primary care visits to the emergency room to inpatient or intensive care admission, causing associated health burdens and mounting costs in COPD management. Recognition of COPD exacerbation in its emerging stages could potentially aid to prevent the rapid decline in lung function, perhaps the critical consequences if acted upon.

Chapter 23 - Chronic Obstructive Pulmonary Disease (COPD) exacerbations are frequently underdiagnosed as a significant part of patients do not seek medical attention to treat their symptoms. When medical intervention is required, it is crucial to define a plan and start treatment as soon as possible.

The authors should always start with assessing severity and defining the most appropriate treatment setting to decide whether the patient should be admitted to the hospital or if an ambulatory treatment is possible.

To delineate a good treatment strategy, it is important to determine the presence or absence of respiratory failure and infection and the coexistence of comorbidities. An appropriate antibiotic therapy considering local resistance patterns is required when an infection is suspected. In the presence of respiratory failure, the gas exchange must be guaranteed through the use of supplementary oxygen or high flow nasal therapy or ventilatory support, invasive or not invasive. The hallmark of treatment in every patient with an acute exacerbation of COPD is bronchodilators and systemic corticosteroids, as they help alleviate symptoms, shorten recovery time, and improve lung function (FEV_1) and hypoxemia and reduce the risk of early relapse, treatment failure, and length of hospital stay. After an exacerbation is appropriately managed, a suitable discharge plan should be prepared. This will depend on the severity of the exacerbation but should generally include reclassification of the patient according to the GOLD criteria, optimization of pharmacological treatment and reassessment of inhaler technique, and management of comorbidities. After discharge and during follow-up, it is also essential to reinforce smoking cessation and plan influenza and pneumococcal vaccination. Finally, end-of-life shared decisions should be faced with patients and familiars after resolving the exacerbated status, especially in subjects with advanced COPD.

Chapter 24 - Pulmonary rehabilitation (PR), including physical exercise as its main component, is an evidence-based strategy in the management of stable chronic obstructive pulmonary disease (COPD). However, in acute exacerbation of COPD (AECOPD), the indication of an exercise-based PR program is not a consensus, although growing evidence shows that the intervention is safe and leads to benefits in exercise capacity and health-related quality of life. In addition, the lack of practical guidance makes it a challenge to deliver PR during AECOPD, especially for hospitalized patients with severe symptoms. Similarly, to avoid the deleterious effects of immobility and physical inactivity, it is imperative to keep the patient active during hospitalization, as well as to establish safety criteria to mobilize this patient. However, in this context, there are some key questions to answer: 1) How to assess safety before mobilizing the hospitalized AECOPD patient? 2) What instruments and tests should be used to evaluate AECOPD inpatients before and after a PR program? 3) What does the evidence show about exercise prescription (type, frequency and intensity) as part of the PR program for this population? Considering this background and in light of scientific evidence, this chapter aims to address the role of exercise-based PR during AECOPD.

Chapter 25 - Acute exacerbation in chronic obstructive pulmonary disease (COPD) is characterized by an acute deterioration in respiratory symptoms that negatively impacts the disease progression, quality of life, and mortality. Self-management interventions in chronic illness such as COPD are intended to help individuals to better self-manage their condition and prevent exacerbation events. These self-management interventions have varied throughout the years from conventional interventions where patients received educational material and coaching to best manage their condition on their own, to tele-monitoring where patients record their health data automatically and transmit it to a healthcare provider via the web. This approach is anticipated to help patients and their healthcare providers detect early symptoms of acute exacerbation and intervene as early as possible to avoid deterioration and hospitalization, however, the efficacy of these interventions is still undetermined. In this paper, the authors reviewed the available evidence in the literature for conventional and telehealth interventions for self-management of acute exacerbation of COPD (AECOPD) to assess the clinical effectiveness of both approaches. The authors conducted a literature search on April 1st, 2022, using OVID Medline, PubMed, Cumulative Index to Nursing and Allied Health Literature (CINAHL), the Wiley Cochrane Library, and Google Scholar for articles published from January 2012 until April 2022. The authors included all study designs that investigated self-management interventions (conventional and telehealth) for AECOPD. Seven studies for the conventional intervention and eight study for the telehealth intervention met the criteria and were included in this review. The authors conclude that the consensus on which components of self-management interventions are still controversial. The telehealth intervention can be promising to achieve self-management of AECOPD, however the optimal solution requires integration of several elements along with the advanced technology such as personal skills, digital literacy, and availability of remote monitoring capabilities.

Chapter 26 - The application of digital health approaches in chronic obstructive pulmonary disease (COPD) management is increasing, providing considerable opportunities in helping with symptom management, reduce health resource utilisation, and improve health status. Optimisation the accessibility and quality of digital health approaches in COPD management requires the identification and integration of context, mechanism, and intended outcome. Current digital health solutions in COPD care vary in terms of context of application, mechanisms of impact, and intended outcomes/impacts. Context refers to the intervention settings which the digital health solutions are proposed, the components of those solutions, and the populations targeted. Digital health mechanisms of impact are shaped by factors such as content, mode of delivery, strategy, intensity, and level of professional support. Additionally, the consideration of other factors, including patient engagement and co-creation, are required for effective intervention development. Optimisation of implementation has four central determinants and consideration, namely patient needs, familiarity with the technology, healthcare professional support, and data privacy. Current research suggests digital health solutions for COPD can be improve symptom management, detecting exacerbations, and improving physical activity and quality of life.

Chapter 27 - Patients with asthma and chronic obstructive pulmonary disease (COPD) have been recognised as populations vulnerable to COVID-19 incidence and death. Because most COPD patients are old and have other comorbidities, those diagnosed with COVID-19 suffer worse outcomes, such as a greater rate of hospitalisation, admission to intensive care unit (ICU), and mortality. The COPD prevalence among COVID-19 patients varies by country, ranging from 0% to 14% worldwide, while data from ICUs range from 4% to 38%. Adults with COPD and asthma have greater rates of anxiety and depression symptoms, and they are more likely to seek medical treatment, putting them at risk for COVID-19 morbidity. It has been suggested to provide educational interventions for people with chronic respiratory diseases to aid them in symptom tracking, early diagnosis of COVID-19, and improved mental health support during the pandemic.

Chapter 28 - It is estimated that there are approximately 300 million cases of COPD worldwide, considering it a vulnerable population for the development, worsening of symptoms and greater complications in SARS-CoV2 infection. The suspected diagnosis, approach, treatment and follow-up of the population diagnosed with COPD and the development of COVID-19 represents a challenge for healthcare personal.

There is limited evidence whether COPD is an independent risk factor for the worsening of COVID-19, or whether the various comorbidities of patients with COPD determine a poor response to the SARS-CoV2 infection.

The authors present a brief summary of the main interventions carried out in the management of patients diagnosed with chronic obstructive pulmonary disease during the COVID-19 pandemic.

Chapter 1

Definition and Epidemiology of COPD

Ahmet Cemal Pazarlı[1,*] and Hakan Şıvgın[2]
[1]Gaziosmanpaşa University, Faculty of Medicine,
Department of Pulmonary Diseases, Tokat, Turkey
[2]Gaziosmanpaşa University, Faculty of Medicine,
Department of Internal Medicine, Tokat, Turkey

Abstract

Chronic Obstructive Pulmonary Disease (COPD) is one of the most common chronic diseases of the lungs; it is among the leading causes of death and health problems worldwide. The definition of the disease has been clearly presented in the current international guidelines, and early diagnosis and treatment of cases suffering from this disease help avert significant morbidities and ultimately mortality. Health expenditures allocated to this disease are ever-increasing worldwide, and this, in turn, leads countries to attach importance to awareness-raising efforts on its prevention and treatment. Annually, approximately 3 million people lose their lives due to COPD and the loss of Disability Adjusted Life Years (DALY) occurs in 29 million lives. In this section, the international definitions and epidemiological data of the disease will be discussed with current literature.

Keywords: chronic obstructive pulmonary disease, prevalence, incidence

Introduction

COPD is considered one of the leading causes of mortality and morbidity among chronic respiratory illnesses, affecting roughly 600 million people worldwide and causing around 3 million deaths each year. However, despite being an important public health problem all over the world, COPD is a disease that is not known enough by the public and physicians, is not sufficiently diagnosed and is usually mistreated. Definitions of the disease are available that have been made so far and published in international guides. The common consensus in these definitions is that smoking, which is the best-known risk factor for the disease, is held as one of the main causes of the disease. In the epidemiological studies that have been conducted on COPD until now, there is sufficient information about the incidence and prevalence of the

* Corresponding Author's Email: drcemalpazarli@gmail.com.

In: Chronic Obstructive Pulmonary Disease
Editor: Jaber S. Alqahtani
ISBN: 979-8-88697-333-4

disease. Through these epidemiological studies, knowing the actual number of patients exhibits the importance of the disease in terms of public health, as well as will help in the planning of health services aiming at diagnosis, preventive measures and treatment.

Definition of COPD

Until recently, COPD has been defined as a lung disease characterized by progressive and irreversible airflow limitation. However, lately, asserting that airflow limitation is associated with an abnormal inflammatory response, and even that it has systemic effects that are not limited to the lungs has led to a change in the definition of COPD. In the first international workshop, including 50 British chronic obstructive pulmonary disease specialists, organized on 24-26 September 1958 to clarify the potential uncertainties that hindered the formulation of a satisfactory classification system until that year, provisional definitions, classifications and terminology of COPD were explored. In this workshop, known as the CIBA Guest Symposium, the experts published a report of conclusions to compare the results of different assessment types with each other to determine their importance and validity, to encourage the use of defined terms when making pathological, clinical and functional assessments, and to investigate the reproducibility of these assessments in the hands of observers [1]. Nevertheless, it took almost forty-two years for the international respiratory community to implement and commence new actions and initiatives, and eventually towards the end of the 1990s, COPD was recognized as an important public health problem.

It was first stated by the organization, which was created by Romain Pauwels and the group of experts he worked with, by bringing together people interested in respiratory diseases, that it was time to make a great effort against this disease [2]. Suzanne S Hurd [3] encouraged the U.S. National Heart, Lung, and Blood Institute (NHLB) and the World Health Organization (WHO) to establish and develop a global think tank organization, which is known as the Global Initiative for Chronic Obstructive Lung Disease (GOLD). Although many definitions of this disease have been made so far by national, regional and even continental organizations, the definitions made by the Global Initiative for Chronic Obstructive Lung Disease (GOLD), the American Thoracic Society (ATS), and the European Respiratory Society (ERS) are those most widely used. In the first COPD definitions made in 1995, the ATS described COPD as the limitation of expiratory airflow depending on chronic bronchitis or emphysema, which is usually progressive, can be accompanied by airway sensitivity and be partially reversible [4], whereas it was reported by the ERS that it is the condition of decreased maximum expiratory flow and slow forced emptying of lungs, which progress slowly, and is mostly irreversible with current medical treatment [5]. The GOLD, on the other hand, defined COPD in 2001 as the disease state characterized by the limitation of airflow which is not completely reversible. According to this definition, the limitation of airflow is usually both progressive and associated with abnormal inflammatory response given by the lungs against harmful particles and gases [6].

The GOLD published the first guideline strategy report in 2001 and has updated its strategies at regular intervals every year since 2011. It published 2022 COPD guidelines at the end of 2021. In this last guide, based on the results of scientific studies conducted on COPD; it is defined as a common, preventable and treatable disease characterized by persistent airflow limitation and respiratory symptoms depending on airway and/or alveolar disruption, usually caused by severe exposure to harmful particles or gases, and by host factors, including abnormal lung development. In addition, the guideline has stated that serious comorbid conditions may influence morbidity and mortality [7].

Epidemiology of COPD

Epidemiology examines the frequency of any disease in the population. As a measure of this frequency, prevalence defines the proportion of the population with the disease investigated in a certain period of time, and incidence defines the proportion of newly diagnosed people in a certain period of time. In epidemiological studies, the factors that are associated with disease prevalence and development and play a role in the etiology are identified, screening initiatives proposed for early diagnosis as well as drugs and interventions recommended in treatment are investigated. The prevalence of COPD varies between 0.2-37%. The reason for this wide range is that COPD diagnosis and classification methods show a great variation between countries and populations [8]. Considering the data of 29 countries in the "Burden of Obstructive Lung Disease (BOLD)" study conducted using the standard methodology, it was estimated that the number of COPD cases in 2010 was 384 million and the global prevalence was 11.7% [9]. Despite different prevalence studies, it has been reported that there were 544 million cases of chronic respiratory diseases worldwide in which the burden of COPD accounts for 55.1% of cases in males and 54.8% in females [10], and that COPD, the third leading cause of death worldwide after ischemic heart disease and neoplasms, caused 3.23 million deaths in 2019 [11].

A 2018 study by the American Lung Association indicated that 6.6% of 16.4 million adults were diagnosed with any type of COPD (chronic bronchitis, emphysema, or COPD) and that the number and proportion of people with any type of COPD have remained relatively stable from 2014 to 2017 before increasing in 2018. Nevertheless, it varies from country to country and the death rate per 100,000 population has been reported to be less than 20 in Sweden, Iceland and Norway, but more than 80 in Ukraine and Romania [12]. The prevalence of COPD is known to be higher in males than in females. Besides, all studies indicate that the prevalence clearly increases with age. The prevalence of COPD goes up to about 20% in males and 15% in females in people aged over 70 years [13]. In the 2007–2012 self-reported prevalence study associated with chronic obstructive pulmonary disease, the National Health and Nutrition Examination Survey reported that 5.2% of US adults aged 40-79 years were diagnosed with COPD [14]. Finally, it is estimated based on the GOLD 2020 report that the prevalence of COPD will continue to increase in the next 40 years and associated deaths will reach 5.4 million in 2060 [15].

Incidence

Various incidence studies conducted by many international researchers on COPD are available in the literature. According to the Rotterdam study, the overall incidence rate (IR) of COPD was 8.9/1,000 person-years (PY) with a 95% confidence interval (CI) of 8.4-9.4. The IR was higher in males and smokers. The proportion of female COPD patients without a history of smoking was 27.2%, while this proportion was 7.3% in males (13). Also, Marco et al., reported that the incidence rate of COPD was 2.8 cases/1,000/yr (95% CI: 2.3–3.3) in 2006, and that the incidence of COPD was high even in young adults (16). It is seen that the annual incidence of COPD patients in the respectable studies [13-19] range between 2.8 and 15.5 per 1,000 patients (Table 1).

Table 1. Incidence rate of COPD

Author	Year	Cohort size	Median follow-up period	Number of COPD cases	Age of patients (years)	Incidence rate (per 1,000 PY)
Terzikhan et al.	1989 -2009	14,926	10.7	1993	> 45	8.9
de Marco et al.	1991-2002	5,002	8.9	123	20–44	2.8
Afonso et al.	2000-2007	185,325	3.4	7308	> 40	2.92
Young et al.	2001-2006	6,517	4	329	40–69	15.5

Mortality

The number of patients who died from COPD have been increasing in the 20th century, although they vary between countries according to patients' demographic characteristics, smoking habits and living conditions. However, the increase in life expectancy and care services contributes to the increase in the incidence of patients with COPD, as in all chronic diseases. Studies investigating mortality rates related to COPD strive to draw attention to the increasing importance of the disease. Between 1990 and 2010, chronic obstructive pulmonary disease (COPD) has risen from the fourth most common cause of death worldwide to the third place. In 2010, 2.8 million people worldwide died due to COPD and there was a decreasing trend compared to previous years [19]. Globally, since 2006, modeled COPD death rates have decreased by 21% [20]. On the other hand, little is known still about the trends observed in COPD mortality in Latin America and more recently in Oceania and Europe. The importance of COPD is exacerbated by the increasing global burden of this disease with an estimated increase in mortality through 2060. According to the WHO report, the annual estimated number of mortality cases until 2030 is 4.5 million and over 5.4 million by 2060 [21].

Economic and Morbidity Burden

Chronic obstructive pulmonary disease (COPD) is a progressive and debilitating respiratory disease that affects millions of people worldwide, causing significant morbidity and mortality and a significant medical and financial burden. In a meta-analysis of 18 studies, it has been emphasized that the highest reported costs in COPD are due to hospitalizations and related pharmacological treatment, and the COPD patient profile is the main cause of lost productivity and indirect costs of disease due to early retirement [22]. In another systematic literature review on the economic burden of COPD; it has been emphasized that despite the availability of comprehensive guidelines in terms of effective treatments, the disease poses a significant economic burden to society and that more research is needed to provide cost-effective COPD management, improve treatments and alleviate budgetary pressures [23].

Conclusion

COPD is common, causes many deaths and limits the comfort of daily life. In the detection of patients with COPD, it is also an undeniable fact that performing objective spirometric measurements will reveal the true prevalence and incidence of the disease. In all countries, the use of COPD standard definitions by clinicians would be beneficial in the prevention and early treatment of this chronic respiratory disease-causing serious mortality and morbidity. In addition to the definitions of COPD, ongoing epidemiological studies are also highly important in terms of contributing to the reduction of the international health expenditure burden of the disease.

Key Points

- COPD is still one of the major chronic respiratory diseases worldwide.
- The disease is considered among the important causes of mortality and morbidity and continues to cause significant health costs.
- The availability of effective treatment guidelines for COPD contributes to disease management.
- The importance of epidemiological data on COPD will contribute to a clearer understanding of the disease and to take necessary precautions.
- It is obvious that the early diagnosis and treatment of the disease will make a positive contribution to reducing the burden of the disease. Therefore, national and international programs should be given importance to increase the awareness of the disease.

References

[1] Heard B E. Further observations on the pathology of pulmonary emphysema in chronic bronchitics. *Thorax* 1959;14:58-70.

[2] Pauwels R. Global initiative for chronic obstructive lung diseases (GOLD): time to act. *Eur. Respir. J.* 2001;18:901-2.

[3] Hurd S S, Lenfant C. COPD: good lung health is the key. *Lancet* 2005;366:1832- 4.

[4] American Thoracic Society. Standards for the diagnosis and care of patients with COPD. *Am. J. Respir. Crit. Care Med.* 1995;152:S77-S121.

[5] Siafakas N M, Vermeire P, Pride N B. Optimal assessment and management of COPD: European Respiratory Society Task Force. *Eur. Respir. J.* 1995;8:1398- 1420.

[6] World Health Organisation. *The GOLD Global Strategy for the Management and Prevention of COPD.* HHLBI/WHO Work Shop Report 2001.

[7] Global Initiative for Chronic Obstructive Lung Disease (GOLD). *Global Strategy for the Diagnosis, Management, and Prevention of Chronic Obstructive Pulmonary Disease 2021 Report.* http://goldcopd.org.

[8] Rycroft Catherine, Heyes, Lanza, and Karin. Epidemiology of chronic obstructive pulmonary disease: a literature review. *Int. J. Chron. Obstruct. Pulmon. Dis.* 2012;7:457-94. https://doi.org/10.2147/COPD.S32330.

[9] Burney P, Jithoo A, Kato B. Chronic obstructive pulmonary disease mortality and prevalence: the associations with smoking and poverty—a BOLD analysis. *Thorax* 2014;69:465-473.

[10] GBD Chronic Respiratory Disease Collaborators Prevalence and attributable health burden of chronic respiratory diseases, 1990–2017: A systematic analysis for the Global Burden of Disease Study. 2017. *Lancet Respir. Med.* 2020;8:585–596. https://www.doi.org/10.1016/S2213-2600(20)30105-3.

[11] World Health Organization. *Assessing National Capacity for the Prevention and Control of Noncommunicable Diseases: Report of the 2019 Global Survey*. Geneva: World Health Organization; 2020.

[12] Raherison C, Girodet P.O. Epidemiology of COPD. *Eur. Respir. Rev.* 2009;18:213–221. https://www.doi.org/10.1183/09059180.00003609.

[13] Terzikhan, Natalie, Katia M. C. Verhamme, Albert Hofman, Bruno H. Stricker, Guy G. Brusselle, and Lies Lahousse. Prevalence and incidence of COPD in smokers and non-smokers: the Rotterdam Study. *Eur. J. Epidemiol*. 2016;31(8):785-792. https://www.doi.org/10.1007/s10654-016-0132-z.

[14] Tilert Timothy, Ryne Paulose-Ram, Donna Howard, James Butler, Sunmin Lee, Min Qi Wang. Prevalence and factors associated with self-reported chronic obstructive pulmonary disease among adults aged 40-79: the National Health and Nutrition Examination Survey (NHANES) 2007-2012. *EC Pulmonol. Respir. Med.* 2018;7(9):650-662.

[15] Global Initiative for Chronic Obstructive Lung Disease (GOLD).*Global Strategy for the Diagnosis, Management, and Prevention of Chronic Obstructive Pulmonary Disease (2021 Report).* https://goldcopd.org/wp-content/uploads/2020/11/GOLD-Report-2021-v1.1.

[16] de Marco, R., Accordini, S., Cerveri, I., Corsico, A., Antó, J. M., Künzli, N., Janson, C., Sunyer, J., Jarvis, D., Chinn, S., Vermeire, P., Svanes, C., Ackermann-Liebrich, U., Gislason, T., Heinrich, J., Leynaert, B., Neukirch, F., Schouten, J. P., Wjst, M., & Burney, P. (2007).Incidence of chronic obstructive pulmonary disease in a cohort of young adults according to the presence of chronic cough and phlegm. *Am. J. Respir. Crit. Care Med.* 2007;175(1):32-9. https://www.doi.org/10.1164/rccm.200603-381OC.

[17] Afonso, A. S. M., Verhamme, K. M. C., Sturkenboom, M. C. J. M., & Brusselle, G. G. O. (2011). COPD in the general population: prevalence, incidence and survival. *Respir Med.* 2011;105(12):1872-84. https://www.doi.org/10.1016/j.rmed.2011.06.012.

[18] Leem Ah Young, Boram Park, Young Sam Kim, Ji Ye Jung, Sungho Won. Incidence and risk of chronic obstructive pulmonary disease in a Korean community-based cohort. *Int. J. Chron. Obstruct. Pulmon. Dis.* 2018;13:509-517. https://www.doi.org/10.2147/COPD.S148618.

[19] Burney Peter G J, Jaymini Patel, Roger Newson, Cosetta Minelli, Mohsen Naghavi. Global and regional trends in COPD mortality, 1990-2010. *Eur. Respir. J.* 2015;45(5):1239-47. https://www.doi.org/10.1183/09031936.00142414.

[20] GBD Causes of Death Collaborators. Global, regional, and national age-sex specific mortality for 264 causes of death, 1980–2016: a systematic analysis for the Global Burden of Disease Study 2016. *Lancet* 2017; 390: 1151–1210.

[21] World Health Organization. *Projections of Mortality and Causes of Death*, 2016 and 2060. https://www.who.int/healthinfo/global_burden_disease/projections/en/.

[22] Gutiérrez Villegas, C., Paz-Zulueta, M., Herrero-Montes, M., Parás-Bravo, P., & Madrazo Pérez, M. Cost analysis of chronic obstructive pulmonary disease (COPD): a systematic review. *Health Econ. Rev.* 2021;11(1):31. https://www.doi.org/10.1186/s13561-021-00329-9.

[23] Iheanacho I, Shiyuan Zhang, Denise King, Maria Rizzo, Afisi S Ismaila. Economic Burden of Chronic Obstructive Pulmonary Disease (COPD): A Systematic Literature Review. *Int. J. Chron. Obstruct. Pulmon. Dis.* 2020;15:439-460. https://www.doi.org/10.2147/COPD.S234942.

Chapter 2

Risk Factors for Developing COPD

Madhuragauri Shevade*, MS, RRT-NPS, PhD Scholar
Symbiosis Center for Research and Innovation,
Faculty of Health Sciences,
Symbiosis International (Deemed) University, Pune, India
Indian Association of Respiratory Care,
Manipal, Udipi, Karnataka, India

Abstract

Chronic obstructive pulmonary disease (COPD) is a chronic, progressive and irreversible lung disorder. COPD is one of the leading causes of suffering and death in the world, affecting millions of people globally. It is not a curable disease, but it can be prevented with proper measures. Many factors contribute to the development or the worsening of COPD. The most commonly known risk factor is tobacco smoking, and long-term exposure has been shown to affect the lung parenchyma and the airways. In recent years it has been noted that a large number of patients develop COPD who have never smoked tobacco in their whole lives. Factors such as air pollution, genetics, age, gender, ethnicity, socioeconomic status, lung growth and exposure during childhood, and other diseases such as Asthma, tuberculosis, and Human Immunodeficiency Virus (HIV) infection also contribute to the development of COPD. It is essential for clinicians to know the factors that lead to COPD development to strategize ways to reduce the burden of the disease, lessen the suffering of patients, and understand and select the appropriate management plan. This chapter discusses all of these risk factors in detail.

Keywords: COPD, risk factors, smoking, air pollution

Introduction

Chronic obstructive pulmonary disease (COPD) is a chronic, progressive and irreversible lung disorder. COPD is the third leading cause of suffering and death in the world [1]. COPD is preventable and manageable, yet it remains one of the leading causes of chronic suffering and death among patients. The disease progression often leads to poor quality of life and an early onset of death [3]. COPD also comes with comorbid conditions and problems associated with it.

---

* Corresponding Author's Email: madhuragauri@gmail.com.

In: Chronic Obstructive Pulmonary Disease
Editor: Jaber S. Alqahtani
ISBN: 979-8-88697-333-4

It primarily affects the smaller airways of the lungs and occurs due to toxic injury to the airways and lung parenchyma to harmful environmental substances. It is characterized by chronic respiratory symptoms and airflow limitations. Oxidative stress is the primary driver of damage that occurs in the airways and lung parenchyma [3]. The oxidants are present in the pollutants (tobacco smoke or biomass smoke, or occupational smoke) in large numbers. In addition, oxidants are also released from the inflammatory cells such as macrophages and neutrophils. The oxidative stress overpowers the antioxidant defense present in the lungs and causes extensive and chronic damage.

The causative factors of COPD are many and have been studied well. They are generally divided into smoking-related, which includes smoking tobacco in various forms, and non-smoking-related factors such as indoor-outdoor air pollution, genetics, and occupational exposures. Tobacco smoking is commonly regarded as a risk factor for the development of COPD. However, non-smoking-related risk factors have also been acknowledged recently as substantial contributors to disease burden. About 50% of COPD cases in the world have a non-smoking-related cause for development [2]. Millions of patients do not know that they have COPD, as many still remain undiagnosed or underdiagnosed. Due to limited resources, many hospitals and clinical setups are not equipped with the correct infrastructure to diagnose and manage patients with COPD. The large doctor-to-patient ratio remains a significant challenge to handle the patient load successfully.

To strategize ways to reduce the burden of the disease, lessen the suffering of patients, and understand and select the appropriate management plan, it is essential for clinicians to know the factors that lead to the development of COPD. This chapter discusses all of these risk factors in detail.

Risk Factors for Developing COPD

COPD is predominantly caused by insult to the airways and lung parenchyma when exposed to noxious gases and particles. However, other resultant factors such as genetics, environmental exposure, airway hyperresponsiveness, and poor lung growth during childhood also play an important role. The effect of these risk factors varies from person to person and is different based on geographical locations as well. Often there is chronic exposure to these factors. The risk factors for the development of COPD are given in Table 1.

Smoking-Related COPD

Smoking is the most commonly known cause of COPD. Smoking tobacco in different forms, such as cigarettes, bidi, hookah, etc., is detrimental and long-term exposure to the toxic gases and particles causes inflammation in the airways leading to respiratory limitation and the development of COPD. Chronic exposure to smoke damages the cilia, causes inflammation, and increases the likelihood of getting infections. The alveoli are also affected, causing a defect in the diffusion mechanism of the respiratory system. This leads to dyspnea and chronic cough. Not all patients who smoke develop COPD; however, 10%-25% of those who have COPD do so because of smoking [4].

Table 1. Risk factors for developing COPD

Smoking-related risk factors
Tobacco Smoking – Cigarette – Bidi or rolled cigarettes – Hookah or water pipe – Chillum – Cigar – Pipe – Electronic cigarettes or vaping
Non-Smoking related risk factors
Genetic (Alpha-1 Antitrypsin Deficiency)
Air Pollution – Indoor Air pollution. Biomass, coal, wood, mosquito coils – Outdoor Air pollution. Industries, fires, power plants, burning of trees and wood, and motor vehicles exhaust, crackers.
Exposure during childhood and impaired growth of the lungs
Occupational exposure – Leather tanning – Farming (Crop and animal) – Construction – Mining – Road Sweeping
Demographic Characteristics – Age – Gender – Ethnicity
Socioeconomic status
Asthma
Tuberculosis
Human Immunodeficiency Virus (HIV) infection

Exposure to harmful smoke could be in the form of first-hand or direct exposure through inhalation of the smoke, or it could be due to second-hand exposure where the patient is around those who smoke. Both first and second-hand exposure to tobacco smoke leads to 8 million deaths in the world [5]. Unfortunately, the majority of these users, about 1.2 billion, live in low-middle income countries (LMICs) [5].

Smoking various forms of tobacco is a major concern in the world due to its addictive properties. They contain nicotine which is highly addictive. In addition to nicotine, cigarettes contain 600 different ingredients that create 7000 toxic and carcinogenic chemicals having a direct impact on the lungs [6].

Other forms of tobacco smoking in the form of "Bidi," or an inexpensive cigarette made of rolled tobacco leaves and chillum pipe smoking, are more harmful than modern cigarette smoking. Further, smoking hookah or water pipes is dangerous as well. Research has shown that one session of hookah or waterpipe smoking is 4.7 times more puffs and 48.6 times the amount of smoke as compared to smoking cigarettes [7]. One puff of the water pipe is equivalent to twelve puffs of the cigarette [7].

Electronic cigarettes, or "vaping," is another form of smoking that increasingly being studied in the last few years. Electronic cigarettes are hand-held devices containing a cartridge that comprises chemicals that are heated and passed through a vaporizer to create the vapor of the chemical for inhalation. Although there is not enough data to show that vaping causes COPD, its damaging effects are now being studied and understood in depth. There are reports that suggest electronic cigarettes significantly increase the chances of development of Asthma and COPD [8]. However, more large-scale and long-term studies are needed on the association between the use of electronic cigarettes and COPD.

Smoking cessation is the most crucial step in the management of COPD. No matter how long the patient has smoked, smoking cessation at any point in time is beneficial. Lung function values gradually decline with aging in a normal healthy person or a person who is not susceptible to smoking. For those who smoke, lung function values decline rapidly, leading to COPD. When an individual stops smoking, the rate of decline of lung function reduces. If the same individual has quit smoking for a long time, the rate of decline in lung function may come close to that of a normal person. Hence it is crucial to understand the harm caused by smoking and the importance of smoking cessation.

Non-Smoking-Related COPD

As mentioned above, there are several non-smoking-related factors that cause COPD. About 50% of COPD cases in the world have a non-smoking-related risk factor [2]. The risk of developing COPD varies based on geographical locations and exposures [2]. Hence it is important to understand all the risk factors that could be generalizable to the entire world as well as specific to the represented region.

Genetic

Genes play a vital role in the occurrence of a lot of diseases. For COPD, it is the deficiency of Alpha -1 antitrypsin (A1AT). A1AT is a protease inhibitor produced by the Liver that inactivates elastase, thereby protecting the lungs from the damaging effects and loss of elasticity [9]. In patients who have a deficiency or an absence of A1AT, elastase breaks down elastin leading to damage to the lungs. The alveoli are affected, making the lungs emphysematous. Loss of elastin leads to inflammation and susceptibility to infections. Thus, the patient develops COPD with symptoms of dyspnea and chronic cough.

A1AT deficiency is not curable, which in combination with exposure to noxious gases could be detrimental and hence is considered a risk factor. Thus, it is crucial to test the patients for A1AT deficiency who have no history of exposure to smoke or other risk factors yet present with symptoms of COPD. Only a small number of populations are affected by it around the world.

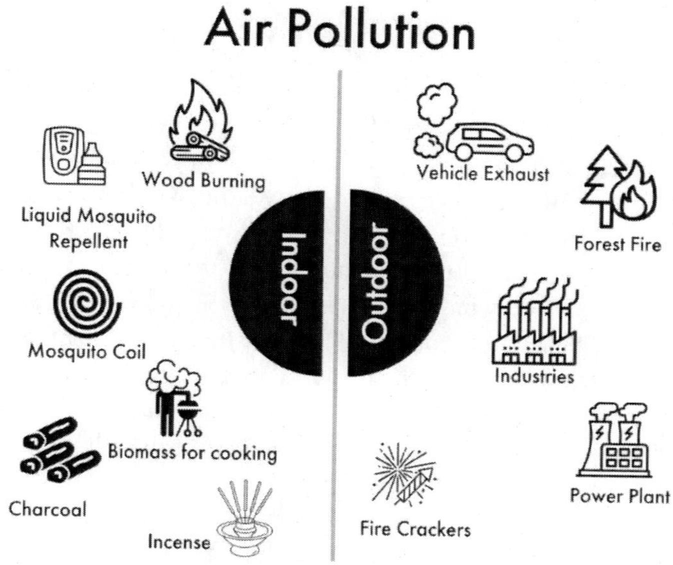

Figure 1. Types of indoor and outdoor air pollution.

Air Pollution

The increasing burden of air pollution has been an issue for healthcare systems across the world. Air pollution affects the majority of organs of the human body, including the heart, lungs, brain, urinary system, and digestive system [10]. It is a risk factor for developing various cardiopulmonary diseases, including COPD. Both indoor and outdoor air pollution contribute to the disease development and progression if exposure is not controlled (Figure 1).

The use of charcoal or biomass fuel for cooking is one of the most widely recognized non-smoking risk factors for COPD. About 2 billion Kg of biomass is burnt every day worldwide for cooking and other household activities [2]. Compared to the number of smokers in the world, a significantly higher number of people are exposed to high levels of biomass smoke pollutants [11]. This is because almost half the world's population (Asia, Africa, and South America) use biomass fuel for cooking and heating purposes. We can therefore argue that biomass smoke exposure is a more significant risk factor for COPD globally than tobacco smoking.

Biomass burning for cooking purposes is used by the majority of the homes in the LMICs [3]. Many women develop this COPD, and unfortunately, many of them are not aware that their disease is caused by this exposure to smoke. To take an example, an average Indian lady who cooks for the family spends anywhere between 2-8 hours in front of the fire. She ends up breathing a very large volume of highly polluted air during her lifetime. It is therefore not surprising that biomass smoke exposure then becomes a significant risk factor for COPD in the Indian population. Reduced exposure to the biomass smoke is, therefore, a crucial part of advice and treatment.

In tropical LMICs, with high incidences of malaria and dengue, the use of mosquito coils is prevalent. Unfortunately, in a room with doors and windows closed, burning mosquito coils produces very high levels of smoke and particulate matter pollution. Research shows that burning one mosquito coil for seven hours produces smoke that is equivalent to smoking 75-137 cigarettes [12]. *In-vivo* experiments have shown that the use of other mosquito repellents, such as liquid repellents, are equally harmful to the lungs as they too damage the lung and emit noxious substances into the environment [13].

Outdoor or ambient air pollution is a growing concern contributing to various respiratory diseases across the world. It contributes significantly to the worsening morbidity and mortality of chronic respiratory diseases [14]. Research suggests that long-term exposure to particulate matter and gaseous air pollutants can be a contributor to the development of COPD [14].

Particulate matter emitted by industries, fires, power plants, burning of trees and wood, and motor vehicles all contributes to air pollution [10]. The gaseous and particulate exhaust emitted by vehicles that run on diesel is one of the biggest contributors to pollution. Inhalation of these particles causes intense cellular and mediator airway inflammation. It may lead to worsening of asthma and COPD exacerbations [10]. It is also associated with the development of Lung Cancer.

In countries that allow the bursting of crackers or fireworks on festivals and holidays, people are impacted by an additional form of air pollution. These crackers emit many different types of harmful gaseous and particulate pollutants that give the cracker its color, sound, or visual appearance. These particles are of various sizes, small enough to affect the different parts of the lungs, including the small airways. Inhaling these affects the lungs, and patients present with various respiratory symptoms. It also leads to the development of or exacerbation of COPD [15].

Exposure during Childhood and Impaired Growth of the Lungs

Air pollution has an impact on the lungs of growing children [2]. The risk of development of COPD in adult life increases if the child is exposed to risk factors in utero with maternal smoking or at a young age of development. Children who spend significant amounts of time with their mothers are exposed to large amounts of biomass smoke pollutants and become more vulnerable to developing COPD later in life [2, 3, 11]. It increases the incidences of recurrent respiratory tract infections, and it also may give rise to Asthma or early COPD. Research indicates that other factors such as premature birth, low birth weight, poor nutrition, and socioeconomic status may be associated with the development of COPD later in life [2, 3, 11]. Large cohort studies reported that COPD patients who were non-smokers had a low baseline lung function; however, the rate of decline of FEV_1 was not rapid, and they attributed it to exposure during childhood and lungs that had not attained complete growth [16].

Occupational Exposure

Apart from the above-mentioned risk factors, certain occupations are also considered as a risk for the development of COPD in non-smokers [2]. Such patients with COPD have had long-term exposure to harmful particles, chemicals, and gases that result in damage to the lungs. Based on patients' personal history, it is always a good idea to understand the background well for a better treatment strategy.

Farming - either animal or crop farming, use of pesticides, mining industry, leather industry, and construction or road sweeping are all established risk factors for COPD. Occupational COPD is responsible for around 20% of all COPD cases and is due to chronic exposure to dust, smoke, and chemicals at workplaces [17]. Not only that, other sources like a persistent exposure to sensitizers (such as nanofibres, animal fur, etc.) may also contribute to allergic hyper-responsiveness, which, if untreated, may lead to COPD in the later stage of life. Organic solvents such as benzene and toluene also damage the alveolar parenchyma if used without proper protection. Continuous exposure to polluted workplace air (such as in leather industries where the air is not at all worthy of breathing) may also increase the risk of COPD.

Demographic Characteristics

Globally, higher age is associated with many chronic respiratory diseases [3, 18]. Due to the advancement in healthcare systems and technologies, people are living longer than they would have a few decades ago. COPD occurs after years of exposure to smoke or other pollutants. The symptoms start showing later in life, and the disease gets more common in patients who are older [3, 18]. Our lung function declines naturally with age, and when exposed to smoke and other pollutants, its rate of decline increases drastically. COPD is more commonly seen in women than in men, and the mortality is also high in women due to the disease and its complications [3, 18]. Lung function is diverse for populations of different countries. The Europeans tend to have a higher lung function when compared to that southeast Asians [19]. The susceptibility of these people also varies. Hence, there is a difference found in the prevalence of COPD in different races and ethnicities [20].

Socioeconomic Status

Low socioeconomic status is associated with the development of COPD [2]. Research indicates that a low household income, low educational level, and the type of residence, especially in the rural area, was associated with a higher prevalence of COPD [2]. Perhaps this is because of the use of smoke generating alternative cooking fuels or biomass, higher exposures to particulate matter, lack of ventilation in houses, lack of proper healthcare, dearth of awareness, and undernutrition [2].

Asthma

According to the latest GOLD guidelines, the presence of Asthma may be a risk factor for the development of COPD [3]. The report suggests that a patient with Asthma is 12 times more likely to develop COPD as compared to those who did not have Asthma [3]. Several other studies have also reported a high prevalence of Asthma in patients with COPD. The airflow limitation is consistent with both Asthma and COPD, and so are the risk factors. Under controlled Asthma and airway remodeling that is associated with it may be consistent with the development of COPD [2, 3].

Tuberculosis

Patients with a history of treated tuberculosis (TB) infection are at risk of developing COPD [2]. Post-infection, they develop airflow obstruction or restriction, which can be seen in the spirometry report. Patients who have had a Multidrug-resistant TB infection are at a higher risk of developing COPD because of greater lung damage during the infection phase. In countries that have a high prevalence of TB, the risk of developing COPD is high.

HIV Infection

Patients with human immunodeficiency virus (HIV) infection are at risk of developing COPD. Studies have shown that one in every ten people with HIV develops COPD [21]. In patients who have an HIV infection, the presence of low body weight, respiratory symptoms, and a history of TB was associated with the development of COPD [2]. The risk of COPD in HIV patients is further increased with a history of use of tobacco. A report suggests that the level of income of a country has an association with the incidence of COPD in HIV patients; the richer the country, the higher the incidence [22].

Conclusion

COPD is a chronic disease that is the third leading cause of death in the world. Although it is not curable, it is preventable if the correct steps are taken to avoid risk factors that lead to the disease. Tobacco smoking is the most commonly known risk factor, however, new information highlights the rise in the incidence of COPD due to factors not associated with smoking. Air pollution, genetics, impaired lung development, age, gender, ethnicity, and other diseases such as Asthma, HIV, and TB play an important role in the development of nonsmoking COPD. Considering the growing burden, it is important for clinicians to understand the disease process well and manage the patients optimally.

Key Points

- COPD is the third leading cause of suffering and death in the world with majority of the patients in LMICs.
- In various forms with high nicotine content, tobacco smoking is the most commonly known risk factor for COPD. Cigarettes, bidis, chillum, hookah are some of the typical methods of tobacco smoking.
- 50% of all the cases of COPD are due to a nonsmoking risk factor.
- Indoor and outdoor Air pollution in the form of biomass, vehicular exhaust, mosquito repellants, and industrial waste contribute significantly to the disease.
- Asthma, TB, and HIV can lead to the development of COPD.
- Childhood exposure to smoke and other noxious pollutants and impaired lung growth may lead to the development of COPD in the older age.

References

[1] World Health Organization. Global Health Estimates: Life expectancy and leading causes of death and disability [Internet]. *The Global Health Observatory*. 2022 [cited 2022 May 7]. Available from: https://www.who.int/data/gho/data/themes/mortality-and-global-health-estimates.

[2] Yang IA, Jenkins CR, Salvi SS. Chronic obstructive pulmonary disease in never-smokers: risk factors, pathogenesis, and implications for prevention and treatment. *Lancet Respir. Med.* [Internet]. 2022;2600(21):1-15. Available from: http://dx.doi.org/10.1016/S2213-2600(21)00506-3.

[3] GOLD. *Global Strategy for Prevention, Diagnosis and Management of COPD. 2022*. Last Accessed 7th May 2022.

[4] Duan, P., Wang, Y., Lin, R., Zeng, Y., Chen, C., Yang, L., Yue, M., Zhong, S., Wang, Y., & Zhang, Q. (2021). Impact of early life exposures on COPD in adulthood A systematic review and meta-analysis. *Respirology*. 2021;26(12):1131-51.

[5] World Health Organization. Tobacco [Internet]. *Fact Sheets. 2021* [cited 2022 May 7]. Available from: https://www.who.int/news-room/fact-sheets/detail/tobacco.

[6] American Lung Association. What's In a Cigarette? [Internet]. *Quit Smoking*. 2020 [cited 2022 May 7]. Available from: https://www.lung.org/quit-smoking/smoking-facts/whats-in-a-cigarette.

[7] Eissenberg T, Shihadeh A. Waterpipe tobacco and cigarette smoking: direct comparison of toxicant exposure. *Am. J. Prev. Med.* 2009 Dec;37(6):518-23.

[8] Osei AD, Mirbolouk M, Orimoloye OA, Dzaye O, Uddin SMI, Benjamin EJ, et al. Association Between E-Cigarette Use and Chronic Obstructive Pulmonary Disease by Smoking Status: Behavioral Risk Factor Surveillance System 2016 and 2017. *Am. J. Prev. Med.* 2020;58(3):336-42.

[9] Sandhaus, R. A., Turino, G., Brantly, M. L., Campos, M., Cross, C. E., Goodman, K., Hogarth, D. K., Knight, S. L., Stocks, J. M., Stoller, J. K., Strange, C., & Teckman, J. (2016). The Diagnosis and Management of Alpha-1 Antitrypsin Deficiency in the Adult. *Chronic Obstr. Pulm. Dis. J. COPD Found.* 2016;3(3):668-82.

[10] Jiang XQ, Mei XD, Feng D. Air pollution and chronic airway diseases: What should people know and do? *J. Thorac. Dis.* 2016;8(1):E31-40.

[11] Salvi S, Barnes P. Chronic obstructive pulmonary disease in non-smokers. *Lancet*. 2009;374(9691):733-43.

[12] Liu W, Zhang J, Hashim JH, Jalaludin J, Hashim Z, Goldstein BD. Mosquito coil emissions and health implications. *Environ. Health Perspect.* 2003;111(12):1454-60.

[13] Andini A, Hasanah M, Azizah SN, Rosyadahan AR, Rimasari D, Triapadma W, et al. The effect of insect repellent exposure on leukocyte profile and histopathologic findings in lungs. *Biointerface Res. Appl. Chem.* 2022;12(6):7796-803.

[14] Park J, Kim HJ, Lee CH, Lee CH, Lee HW. Impact of long-term exposure to ambient air pollution on the incidence of chronic obstructive pulmonary disease: A systematic review and meta-analysis. *Environ. Res.* [Internet]. 2021;194:110703. Available from: https://doi.org/10.1016/j.envres.2020.110703.

[15] Shah R, Sneha Limaye, Dhammasagar Ujagare, Sapna Madas, Salvi S. Personal exposures to particulate matter <2.5 μm in mass median aerodynamic diameter (PM2.5) pollution during the burning of six most commonly used firecrackers in India. *Lung India*. 2019;36(4):324-9.

[16] Gordon, S. B., Bruce, N. G., Grigg, J., Hibberd, P. L., Kurmi, O. P., Lam, K. H., Mortimer, K., Asante, K. P., Balakrishnan, K., Balmes, J., Bar-Zeev, N., Bates, M. N., Breysse, P. N., Buist, S., Chen, Z., Havens, D., Jack, D., Jindal, S., Kan, H., Martin, W. J. (2014). Respiratory risks from household air pollution in low and middle income countries. *Lancet Respir. Med.* [Internet]. 2014 Oct 1;2(10):823-60. Available from: https://doi.org/10.1016/S2213-2600(14)70168-7.

[17] Boschetto P, Quintavalle S, Miotto D, Lo Cascio N, Zeni E, Mapp CE. Chronic obstructive pulmonary disease (COPD) and occupational exposures. *J. Occup. Med. Toxicol.* 2006;1(1):1-6.

[18] MacNee W. Is chronic obstructive pulmonary disease an accelerated aging disease? *Ann. Am. Thorac. Soc.* 2016;13:S429-37.

[19] Duong, M., Islam, S., Rangarajan, S., Teo, K., O'Byrne, P. M., Schünemann, H. J., Igumbor, E., Chifamba, J., Liu, L., Li, W., Ismail, T., Shankar, K., Shahid, M., Vijayakumar, K., Yusuf, R., Zatonska,

K., Oguz, A., Rosengren, A., Heidari, H., Yusuf, S. (2013). Global differences in lung function by region (PURE): an international, community-based prospective study. *Lancet Respir. Med.* [Internet]. 2013 Oct 1 [cited 2018 Dec 27];1(8):5990609. Available from: http://www.ncbi.nlm.nih.gov/pubmed/24461663.

[20] Gilkes, A., Ashworth, M., Schofield, P., Harries, T. H., Durbaba, S., Weston, C., & White, P. (2016). Does COPD risk vary by ethnicity? A retrospective cross-sectional study. *Int. J. COPD*. 2016; 11(1):739-46.

[21] Alcorn K. Chronic obstructive pulmonary disease (COPD) increases the risk of heart attack in people with HIV [Internet]. *NAM aidsmap*. 2019 [cited 2022 May 7]. Available from: https://www.aidsmap.com/news/mar-2019/chronic-obstructive-pulmonary-disease-copd-increases-risk-heart-attack-people-hiv#:~:text=COPD is one of the,risk of suffering from COPD.

[22] Bigna JJ, Kenne AM, Asangbeh SL, Sibetcheu AT. Prevalence of chronic obstructive pulmonary disease in the global population with HIV: a systematic review and meta-analysis. *Lancet Glob. Heal.* [Internet]. 2018;6(2):e193-202. Available from: http://dx.doi.org/10.1016/S2214-109X(17)30451-5.

Chapter 3

Pathophysiology of COPD

Asma Falah Alharbi*, MSc

Department of Respiratory Care,
Prince Sultan Military College of Health Sciences,
Dammam, Saudi Arabia

Abstract

Chronic obstructive pulmonary disease (COPD) is a group of diseases characterized by progressive irreversible airflow limitation. The major risk factor for developing COPD is smoking. The pathophysiology of COPD is not fully understood; however, the current hypothesis is that chronic exposure to tobacco or other noxious particles triggers the immune system leading to an extensive inflammation process. The inflammatory cell infiltration and the release of different cytokines result in pathological changes in airway epithelium, lung parenchyma, and blood vessel walls. These pathological changes result in increased mucus production, mucociliary dysfunction, airway narrowing, mucus plugging, airway fibrosis, and alveolar destruction. This leads to an increase in peripheral airway resistance and an increase in lung compliance, which affect ventilation/perfusion ratios and may lead to dynamic hyperinflation.

Keywords: COPD pathophysiology, chronic bronchitis, emphysema, pulmonary mechanics, lung hyperinflation

Introduction

Chronic obstructive pulmonary disease (COPD) is a group of diseases characterized by airflow limitation that is usually progressive and irreversible [1, 2]. The disease affects different structures of the lungs which leads to abnormal lung mechanics [2]. Eventually, the disease may affect ventilation/perfusion ratios and increase the work of breathing [3].

Normal Airway Anatomy

The respiratory airways begin from the trachea which divides into two mainstem bronchi [4-6]. Each bronchus then divides into two smaller branchings; the continuous branching creates

* Corresponding Author's Email: asma@psmchs.edu.sa.

In: Chronic Obstructive Pulmonary Disease
Editor: Jaber S. Alqahtani
ISBN: 979-8-88697-333-4

the airway structure known as the tracheobronchial tree [4]. The tracheobronchial tree has a semi-dichotomous branching [5]. As the tracheobronchial tree continues to branch, the number of airways increases, and the airways' internal diameters decrease [2]. The branching continues to the level of gas exchange units or acini [4]. Each acinus arises from a single terminal bronchiole which then divides into respiratory bronchioles [2, 6]. At the level of respiratory bronchioles, alveoli begin to appear [2, 6].

Airways continue to branch and gradually become smaller in diameter. Small airways are defined as airways with an internal diameter of less than 2 mm [4]. Despite their small individual diameter, the cross-sectional area of the small airways is larger than the cross-sectional area of the trachea and larger airways [4]. Airways' cross-sectional areas increase gradually toward the gas exchange area. This increase is attributed to the rapid increase in the number of smaller airways with the continuous branching of the tracheobronchial tree [7].

Resistance to airflow is inversely related to the fourth power of the total cross-sectional area. Therefore, airway resistance decreases at the level of small airways [4]. The central conducting airways with an internal diameter of more than 2 mm account for 75% of the lower airway resistance, while smaller airways account for only 25% of the lower airway resistance [6]. When airway resistance is measured at the mouth, 50% of the airway resistance is attributed to the airways below the larynx, thus the small airways account for only 10-15% of the total airway resistance in healthy subjects [6].

Airway resistance and lung compliance determine the bulk gas movement between the atmosphere and the lungs [7]. The total resistance to airflow is a combination of the airways' resistance to airflow and the resistance to lungs and chest wall movement [7]. The airways are enlarged during inhalation due to the forces exerted by the inspiratory effort, which decreases the resistance to airflow [7]. Exhalation is a passive process that depends on the lungs' elastic recoil. During exhalation, the intrathoracic airways are compressed by the expiratory effort [7]. Therefore, airway resistance and lung compliance increase during exhalation due to the decrease in the lungs' elastic recoil and the decrease in intraparenchymal airway diameter [7].

The large proximal airway walls are composed of cartilage and smooth muscle [8]. The cartilage gradually decreases until it disappears at terminal bronchioles [8]; small airways contain no cartilage in their walls; hence they collapse easily [4]. Large proximal airway lumens are lined with ciliated pseudostratified columnar epithelial cells, goblet cells, and basal and club cells. Also, submucosal glands are extensively present beneath the epithelium of the large airways [7, 8]. Goblet cells and submucosal glands produce mucus which along with the cilia create the mucociliary clearance system of the lungs. The ciliated cells and goblet cells gradually decrease in number until they disappear in smaller airways [7].

COPD Pathogenesis

COPD is a group of diseases characterized by gradually progressive irreversible airflow limitation. The airflow limitation is mainly due to the inflammatory response in airways to noxious gases or particles [1, 16]. Studies have shown that lung inflammation is present in all smokers; however, not all smokers develop COPD [6]. Therefore, smokers who develop COPD may have an abnormal immune response to noxious particles [3]. The abnormal inflammatory response leads to pathological changes in the lungs' parenchyma, airways wall, and vascular structure which result in the development of airflow limitation [2].

Immune Response

Long-term exposure to noxious gases or particles such as tobacco smoke triggers the innate and adaptive immune response [3, 11]. The innate immune system in the lungs includes airway mucociliary clearance that removes foreign particles from the respiratory system. The macrophage/monocyte system takes up deposited foreign particles from the bronchial and alveolar surfaces. Also, tight junctions connect lung epithelial cells which create a physical barrier between the tissue and the airspace inside the alveoli [6, 11]. The adaptive immune system includes cellular and hormonal immune components that have memory for the previous antigen that is inhaled or aspirated in the lungs [6, 11].

Normally an acute injury to the airways triggers a physiological process to control the injury site. The inflammatory process is then initiated by sending macrophages to the injury site. Macrophages protect the site against infection and clear the site of any debris that may result from dead tissue. These cells will leave the site before the fibroblast and fibrocyte are activated and migrate into the cells [7]. The fibroblast and fibrocyte create a scar in the injury site by remodeling collagenous and non-collagenous tissues. However, in repetitive injuries, such as exposure to tobacco smoke, the inflammatory process persists during the tissue remodeling which may increase the potential for an abnormal tissue repair process and abnormal scar tissue formation. This may lead to further injury and permanent remodeling of the tissue [7].

Atmospheric particles smaller than 2.5 μm in size can reach and deposit in the lower lung region [7]. These particles are removed by macrophages through the process of phagocytosis. This process induces a local and systemic inflammatory response, which leads to an increase in the cycling of leukocytes [7]. Alveolar macrophages and epithelial cells generate inflammatory mediators when exposed to atmospheric particles and cigarette smoke [7, 16]. Moreover, cigarette smoke induces the release of reactive oxygen species (ROS) by macrophages and neutrophils leading to the disruption of cellular membranes and the inactivation of receptors and enzymes [7, 16].

Moreover, inhalation of noxious gasses damages the epithelial wall leading to reduced mucociliary clearance and increased epithelial cell membrane permeability [7]. In bronchi, the goblet cell and squamous epithelial cells change in form, cilia decrease in number, and submucosal glands become hypertrophied. These changes lead to the production of a continuous layer of mucus covering the airway surface in patients with chronic bronchitis [7].

COPD Pathology

COPD includes three main pathological entities: chronic bronchitis, small airway disease, and emphysema [10]. Figure 1 shows a summary of the potential mechanisms that lead to the development of COPD entities.

Chronic Bronchitis

Chronic bronchitis is a condition associated with chronic cough and mucous production [6]. Patients are diagnosed with chronic bronchitis when they have "chronic cough and sputum production in most days of the month for at least three months in the last consecutive two years" [11, 12].

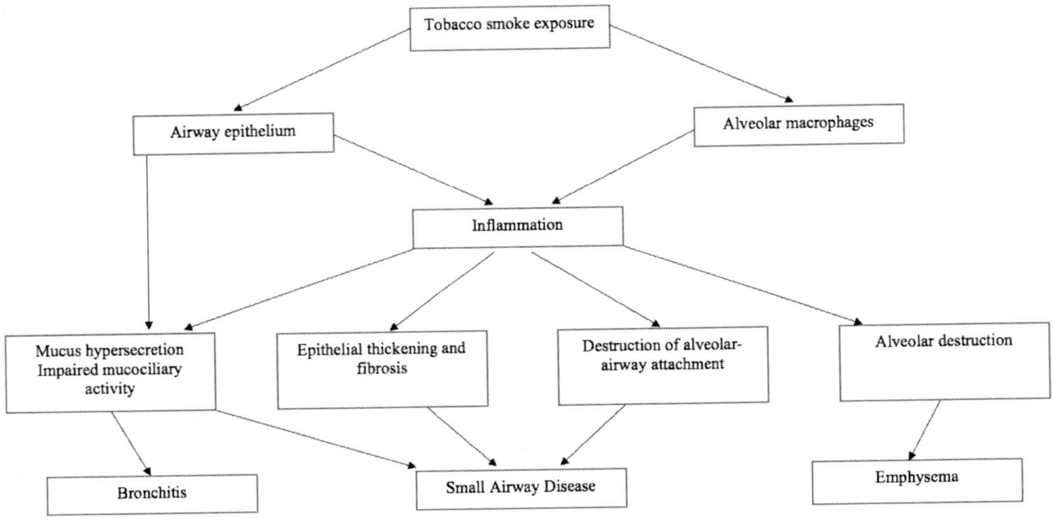

Figure 1. Summary of the potential mechanisms lead to different COPD entities.

Pathological Changes

The inflammation process triggered by exposure to atmospheric particles or tobacco smoke affects larger central cartilaginous airways (airways with a diameter larger than 4 mm). It affects the epithelial cells lining the central airway lumen and extends below to the mucus-producing glands [6, 11]. This inflammation process disrupts the innate and adaptive immune system [3], as described above. This results in an increased number of macrophages and T lymphocytes, enlargement of submucosal glands and goblet cell metaplasia, squamous epithelial cell metaplasia, ciliary clearance dysfunction, and smooth muscle and connective tissue hypertrophy [3, 6, 11]. These pathological changes lead to airway obstruction due to excessive mucus production and mucus plugging in small airways [6, 12]. Bronchial wall thickening is also associated with chronic bronchitis which can be related to the increased deposition of connective tissue [6]. Studies following bronchitis patients with normal pulmonary function have shown that not all patients progress to develop COPD.

Small Airways Disease

Small airways are those of internal diameters less than 2 mm. Airway remodeling and destruction in small airways is a result of an abnormal inflammatory response [2]. Lung exposure to foreign particles (mainly tobacco smoke) triggers the innate and adaptive immune response [3]. The main pathological changes in small airways are inflammation, epithelium damage, fibrosis, and loss of alveolar and bronchiole attachment, which all lead to airway narrowing [2, 17].

Inflammatory cell infiltration is present not only in small peripheral airways but also in central airways lumen, the lung parenchyma, and the adventitia of pulmonary vessels. There is evidence of an increase in the number of macrophages, T lymphocytes, and B lymphocytes in COPD patients. Also, the presence of lymphoid follicles, fibroblasts, and inflammatory exudates is observed in severe COPD. These inflammatory cells and the inflammatory mediators released by some of these cells have an important role in all pathological changes observed in small airways [3-5].

Pathological changes induced by smoking involve damaging the airway epithelium. Epithelium damage leads to squamous cells and goblet cell metaplasia [5, 7, 17]. The presence of goblet cells in small airways is usually rare; however, they pathologically extend in this area in patients with COPD. Moreover, cilia lining the airway walls may disappear, and the remaining cilia may become dysfunctional [7, 17]. Additionally, the composition of airway mucus in COPD patients changes to become viscous and difficult to clear. Increased production of abnormally viscous mucus and decreased airway clearance due to destruction of the airway epithelium and dysfunction of cilia lead to the accumulation of secretions in small airways [7]. This would initially narrow the small airways, then lead to airway obstruction [7]. Small airway mucus plugging is common in COPD patients [7]. Airway obstruction and accumulation of secretions may provide an opportunity for bacterial replication, which increases the possibility of infection [7].

Any increase in the layer between the airway lumen and the smooth airway muscle may decrease the airway caliber and increase airway resistance. Some of the cells participating in the immune response are located at the subepithelial level, which leads to increased airway thickening [6]. Also, smooth muscle hypertrophy is observed in COPD patients, which may be due to the direct effect of inflammatory mediators or due to increased muscle tone in these patients [5]. Moreover, the interaction between inflammatory cells and fibroblasts may lead to fibrotic remodeling of the airway wall [5]. Histological studies have shown evidence of inflammation and fibrosis in the peripheral airways in COPD patients. Moreover, deposition of connective tissue in the adventitia of airways in patients with advanced emphysema was observed in a study by Matsuba and Thurlbeck [6]. Thickening of the epithelium and the adventitia and smooth muscle hypertrophy leads to airway wall thickening and decrease airway caliber. This may be amplified by the contraction of the airway smooth muscle as a result of airway hyper-responsiveness that may be observed in COPD [5, 6].

The alveolar wall is directly attached to the adjacent small airway wall. These attachments between alveoli and small airways provide support to the small airways by providing a tethering effect that stabilizes and holds small airways open during exhalation [6]. Airway thickening due to inflammation, fibrosis, and muscle hypertrophy may facilitate alveolar wall detachment from airway walls [5]. Additionally, the inflammation process in the adventitia may destroy the alveolar attachment to the small airways, which may play a role in the obstruction of the small airways [5, 6].

All aforementioned pathological changes result in airway narrowing or even obstruction. Bronchograms of post-mortem lungs and histological studies have shown that smaller bronchi and bronchioles lumen become narrow and deformed in COPD [7]. Moreover, radiological studies demonstrated both narrowing and a decrease in the number of the small airways (peripheral and respiratory bronchioles), usually prior to emphysematous changes [2]. Airway obstruction is responsible for increasing airflow resistance, mainly in the peripheral airways in COPD patients. Although normally small airways account for the least airway resistance in the tracheobronchial tree, only 10% of the total airway resistance is attributed to small airways less than 2 mm in diameter [7]; these airways become the major site for airway resistance in COPD [6]. However, due to the large surface area at the level of small airways, airway resistance does not markedly increase until later in the disease progression [4]. Therefore, the disease can accumulate in the small airways (<2 mm internal diameter) for a long time before showing symptoms or causing a change in pulmonary function tests (PFT). Thus, these areas in the lungs are called the quiet zone [6, 7].

Emphysema

Emphysema is a pathological term [9] that is defined as "a condition of the lung characterized by permanent, abnormal enlargement of the respiratory airspaces, accompanied by destruction of their walls without obvious fibrosis" [2, 11]. It is also described as "dilation and destruction of the lung tissue beyond the terminal bronchiole" [6].

Pathogenesis

The theory of protease/antiprotease imbalance was classically used to describe emphysema pathogenesis [2]. Proteases including elastase are proteins produced by leukocytes and macrophages during an immune response to noxious gases or foreign particles. Elastase is capable of damaging elastin, connective tissue protein, and epithelial cells' basement membrane. However, normally elastase is counterbalanced by an elastase inhibitor namely, Alpha-1 antitrypsin (AAT) [9]. AAT is a protein produced by the liver to protect the lungs and other body tissue from damage produced by proteases that are released by the immune response. AAT deficiency was associated with the development of emphysema [9].

Although data suggest that tobacco smoke inactivates AAT, the protease/antiprotease theory does not explain smoking-induced emphysema completely. This leads to the current theory that emphysema can be related to the inflammation and tissue repair process. Alveolar macrophages are present in COPD abundantly and their presence has been correlated with tissue destruction in histological studies. Alveolar macrophages and neutrophils release metalloproteinase (MMP-12) and protease respectively, which have a role in elastin and collagen destruction. Following tissue destruction, the repair process should be initiated to restore the normal tissue structure. However, emphysema may develop due to failure of the repair process [9]

Pathological Changes

The main part of the lung that is involved in the pathological changes in emphysema is the acinus. Lung acinus is defined as a "lung unit supplied by one terminal bronchiole" [2]. The lung acinus is composed of respiratory bronchioles, alveolar ducts, alveolar sacs, and alveoli [9]. The lung acinus is the region of the lung where gas exchange between alveoli and capillary appears [9]. The emphysematous changes are described based on their histological appearance, and there are many forms of emphysema [9].

The main forms of emphysema are *centriacinar* and *panacinar* emphysema. The *centriacinar* or *centrilobular* type of emphysema is mostly associated with tobacco smoking and is usually located in the upper lung zones (proximal acinar emphysema) [2, 6]. It is characterized by dilation of the respiratory bronchiole and destruction of the adjacent airspace wall [2]. Airspace destruction involves respiratory bronchioles with relatively unchanged alveolar ducts and alveoli. Separate emphysematous lesions in the lungs may merge to produce one large cavity. The emphysematous lesion in this form of emphysema appears in the center of the acini, which generates the name centriacinar [6]. On the other hand, the *panacinar* or *panlobular* form of emphysema is usually associated with AAT deficiency [2] and is mostly located in the lower lung zone. It is characterized by a widespread dilation and destruction of the entire acinus [2, 6].

Either type of emphysema can be prominent in severe COPD; however, the centrilobular or centriacinar type is associated with more severe small airway obstruction. There is an evident relationship between smoking and the development of emphysema; however, only 40% of heavy smokers develop severe emphysema and only 15% develop airflow limitation. This indicates that emphysematous changes can be seen in patients before developing a decline in pulmonary function [6]. Airflow limitation in emphysema is mainly due to the loss of lung elastic recoil forces, which develop as a result of the destruction of the alveolar space and loss of lung surface area.

COPD Pathophysiology

Airflow Limitation

Airflow limitation in COPD is mainly due to increased airway resistance or loss of lung compliance as described above [11]. It affects the lungs' volume compartment and may lead to air-trapping and dynamic hyperinflation [13]. Figure 2 shows a comparison between normal lung volumes and lung volumes in COPD with air-trapping.

Lung Volumes

Airflow limitation due to airway obstruction or loss of the lungs' elastic recoil affects the lung volumes compartment. Functional residual capacity (FRC) is the volume of air that remains in the lungs after normal exhalation; it is determined by the balance between the elastic recoil of the lungs and the chest wall recoil [13]. The lungs recoil inward, and the chest wall recoils outward. When the lungs' elastic recoil and the chest wall recoil are equal and in opposite directions, the respiratory system is in equilibrium and the normal FRC is established. Thus, the loss of elastic recoil results in increased FRC, and a new equilibrium point is established. Moreover, severe airway obstruction may increase FRC; exhalation is a passive process that depends on the lungs' elastic recoil [13]. Airway obstruction increases the exhalation time required to reach the point of equilibrium. When the exhalation time exceeds the time between breaths, exhalation is interrupted by the initiation of the next breath before the exhaled volume is emptied completely. Thus, air remains in the lungs after normal exhalation increases.

However, FRC increases in emphysema more than in bronchitis; in bronchitis, the obstruction should be severe to increase FRC [13].

Residual volume (RV) is the volume of air that remains in the lungs after maximal exhalation; it is established at the point where the chest wall recoil limits the exhalation. At this point, all airways are almost closed, and the volume trapped in the lungs is the RV [13]. The loss of the lungs' elastic recoil and airway obstruction may lead to early closure of airways at higher lung volumes which increases the amount of air trapped at the end of maximum exhalation, thus increasing RV [13]. Increased RV is one of the earliest changes seen in PFT in patients with bronchitis. These changes may reflect the early closure in the airways at higher-than-normal lung volumes. This is mainly attributed to airway obstruction rather than loss of lung recoil, which remains normal in bronchitis [13].

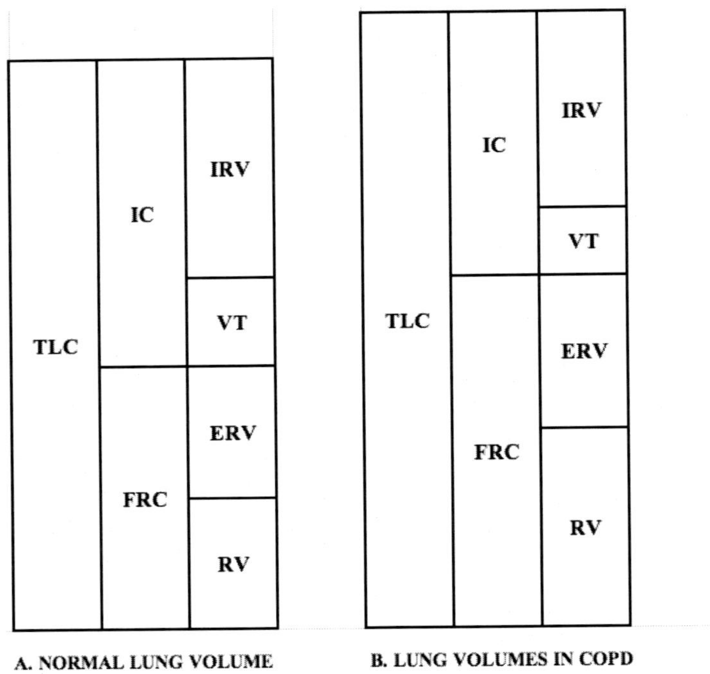

Figure 2. Comparison of the lungs compartment in normal lung and in COPD lung. (A) shows the normal lungs volume distribution. (B) shows the COPD lungs volume distribution; RV and FRC increase which compromise the VT and IC.
TLC: total lung capacity, IC: inspiratory capacity, FRC: functional residual capacity. IRV: inspiratory reserve capacity, VT: tidal volume, ERV: expiratory reserve volume, RV: residua; volume.

Total lung capacity (TLC) is the volume of air contained in the lungs after maximal inhalation; it is established when the inspiratory muscle strength is depleted to overcome the lung elastic recoil. Loss of elastic recoil allows the inspiratory muscle to stretch, further increasing the TLC [13]. However, this increase is limited because the inspiratory muscle stretch reaches a limit at high lung volumes. Airway obstruction without loss of lung recoil does not result in increased TLC. Therefore, emphysema may lead to hyperinflation as a result of increased FRC, and to a lesser extent TLC, and air trapping as a result of increased RV. At the same time, vital capacity (VC) is usually reduced because the increase in RV exceeds the increase in TLC. Bronchitis without emphysema may result in air trapping due to increased RV and normal TLC. Moreover, FRC may increase in cases of severe airway obstruction [13].

Air-Trapping and Hyperinflation

The changes in lung volumes as described previously results in establishing a new balance point (FRC), which is also known as end-expiratory lung volume (EELV). This volume is the baseline for normal tidal breathing (i.e., lung volume returns to this point after each breath) [14, 15]. Expiratory airflow limitation, either due to loss of elastic recoil or airway obstruction, increases EELV, which is dynamically determined and maintained. EELV fluctuates with changes in breathing pattern and effort; it is influenced by the time constant (a product of lung compliance and airway resistance), tidal volume, expiratory time, and respiratory frequency [14, 15]. As EELV increases in COPD patients, tidal breathing must be achieved at higher lung volumes near TLC. Lung compliance is low near TLC because most alveoli are already full and cannot distend further, which results in reduced ventilation. Breathing at higher EELV reduces the inspiratory reserve volume, limiting the expansion in tidal volume. This effect is amplified by any increases in respiratory frequency, such as during exercise. Respiratory frequency and tidal volume increase to meet increased metabolic demands due to exercise. Higher respiratory frequencies reduce the time between breaths, leading to less time for lung emptying. This may further increase EELV, which then further reduces ventilation. This process is known as dynamic hyperinflation (DH) and is responsible for exercise intolerance and dyspnea in COPD. Moreover, DH is believed to be one of the major mechanisms in the development of hypercapnia during exercise [14, 15].

Ventilation/Perfusion Ratio

The alveoli in the lungs fill and empty simultaneously. The speed of filling and emptying of the alveoli is the function of their time constant which reflects the speed of volume changes as a result of pressure change [13]. The time constant is defined as the time required by a lung unit to reach equilibrium after a change in pressure either during inhalation or exhalation (i.e., the time required by lung units to fill or empty). The time constant is the product of airway resistance and lung compliance of lung units (time constant = lung compliance X airway resistance) [7]. When airway resistance and lung compliance are low, the time constant is short. A short time constant means the alveoli change volume rapidly in response to a change in pressure. When airway resistance and lung compliance are high, the time constant is long. A long-time constant means the alveoli change volume slowly in response to a change in pressure [13].

Normally, time constant differences between various alveoli are not large enough to create asynchrony at normal physiological respiratory frequencies. However, in peripheral airway obstruction, the time constant varies significantly between alveoli. Alveoli with a long-time constant receive less ventilation than alveoli with a short time constant. This ventilation variation becomes more obvious with changes in respiratory frequency [13]. Higher respiratory frequency reduces the alveoli filling time, so the volume received by alveoli with a long-time constant is reduced. Alveoli receiving inadequate ventilation have higher PCO_2 and lower PO_2

than alveoli receiving normal ventilation. If perfusion remains equal in all alveoli, gas exchange will be impaired. In chronic bronchitis, gas exchange impairment and abnormal distribution of ventilation occur prior to the increase in airway resistance [13].

Time constant variation not only leads to receiving less volume by alveoli with a long time constant but may also lead to slow emptying of these alveoli. Alveoli with a slow emptying lag behind other alveoli. At the end of exhalation, these alveoli have different pressure than alveoli with intact airways. The pressure difference between adjacent alveoli results in gas flow through collateral channels [13]. Loss of lung elastic recoil due to alveolar destruction results in hyper-compliant airspaces. High compliance leads to a long time constant in these airspaces, which may lead to a time constant variation throughout the lungs. Emphysematous airspace will receive less ventilation than normal airspace leading to gas exchange impairment. However, alveolar wall destruction in emphysema may also destroy capillary beds, hence perfusion rate is reduced. Therefore, the gas exchange impairment is less significant in emphysema than in airway obstruction [13].

Pulmonary Hypertension

The vascular system in the lungs is affected by the inflammation process that ensues after exposure to noxious particles. The pathological changes observed in small arteries and arterioles include thickening of the intima, deposition of elastin and collagen, endothelial dysfunction, and smooth muscle hypertrophy [2, 9]. These changes result in vessel lumen narrowing and reduced vessel distensibility [2]. These factors along with hypoxemia in severe COPD may lead to vasoconstriction that increases pulmonary vascular resistance. Eventually, pulmonary hypertension may develop as a result of increased pulmonary vascular resistance [2, 9].

Conclusion

COPD is a group of diseases that results from a wide variety of pathological changes due to abnormal inflammatory responses to tobacco exposure. The pathological changes include epithelial damage, mucus hypersecretion, mucociliary impairment, epithelial thickening and fibrosis, and alveolar destruction. These changes lead to abnormal lung mechanics; airway resistance increases due to mucus plugging, airway narrowing, and fibrosis, while lung compliance increases due to alveolar destruction. Airflow limitation is the main pathophysiological consequence of COPD and may reduce both inspiratory ventilation and expired volume. This may lead to ventilation impairment and increased work of breathing. If airflow limitation is severe, air-trapping and dynamic hyperinflation may develop.

Key Points

- Smoking is the main risk factor for COPD which triggers an inflammatory process. This inflammatory process results in epithelial damage, goblet cell metaplasia, enlargement of submucosal glands, and airway fibrosis.

- In bronchitis, goblet cells metaplasia, enlargement of submucosal glands, and damage to mucociliary function lead to increased production of mucus and impairment of secretion clearance which leads to airway narrowing.
- Small airway disease developed as a result of epithelial damage, thickening of airway walls, and loss of alveolar-to-airway attachment. All lead to airway narrowing and increased airway resistance.
- In emphysema, the inflammation process may lead to a protease/antiprotease imbalance that initiates alveolar damage and loss of alveolar space and capillary beds. This destruction leads to loss of lung elastic recoil and increases lung compliance.
- The main pathophysiological consequence of all COPD entities is airflow limitation, which leads to air-trapping and dynamic hyperinflation. This results in impaired ventilation, ventilation/perfusion mismatch, and increased work of breathing.

References

[1] Global strategy for the diagnosis, management, and prevention of COPD. Global Initiative for Chronic Obstructive Lung Disease (GOLD) Web site. https://goldcopd.org/2022-gold-reports-2/.

[2] Berg K, Wright JL. The Pathology of Chronic Obstructive Pulmonary Disease: Progress in the 20th and 21st Centuries. *Arch. Pathol. Lab. Med.* 2016 Dec;140(12):1423-1428. https://www.doi.org/10.5858/arpa.2015-0455-RS. PMID: 27922768.

[3] MacNee W. Pathology, pathogenesis, and pathophysiology *BMJ* 2006; 332 :1202 https://www.doi.org/10.1136/bmj. 332.7551.1202.

[4] Bonini M, Usmani OS. The role of the small airways in the pathophysiology of asthma and chronic obstructive pulmonary disease. *Ther. Adv. Respir. Dis.* 2015 Dec;9(6):281-93. https://www.doi.org/10.1177/1753465815588064. Epub 2015 Jun 2. PMID: 26037949.

[5] Baraldo S, Turato G, Saetta M. Pathophysiology of the small airways in chronic obstructive pulmonary disease. *Respiration.* 2012;84(2):89-97. https://doi.org/10.1159/000341382 .Epub 2012 Aug 6. PMID: 22868355.

[6] Hogg JC. Pathophysiology of airflow limitation in chronic obstructive pulmonary disease. *Lancet.* 2004 Aug 21-27;364(9435):709-21. https://doi.org/10.1016/S0140-6736(04)16900-6. PMID: 15325838.

[7] Hogg JC, Paré PD, Hackett TL. The Contribution of Small Airway Obstruction to the Pathogenesis of Chronic Obstructive Pulmonary Disease. *Physiol. Rev.* 2017 Apr;97(2):529-552. https://doi.org/10.1152/physrev.00025.2015. *Erratum in: Physiol. Rev.* 2018 Jul 1;98(3):1909. PMID: 28151425; PMCID: PMC6151481.

[8] Hyde DM, Hamid Q, Irvin CG. Anatomy, pathology, and physiology of the tracheobronchial tree: emphasis on the distal airways. *J. Allergy Clin. Immunol.* 2009 Dec;124(6 Suppl):S72-7. doi: http://doi.org/10.1016/j.jaci.2009.08.048. PMID: 19962039.

[9] Keller CA. Pathophysiology and classification of emphysema. *Chest Surg. Clin. N Am.* 2003 Nov;13(4):589-613. https://doi.org/10.1016/s1052-3359(03)00092-9. PMID: 14682597.

[10] Noujeim C, Bou-Khalil P. COPD updates: what's new in pathophysiology and management? *Expert Rev. Respir. Med.* 2013 Aug;7(4):429-37. https://doi.org/10.1586/17476348.2013.814392. PMID: 23 964630.

[11] Hogg JC, Timens W. The pathology of chronic obstructive pulmonary disease. *Annu. Rev. Pathol.* 2009;4:435-59. https://doi.org/10.1146/annurev.pathol.4.110807.092145. PMID: 18954287.

[12] Kim V, Criner GJ. Chronic bronchitis and chronic obstructive pulmonary disease. *Am. J. Respir. Crit. Care Med.* 2013 Feb 1;187(3):228-37. https://doi.org/10.1164/rccm.201210-1843CI.Epub 2012 Nov 29. PMID: 23204254; PMCID: PMC4951627.

[13] Peter T. Macklem, The Pathophysiology of Chronic Bronchitis and Emphysema, *Medical Clinics of North America,* Volume 57, Issue 3, 1973, Pages 669-679, ISSN 0025-7125,

https://doi.org/10.1016/S0025-7125(16)32266-0. https://www.sciencedirect.com/science/article/pii/S0025712516322660.

[14] D. E. O'Donnell, P. Laveneziana. Physiology and consequences of lung hyperinflation in COPD. *European Respiratory Review* Dec 2006, 15 (100) 61-67; http://doi.org/10.1183/09059180.00010002.

[15] Puente-Maestu L, Stringer WW. Hyperinflation and its management in COPD. *Int. J. Chron. Obstruct. Pulmon. Dis.* 2006;1(4):381-400. https://doi.org/10.2147/copd.2006.1.4.381. PMID: 18044095; PMCID: PMC2707802.

[16] Rodrigues SO, Cunha CMCD, Soares GMV, Silva PL, Silva AR, Gonçalves-de-Albuquerque CF. Mechanisms, Pathophysiology and Currently Proposed Treatments of Chronic Obstructive Pulmonary Disease. *Pharmaceuticals* (Basel). 2021 Sep 26;14(10):979. http://doi.org/10.3390/ph14100979. PMID: 34681202; PMCID: PMC8539950.

[17] Martin C, Frija J, Burgel PR. Dysfunctional lung anatomy and small airways degeneration in COPD. *Int. J. Chron. Obstruct. Pulmon. Dis.* 2013;8:7-13. https://www.doi.org/10.2147/COPD.S28290. Epub 2013 Jan 4. PMID: 23319856; PMCID: PMC3540907.

Chapter 4

Comorbidity and COPD

Amal Al-Somali*, **MSc, RRT, RRT-NPS, RPFT**
Department of Respiratory Care,
Prince Sultan Military Collage of Health Sciences,
Dammam, Saudi Arabia

Abstract

Chronic obstructive pulmonary disease (COPD) occurs alongside other chronic medical conditions called comorbidities. The most frequently occurring concomitant chronic diseases in individuals with COPD include cardiovascular disease, lung cancer, metabolic disorders, psychiatric disorders, skeletal muscle weakness, and osteoporosis. These comorbidities are associated with an increased risk of mortality, and they significantly contribute to morbidity and increased healthcare costs in individuals with COPD. The links between COPD and other chronic illnesses may be partially explained by shared risk factors, including smoking, physical inactivity, and advancing age; systemic inflammatory changes in COPD have also been linked to the development of comorbidities. Comorbidity prevalence does not necessarily correspond with lung disease severity, and the increased risk of various comorbidities is frequently independent of shared risk factors such as cigarette consumption. This chapter focuses on common comorbidities associated with COPD.

Keywords: chronic obstructive pulmonary disease, comorbidity, inflammation, GOLD

Introduction

Chronic obstructive lung disease (COPD) is a serious chronic respiratory illness that is associated with increased mortality rates worldwide. COPD has become the third leading cause of death in the world where the number of deaths has exceeded 3 million per year worldwide [1, 2]. Comorbidity is defined as two or more diseases occurring in the same individual at the same time. Several comorbidities have been linked to COPD. Studies have shown that approximately 86% to 98% of patients with COPD have at least 1 one additional comorbidity with an average of 1.2–4.3 comorbidities per individual [3, 4]. The most prevalent

* Corresponding Author's Email: amalalsomali88@gmail.com.

In: Chronic Obstructive Pulmonary Disease
Editor: Jaber S. Alqahtani
ISBN: 979-8-88697-333-4

comorbidities associated with COPD are cardiovascular disease (CVD), metabolic disorders, anxiety, depression, skeletal muscle weakness, osteoporosis, and lung cancer [5].

When these comorbidities coexist with COPD they impose a negative impact on the prognosis and severity of COPD. The amount of daily physical activities appears to be significantly reduced by the presence of comorbidities, regardless of the type of illness and the degree of airflow limitation [4]. This would result in a declined health-related quality of life, increased mortality rates, and increased hospitalizations which puts a burden on health care systems [6]. The main risk factor for COPD is tobacco smoking; some other environmental exposures such as biomass fuel exposure and air pollution may also cause it. COPD, lung cancer, and cardiovascular disease all share a common risk factor: exposure to cigarette smoking. Other extrapulmonary comorbidities such as anxiety, depression, osteoporosis, metabolic syndrome (MetS), and Diabetes mellitus (DM), have no clear pathophysiological relationship with COPD but the main factor influencing their interaction with COPD are the inflammatory mediators in circulation that come along with chronic systemic inflammation. Increased prevalence of comorbidities among patients with COPD may have other contributing factors such as aging, inactivity, medication interaction, and polypharmacy. Comprehensive care for patients with COPD is needed as these comorbidities make the management of COPD challenging. They may affect patients with mild, moderate, or severe airflow limitation and independently impact death rates and hospitalizations [6]. Therefore, the Global Initiative for Chronic Obstructive Lung Disease (GOLD) in its latest report in 2022 stated that comorbidities should be identified and treated appropriately. Any patient with COPD must be assessed and evaluated for the presence of comorbidities; the goal of this assessment is to determine the risk of future death incidents and hospital admissions. However, the existence of comorbidities should not change COPD management and treatment plans and *vice versa* for comorbid diseases, the usual treatment standards should be followed irrespective of the presence of COPD [6].

Cardiovascular Disease

Cardiovascular disease (CVD) is the most frequent and important comorbidity that affects patients with COPD. Patients with COPD have a substantial risk of a wide range of concurrent cardiovascular diseases such as congestive heart failure (HF), coronary artery disease (CAD), pulmonary artery hypertension (PAH), and peripheral vascular disease. The two most common cardiovascular comorbidities are HF and CAD [7]. Two different cohort studies found that those with airflow obstruction among patients with GOLD grades 3 or 4 had a two-fold increased risk of developing CVD versus those without obstruction [7]. In some studies, the incidence of coronary heart disease among patients with COPD is estimated to be 22%–33.6%, while the prevalence of HF is 13.5%–24.4%. Where other studies have found significant variability in estimates of CVD prevalence, with coronary heart disease ranging from 4.7% to 60%, and HF ranging from 7.1% to 31.3% [7]. According to the GOLD report 2022, HF prevalence in patients with COPD ranges from 20% to 70% [6]. Also, in a large cohort of patients with various severity levels of COPD, 8.8% were diagnosed with peripheral artery disease (PAD), which was a greater frequency than among non-COPD controls (1.8%). Compared to those without PAD, patients with COPD and PAD reported a lower functional ability and health state [6]. CVD and COPD commonly coexist due to their shared risk factors, including aging, a history of cigarette smoking, systemic inflammation, and a sedentary lifestyle [8]. Epidemiological studies have also shown that individuals with COPD had a high rate of mortality from cardiovascular causes, indicating the high burden of concurrent cardiovascular illness in the COPD community. One COPD research study has shown that cardiovascular reasons were responsible for 27% of fatalities [3]. It has also been proven that cardiovascular disease is linked to worse quality of life and health status in patients with COPD, as well as dyspnea and exercise capacity. COPD-related hospitalization, as well as healthcare usage and expenses, have all been linked to CVD [3, 9].

Many processes are assumed to be involved and may interact to explain the link between COPD and CVD, although the exact mechanisms remain unknown. These include lung hyperinflation, hypoxemia, pulmonary hypertension (PH), systemic inflammation and oxidative stress, exacerbations, shared risk factors and genetics, and COPD phenotype as shown in Figure 1 [9].

Hyperinflation, which is characterized by unusually increased residual gas in the lungs after normal exhalation, is a key contributor to COPD burden and death. It is the primary pathophysiological mechanism affecting the mechanics of breathing and can be either *static,* resulting from destruction of lung parenchyma and loss of lung elastic recoil, or *dynamic,* occurring when a patient inhales before exhaling fully, trapping air with each additional breath. Hyperinflation impairs the efficacy of the respiratory muscles and is becoming recognized as a primary cause of dyspnea. Abnormal lung function, especially hyperinflation, may impair heart function. Lung hyperinflation can restrict airflow, causing higher pressure in the cardiopulmonary system, right ventricular dysfunction, poor left-ventricular filling, and reduced cardiac output. Emphysema causes static hyperinflation, which may be a risk factor for CVD in people with emphysema-predominant COPD. Furthermore, patients with COPD experiencing increasing airflow restriction and emphysema have a ventilation/perfusion mismatch, which is a major factor in the development of hypoxemia, which can be aggravated by exercise and sleep-disordered breathing. Hypoxemia in patients with COPD can cause pulmonary vasoconstriction and vascular remodeling, leading to diastolic dysfunction of the right ventricle. Indeed, PH, which is frequent in individuals with severe COPD, can result in right HF, which is then linked to left HF. Moreover, abnormal cardiac repolarization in patients with COPD may be associated with hypoxemia and may increase the risk of ventricular arrhythmias and abrupt cardiac death [7–10].

Chronic or intermittent hypoxia may also enhance systemic inflammation, which is known to play a role in the pathophysiology of CVD and has been associated with the development of arterial stiffness, which is a powerful predictor of cardiovascular events. In patients with stable COPD, markers of pulmonary inflammation (such as surfactant protein D) and systemic inflammation (such as C-reactive protein [CRP]) are elevated, whereas patients with COPD and CVD have higher blood concentrations of inflammatory markers, including fibrinogen, interleukin (IL)-6, and IL-8 than those without CVD. In patients with COPD, coronary artery calcification scores (a measure of coronary atherosclerosis) correspond with indicators of systemic and pulmonary inflammation, including IL-6, IL-8, surfactant protein D, and peripheral blood neutrophil count. These findings show that COPD is either a systemic inflammatory condition or that inflammatory processes from the lungs spill over into the systemic circulation, contributing to the development of CVD [7, 8].

COPD exacerbations have been proven to increase the incidence of recurrent cardiovascular events in individuals with CVD or cardiovascular risk factors which might be linked to increased lung inflammation. In addition, lower respiratory tract infections, a major cause of COPD exacerbation, are associated with elevated inflammatory markers such as fibrinogen and IL-6, which have been related to thrombosis and cardiovascular events. Interestingly, the abrupt rise in airway resistance that occurs during an exacerbation severely restricts lung emptying and expiratory flow. As a result, patients who are having an exacerbation tend to take quick and shallow breaths, creating a vicious loop of decreased lung emptying time and increased dynamic hyperinflation [1, 7–9].

The source of CVD risk may be connected to chronic bronchitis or emphysema dominating the COPD clinical picture. The presence of emphysema may indicate accelerated lung aging, which may also lead to HF due to the downregulation of anti-aging molecules such as sirtuins, whereas the presence of chronic bronchitis may indicate a distinct inflammatory subtype of COPD requiring specific anti-inflammatory interventions. Additionally, the genetic bases of chronic bronchitis and emphysema are different, which may alter the underlying mechanisms that link COPD and CVD [1, 7–9].

The physiological effects of CVD, such as HF-associated dyspnea resulting from pulmonary edema and reduced exercise capacity (due to reduced cardiac output and impaired perfusive and diffusive oxygen transport), may exacerbate the effects of COPD caused by pulmonary mechanisms (dyspnea due to hyperinflation and the resultant exercise avoidance and deconditioning). In HF, cardiomegaly may play a role in producing a restrictive lung pattern and decreased alveolar volume, with alveolar gas diffusion progressively deteriorating as a result of a loss in lung tissue contributing to gas exchange. Ventilatory response to exercise is greater than normal for a given metabolic rate due to an increase in physiological dead space to tidal volume ratio (driven by high ventilation/perfusion mismatching, increased carbon dioxide production relative to oxygen uptake from lactate buffering, and a decrease in carbon dioxide partial pressure). Patients with COPD with ischemic heart disease (IHD) exhibited significantly lower health status, dyspnea, and lower exercise capacity than those without IHD. In addition, although exacerbations were not more common, recovery time was greater in those with IHD. CVD is a primary cause of hospitalization and death among patients with COPD [7, 9].

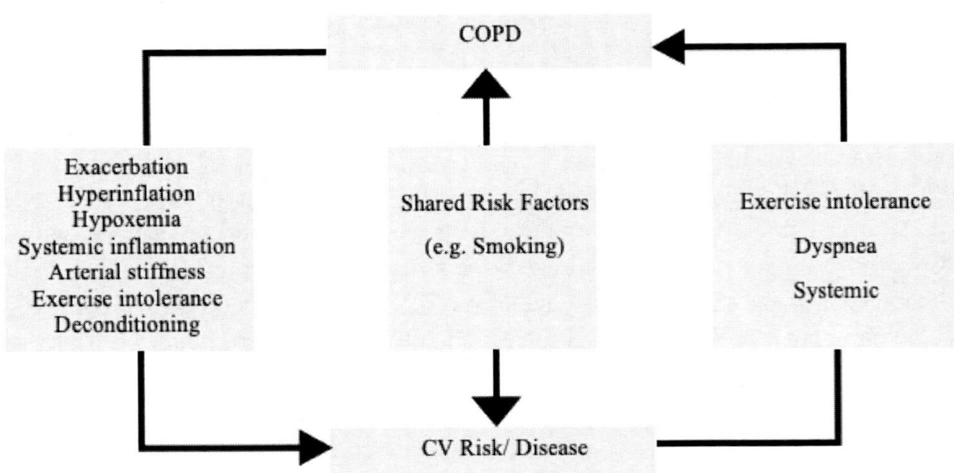

Figure 1. Possible interactions between chronic obstructive pulmonary disease (COPD), cardiovascular risk, and cardiovascular disease (CVD).

Patients with COPD and cardiovascular comorbidity must undergo examinations of their respiratory function, heart function, and systemic inflammatory state. These examinations should be completed differently depending on whether a patient has stable COPD or has an acute exacerbation. Patients with stable COPD need a clinical and functional assessment that includes complete clinical history and physical examination and incorporates the recommended dyspnea and quality of life assessment questionnaires (modified Medical Research Council [mMRC] and COPD Assessment Test [CAT]). Additionally, laboratory assessments must be performed including complete blood count, arterial blood gas analysis, and cardiac biomarkers such as CRP, Brain-type Natriuretic Peptide (BNP), and/or N-terminal proBNP (NT-proBNP). Assessment should also include pulmonary function testing such as spirometry, static lung volumes, and carbon monoxide diffusion capacity (DLCO). Also, it is recommended to do a chest X-ray, a 12-lead electrocardiogram, and if necessary, an echocardiogram evaluation. Additional lab assessments must be performed for those experiencing an acute exacerbation of COPD such as leukocyte count, platelets, fibrinogen, and troponin I to identify the key pathophysiologic processes that caused the exacerbation when multiple diseases coexist: decompensated heart disease, COPD exacerbation, underlying infection, or another concurrent illness [1, 9].

COPD and CVD Pharmacological Treatment

Due to the tight relationship between COPD and CVD, therapy for one condition may likely affect the other, making it vital to treat all disorders appropriately. Better management of COPD and associated comorbidities, including the use of cardiovascular therapies such as angiotensin-converting enzyme inhibitors (ACEIs), angiotensin receptor blockers (ARBs), blockers, and statins, has been attributed to increases in survival following hospital discharge for acute COPD exacerbation. However, the management of cardiovascular problems in patients with COPD presents therapeutic concerns, particularly the co-administration of (selective) β1-blockers and β2-agonists. β-blockers are often recommended for the treatment of cardiovascular disease (CVD), whereas β-agonists are the cornerstone of COPD treatment. However, the two have opposing pharmacological activities, and clinicians may be worried that treating one condition may exacerbate the other [1, 7]

According to the GOLD 2022 report, COPD should be treated as usual as there is no direct evidence that COPD should be treated differently in the presence of Cardiovascular disease or risk factors such as hypertension [6]. Acute heart failure should be treated according to standard heart failure recommendations. Noninvasive ventilation combined with conventional treatment improves outcomes in patients suffering from either hypercapnic respiratory failure owing to a COPD exacerbation or heart failure with acute pulmonary edema. Hypertension should be managed in accordance with standard recommendations. The recent hypertension recommendations place less emphasis on therapy with selective beta-blockers, and there is no evidence that beta-blockers impair the advantages of long-acting beta-blockers (LABA) treatment or raise cardiovascular risk in patients with COPD and elevated cardiovascular risk [6].

Metabolic Disorders (Metabolic Syndrome and Diabetes)

Metabolic disorders, such as type 2 diabetes and metabolic syndrome, are typical COPD comorbidities. Diabetes mellitus (DM) is characterized by inadequate insulin secretion or function [7]. Metabolic syndrome (MetS) is a complicated condition identified clinically by the presence of a cluster of risk factors, such as excess abdominal obesity or body mass index (BMI) > 30, high blood pressure, proatherogenic blood lipid profile, and impaired fasting blood glucose with or without insulin resistance. The prevalence of MetS in patients with COPD is observed to be double that of the general population [11]. According to some studies, the prevalence was estimated to range from 21% to 62%, while the overall prevalence of DM in COPD ranges from 2% to 37% [12]. The effects of DM and MetS on the lungs lead to a restrictive pattern, with significantly lower forced expiratory volume (FEV_1) and forced vital capacity (FVC) values than in people without DM. This restrictive pattern may be caused by a combination of abdominal obesity, decreased pulmonary elasticity owing to non-enzymatic glycosylation of tissue proteins, reduced inspiratory muscle strength, and/or diaphragmatic weakness caused by diabetic neuropathy [7].

Epidemiological investigations have shown that MetS impairs respiratory symptoms and lung function in patients with COPD due to higher systemic inflammation. The elevated blood inflammatory mediators may amplify metabolic problems such as dyslipidemia and insulin resistance. Both the course of COPD and the development of insulin resistance are influenced by systemic inflammation. The likelihood that MetS is a result of COPD is supported by the fact that MetS is a disorder related to lifestyle and diet along with cigarette smoking which is an important modifiable risk factor for MetS. Smoking cessation measures in COPD management have shown beneficial effects on MetS and its individual components [8].

The presence of DM may harm the disease progression of patients with COPD. People with DM and acute exacerbations of COPD (AECOPD) tended to have longer hospital stays and higher death rates compared to those without DM. Hyperglycemia, inflammation, and susceptibility to bacterial infections may exacerbate the course and prognosis of COPD in individuals with DM. A study has found that the absolute risk of worse outcomes went up by 15% for every 1 mmol/l (18 mg/dl) rise in blood glucose in patients with AECOPD who were hospitalized, regardless of other factors like age, gender, history of DM, and COPD severity. Also, poor glycemic management was related to considerably greater mortality rates among patients with COPD hospitalized for mild to moderate exacerbations [8, 13].

Skeletal Muscle Weakness and Osteoporosis

Osteoporosis and skeletal muscle weakness are two comorbidities that often coexist with COPD [13]. Both comorbidities share several risk factors with COPD, including age, limited physical activity, low BMI, smoking, systemic and local inflammation, hypogonadism, vitamin D deficiency, malnutrition, and the use of systemic corticosteroids in patients with exacerbations or severe disease [3, 7, 14]. Among patients with COPD, the prevalence of skeletal muscle weakness was estimated to be 32%, characterized by low muscle strength, low muscle endurance, and fatigue. Independent of lung function, skeletal muscle weakness has been found to lead to lower functional ability, poor quality of life, higher healthcare use, and even death

[3, 14]. Additionally, an increased prevalence of osteoporosis is seen in 21% to 66% of the COPD population [3]. Osteoporosis is characterized by a loss of skeletal resistance due to degeneration of bone tissue microarchitecture, resulting in decreased bone mass and mineral content. Bone fragility and higher fracture risk are the results. Because COPD is a disease that affects people in their later years, comorbidity is to be expected [3, 14]. The pulmonary difficulties of osteoporosis are magnified in COPD because they worsen preexisting physical inactivity and raise the likelihood of vertebral fractures, with total lung capacity decreasing as the number of vertebral fractures rises. These fractures can also cause kyphosis, which restricts breathing movement and reduces lung function (9% reduction in FVC per fracture, and reduced FEV_1) [7]. Non-pharmacological interventions are required for the treatment and prevention of osteoporosis and musculoskeletal weakness in patients with COPD.

Apart from quitting smoking, which is critical, the most important intervention is pulmonary rehabilitation, which has been demonstrated to enhance bone mineral density in exercise retraining programs. Pulmonary rehabilitation programs have been shown to be effective in improving symptoms and health status in patients with COPD by enhancing their muscular strength, exercise capacity, and balance, lowering their chances of falls. Pharmacological interventions in osteoporosis and skeletal muscle weakness include calcium and vitamin D supplementation, and testosterone replacement therapy. Vitamin D and calcium supplementation have demonstrated efficacy in lowering fracture risk, with the benefit being dose-dependent for vitamin D and only present when calcium is also supplemented. Vitamin D has been reported to increase muscle function and postural stability. Testosterone replacement therapy has been demonstrated to boost muscle protein synthesis in older men as well as muscle mass and muscle strength in healthy and hypogonadal men. Testosterone treatment has increased bone mineral density in those males by inhibiting bone resorption and bone remodeling [7, 14]. Regardless of the presence of osteoporosis, COPD should be treated according to standards. However, systemic corticosteroids enhance the risk of osteoporosis and repeated courses for COPD exacerbations should be avoided if possible [6].

Psychiatric Disorders

Depression and anxiety disorders are commonly seen comorbidities in patients with COPD. Depression affects between 20% and 60% of patients with COPD and is more prevalent in elderly patients. The development of depression may be related to aging, poor health status, systemic inflammation, low levels of education, marital status, and/or the effects of low oxygen levels on brain function [3, 5, 7]. In the presence of depression in patients with COPD, worse outcomes are expected such as increased hospital revisits, lower exercise tolerance, and dyspneic sensation; it also hinders daily living activities. Increased risk of death has been estimated at 83% in patients with COPD and depressive symptoms [3]. Additionally, anxiety disorder affects adherence to medication and rehabilitation programs for people with COPD [15].

Similar to depression, anxiety disorders in patients with COPD have adverse effects on their exercise tolerance and quality of life, and it increases health care expenditures [15]. According to the GOLD 2022 report, people with COPD are 1.9 times more likely to commit suicide than those without COPD [6]. Therefore, it is essential to assess the psychological impact of the disorder in patients with COPD. The Hospital Anxiety and Depression (HAD) scale can be used as a rapid and easy screening instrument for anxiety and depressive disorders [7]. In the presence of COPD, management of anxiety and depression should include antidepressants as they have been proven to improve quality of life and alter patients' perception of dyspnea. Similarly, the treatment of COPD should follow the usual guidelines without alteration. However, pulmonary rehabilitation should be emphasized as recent studies highlighted the positive impact of therapeutic patient education and physical exercise on depression [7].

Lung Cancer

Lung cancer continues to be the leading cause of cancer deaths in the world [16]. Multiple epidemiological studies have identified a link between COPD and lung cancer. The prevalence of COPD among patients with lung cancer ranges from 40% to 70%. In a cohort of patients with COPD, the yearly incidence of lung cancer was at least four times that of the general population. Individuals with COPD have a worse prognosis when they are also diagnosed with lung cancer. It is a leading cause of mortality among these patients. In one study, 15% had a 3-year survival rate in the COPD–lung cancer group, compared to 26% in the lung cancer group without COPD [7, 17]. It is known that smoking is one of the major shared factors responsible for lung cancer and COPD [7].

The majority of people with lung cancer have a history of smoking which is one of the factors responsible for the development of cancer, where years of exposure to inhaled carcinogenic substances lead to the development of tumors in the airways or lungs [16, 18] However, the mechanism of this relationship is impacted not just by cigarette smoking, but also by genetic and molecular processes shared by COPD and cancers [7]. According to recommendations for the general population mentioned in the GOLD 2022 report, annual low-dose computed tomography (LDCT) scans are advised for lung cancer screening in patients with COPD who smoke [6]. Cessation of smoking is the cornerstone of COPD treatment. Therefore, it is the most effective method for controlling the development of COPD and reducing the chance of acquiring lung cancer. For patients with COPD, pharmacological therapies such as nicotine replacement therapy and cognitive behavioral therapy have been demonstrated to improve the chances of successful cessation [7].

COPD and Comorbidity Burden

At all stages of the disease, COPD is linked with a significant economic, social, and personal burden, as shown by the high rates of emergency department visits, hospitalizations, and readmissions. Also, there is a clear correlation between COPD severity and the cost of care, which increases as the disease progresses [19]. Despite greater awareness and attention to COPD, the disease continues to be underdiagnosed and under-recognized. It has been found that in the five years preceding their diagnosis, 85% of patients with COPD were found to have missed diagnostic chances [19]. Therefore, it is inevitable that early identification of COPD would be associated with fewer exacerbations, fewer comorbidities, and less health care consumption. It has been found that comorbidities such as CVD, depression, osteoporosis, and

DM are more prevalent in individuals with a late diagnosis of COPD than in those with an early diagnosis [19]. COPD is considered one of the leading causes of death in the United States. Globally, the prevalence of comorbidities in patients with COPD is nearly universal, and their presence is associated with a considerable risk for mortality and worse patient outcomes. Patients with AECOPD and comorbidities were expected to have a longer length of stay, increased readmission rates, and cardiovascular events within one year following hospitalization. As a result, several researchers have sought to create methods for describing the burden of comorbidities in COPD [3, 20].

Several factors, including FEV_1, exercise tolerance measured by walking distance or peak oxygen consumption, weight loss, and reduction in arterial oxygen tension, are used to identify individuals at an elevated risk for death. Using a combination of the majority of the factors described above, a relatively simple method for determining illness severity has been presented. The Body mass index, Obstruction, Dyspnea, and Exercise (BODE) technique provides a composite score that is a more efficient predictor of future survival than any of its individual components. It is considered one of the most effective multidimensional scoring systems [6, 21].

Additionally, the Charlson Comorbidity Index (CCI) is utilized to describe the comorbidity burden. The CCI is perhaps the most extensively utilized measure for determining the impact of comorbidity diseases on overall survival in patients with COPD. A major limitation of this index, however, is that it does not account for some common comorbidities such as depression and anxiety [3]. There is also another test called the COmorbidity TEst (COTE). The COTE index is the first COPD-specific comorbidity index; it estimates the risk of mortality associated with COPD-related comorbidities. This index is based on twelve comorbidities that show strong connections to mortality. In combination with the BODE index, the COTE index might improve prognostication as it adds a more important degree of prediction to mortality. Similarly, given the importance of clinical outcomes in patients with COPD, the Comorbidities in COPD (COMCOLD) index was created to predict the health status of patients with COPD. Descriptions of these indexes can be found in Table 1 [3]. Other indexes for comorbidities include the CODEx index (comorbidity, airway obstruction, dyspnea, and previous exacerbation), and DECAF score (dyspnea, eosinopenia, consolidation, acidemia, and atrial fibrillation). Although multiple indexes have been published that assist in the assessment and prediction of various outcomes in COPD, their predictive accuracy and applicability vary. The decision to choose one index over another should be dictated primarily by the outcome of interest [3, 21].

There is a growing interest in identifying subphenotypes of COPD; a few studies have sought to combine comorbidities to identify distinct COPD phenotypes. Researchers have identified five distinct comorbidity clusters: 1) less comorbidity, 2) cardiovascular cluster with increased hypertension and atherosclerosis, 3) cachectic cluster with lower BMI, muscle wasting, osteoporosis, and renal impairment, 4) metabolic cluster with higher BMI, lipid abnormalities, hypertension, and atherosclerosis, and 5) psychological cluster with increased anxiety and depression as well as a high prevalence of coronary heart disease [21]. Cluster evaluation has shown the asthma/COPD overlap phenotype was linked to morbid obesity and alveolar hypoventilation. The emphysema subtype was linked to cachexia and pulmonary heart disease; and the chronic bronchitis subtype was linked to obesity, DM, and hypertension. Since COPD is a multidimensional complex illness with several disease phenotypes and subphenotypes, some of which entail comorbidities, these cluster analyses and indexes will enable clinicians to optimize COPD management [3, 21].

Table 1. Description of COPD comorbidity indexes

Indexes	Predicted outcome	Score formulation
BODE	Mortality	0–3 points for FEV_1 0–3 points for 6MWD 0–3 points for mMRC 0 or 1 point for BMI
COTE index	Mortality	6 points each: lung, esophageal, pancreatic, and/or breast cancer, anxiety (women only); 2 points each: all other cancers, liver cirrhosis, atrial fibrillation/flutter, DM with neuropathy, pulmonary fibrosis; 1 point each: HF, gastric/duodenal ulcers, coronary heart disease.
COMCOLD index	Health status (feeling thermometer)	6 points for depression; 4 points for anxiety; 3 points each for peripheral artery disease, cerebrovascular disease, symptomatic heart disease (CHF or CHD).

Conclusion

The majority of patients with COPD have coexisting chronic illnesses with shared risk factors. These comorbidities have a significant influence on health and survival. Patients with COPD have a substantial risk of having cardiovascular, metabolic, psychiatric, and skeletal muscle disorders. The existence of comorbidities should not alter the therapy for COPD and should be treated according to conventional protocols regardless of the presence of COPD. Comorbidities in patients with COPD may be underdiagnosed and thus impose a substantial risk on prognosis, health status, and healthcare expenditure. Therefore, early diagnosis is essential to improve clinical outcomes and reduce the economic burden of COPD and its comorbidities. There are several indexes available to describe comorbidity burden, and other methods incorporate comorbidities into clustering models.

Key Points

- It is generally established that COPD is associated with a variety of comorbidities, which may influence the disease's progression, and that COPD can negatively impact the outcome of other conditions.
- Systemic inflammation plays an important role in both the progression of COPD and the development of most associated comorbidities.

- COPD comorbidities such as osteoporosis and depression/anxiety are common, serious comorbidities that are frequently underdiagnosed and are linked to poor health and prognosis.
- Early identification of COPD and its comorbidities has a role in slowing the progression of COPD and improving patient-related outcomes.
- Various methods to assess the burden of comorbidities in COPD are available and the selection of reliable assessment methods would improve clinical outcomes and appropriate management of patients with COPD and comorbidities.

References

[1] Andre S, Conde B, Fragoso E, Boleo-Tome J P, Areias V, Cardoso J, GI DPOC-Grupo de Interesse na Doença Pulmonar Obstrutiva Crónica. COPD and cardiovascular disease. *Pulmonology* 2019 May-Jun; 25(3):168-176.

[2] World Health Organization [Internet]. Geneva CH: WHO; 2022. *Chronic obstructive pulmonary disease (COPD): Key facts;* 2022 May 19 [cited 2022 June 8]. Available from: https://www.who.int/news-room/fact-sheets/detail/chronic-obstructive-pulmonary-disease-(copd).

[3] Putcha N, Drummond M B, Wise R A, Hansel N N. Comorbidities and chronic obstructive pulmonary disease: Prevalence, influence on outcomes, and management. *Semin. Respir. Crit. Care Med.* 2015 Aug;36(4):575-591.

[4] Mantoani L C, Dell'Era S, MacNee W, Rabinovich R A. Physical activity in patients with COPD: the impact of comorbidities. *Expert Rev. Respir. Med.* 2017 Sep;11(9):685-698.

[5] Jureviciene E, Burneikaite G, Dambrauskas L, Kasiulevicius V, Kazenaite E, Navickas R, Puronaitė R, Smailytė G, Visockienė Ž, Danila E. Epidemiology of chronic obstructive pulmonary disease (COPD) comorbidities in Lithuanian National Database: A cluster analysis. *Int. J. Environ. Res.* Public Health 2022 Jan 15;19(2): https://doi.org/10.3390/ijerph19020970.

[6] Global Initiative for Chronic Obstructive Lung Disease, Inc. *Global strategy for the diagnosis, management, and prevention of COPD: 2022 report.* Available from: https://goldcopd.org/2022-gold-reports-2/.

[7] Cavailles A, Brinchault-Rabin G, Dixmier A, Goupil F, Gut-Gobert C, Marchand-Adam S, Meurice J-C, Morel H, Person-Tacnet C, Leroyer C, Diot P. Comorbidities of COPD. *Eur. Respir. Rev.* 2013 Dec;22(130):454-475.

[8] Chan S M H, Selemidis S, Bozinovski S, Vlahos R. Pathobiological mechanisms underlying metabolic syndrome (MetS) in chronic obstructive pulmonary disease (COPD): Clinical significance and therapeutic strategies. *Pharmacol. Ther.* 2019 Jun;198:160-188.

[9] Rabe K F, Hurst J R, Suissa S. Cardiovascular disease and COPD: Dangerous liaisons? *Eur. Respir. Rev.* 2018 Oct 3;27(149): https://doi.org/10.1183/16000617.0057-2018. Print 2018 Sep 30.

[10] Guder G, Stork S. COPD and heart failure: Differential diagnosis and comorbidity. *Herz* 2019 Sep;44(6):502-508.

[11] Charikiopoulou M, Nikolaidis P T, Knechtle B, Rosemann T, Rapti A, Trakada G. Subjective and objective outcomes in patients with COPD after pulmonary rehabilitation—The impact of comorbidities. *Front. Physiol.* 2019 Mar 22;10:286.

[12] Katsiki N, Steiropoulos P, Papanas N, Mikhailidis D P. Diabetes mellitus and chronic obstructive pulmonary disease: An overview. *Exp. Clin. Endocrinol. Diabetes* 2021 Oct;129(10):699-704.

[13] Chatila W M, Thomashow B M, Minai O A, Criner G J, Make B J. Comorbidities in chronic obstructive pulmonary disease. *Proc. Am. Thorac. Soc.* 2008 May 1;5(4):549-555.

[14] Cielen N, Maes K, Gayan-Ramirez G. Musculoskeletal disorders in chronic obstructive pulmonary disease. *Biomed. Res. Int.* 2014;2014:965764.

[15] Recio Iglesias J, Diez-Manglano J, Lopez Garcia F, Diaz Peromingo J A, Almagro P, Varela Aguilar J M. Management of the COPD patient with comorbidities: An experts recommendation document. *Int. J. Chron. Obstruct. Pulmon. Dis.* 2020 May 7;15:1015-1037.

[16] Ferlay J, Soerjomataram I, Dikshit R, Eser S, Mathers C, Rebelo M, Parkin D M,·Forman D, Bray F. Cancer incidence and mortality worldwide: Sources, methods and major patterns in GLOBOCAN 2012. *Int. J. Cancer* 2015 Mar 1;136(5):E359-86.

[17] Kiri V A, Soriano J, Visick G, Fabbri L. Recent trends in lung cancer and its association with COPD: An analysis using the UK GP Research Database. *Prim. Care Respir. J.* 2010 Mar;19(1):57-61.

[18] Bade B C, Dela Cruz C S. Lung cancer 2020: Epidemiology, etiology, and prevention. *Clin. Chest Med.* 2020 Mar;41(1):1-24.

[19] Larsson K, Janson C, Stallberg B, Lisspers K, Olsson P, Kostikas K, Gruenberger J-B, Gutzwiller F S, Uhde M, Jorgensen L, Johansson G. Impact of COPD diagnosis timing on clinical and economic outcomes: The ARCTIC observational cohort study. *Int. J. Chron. Obstruct. Pulmon. Dis.* 2019 May 13;14:995-1008.

[20] Singhvi D, Bon J. CT imaging and comorbidities in COPD: Beyond lung cancer screening. *Chest* 2021 Jan;159(1):147-153.

[21] Negewo N A, Gibson P G, McDonald V M. COPD and its comorbidities: Impact, measurement and mechanisms. *Respirology* 2015 Nov;20(8):1160-1171.

Chapter 5

Mental Disorders and COPD

Rayan A Siraj*
Department of Respiratory Therapy,
King Faisal University, Al Hofuf, Saudi Arabia

Abstract

Mental health disabilities are among the most common comorbidities in patients with chronic obstructive pulmonary disease (COPD), with severe impacts on health, including functional disability, poor adherence to treatment, and increased risk of mortality. While international guidelines recommend identifying mental illnesses in COPD patients, assessing such comorbidities is not part of standard practice. Indeed, the current literature suggests that mental illness in COPD patients remains under-recognized, and thus many patients do not receive appropriate treatment. Several barriers have been proposed to the provision of treatment, including patients, physicians, and systems.

Early and accurate diagnosis of mental health facilitates the development of an appropriate treatment plan that meets patients' needs. Evidence regarding pharmacological interventions in patients with COPD remains limited. However, non-pharmacological interventions remain the first-line approach for managing mental health in patients. While there are also some promising findings on the effect of non-pharmacological interventions in alleviating mental health symptoms in patients with COPD, an integrated approach is recommended to improve clinical outcomes.

Keywords: COPD, mental health, comorbidities, depression, anxiety

Introduction

COPD, a multicomponent disease, is commonly associated with comorbidities. Mental health-related disorders are common comorbidities in COPD patients. The impacts of mental health-related disorders are significant, including functional disability, poor adherence to treatment, increased length of stay, and mortality [1-5]. Nevertheless, mental illness comorbidities remain under-treated or even untreated in patients with COPD and are largely overlooked. This chapter focuses on mental health-related disorders, namely, anxiety and depression.

---

* Corresponding Author's Email: rayan_as18@hotmail.com.

In: Chronic Obstructive Pulmonary Disease
Editor: Jaber S. Alqahtani
ISBN: 979-8-88697-333-4

Epidemiology

Anxiety encompasses a range of disorders, including generalized anxiety disorder (GAD), phobias, panic disorder (PD), agoraphobia, obsessive-compulsive disorder, and traumatic stress disorders [6]. Excessive fear and anxiety, which are key features of anxiety-related conditions, are often associated with other behavioral disturbances, such as avoidance and panic attacks.

There are discrepancies in the anxiety prevalence estimates for COPD patients, which are attributed to the study populations, assessment and diagnostic tools, and methodological designs that have been used. It is estimated that 13%–46% of outpatients with COPD have clinical anxiety, and 10%–55% of those are inpatients [7]. There has also been an association found between COPD severity and increased prevalence of anxiety. In a previous systematic review of 64 studies, anxiety was considerably high, ranging from 50% to 75% in patients with end-stage COPD [8]. Although longitudinal studies on the risk of anxiety disorders have not been conducted, current data suggest that patients with COPD are at a magnified risk of anxiety (by 85%) compared to individuals without COPD. Interestingly, this association remains even after accounting for possible confounding factors [9].

The most frequently anxiety-specific disorders occurring in patients with COPD are GAD, PD, and phobias. Studies indicate that GAD affects 10%–33% of patients with COPD [10, 11] and that patients with COPD are 10 times more likely to experience panic disorders than individuals from the general population [12].

Unless appropriately targeted and adequately treated, anxiety disorders remain disabling and may become chronic, lowering self-esteem, increasing the risk of hospital admissions, and heightening the risk of suicidal thoughts.

Depression, a common comorbidity in COPD, is a mental health illness characterized by feelings of hopelessness, helplessness, sadness, pessimism, and frustration [13, 14]. In addition to having severe impacts on health and COPD prognosis, depression is probably the most frequent psychological disorder in COPD [15], with a spectrum of severity, ranging from minor to major depression.

Depression prevalence estimates range from 27% [16] to 40% [17] in patients exhibiting clinical stability, while the prevalence can be as high as 86% in patients with acute exacerbations [18]. Current evidence indicates that a significant proportion of COPD patients are living with moderate-to-severe depression, and 25% of patients have unrecognized subclinical depression [19]. Depression is also more frequent in patients with more severe COPD than in those with less severe COPD, as shown in previous findings [20].

Increasing evidence suggests that the risk of depression is more significant in COPD patients than in subjects without COPD [21-23]. A recent population-based study conducted by Siraj and colleagues found that patients with COPD have a higher incidence rate of depression (11.4/1000 person-years) than matched controls (5.7/1000 person-years) [24]. In the same study, depression was more significant in patients with more breathlessness than in patients with less breathlessness [24], highlighting the role of COPD severity. Indeed, another study showed that people with more severe COPD have a two-fold increased risk of depression compared to patients with mild COPD [22]. Although depression has a significant effect on patients with COPD, it remains under- or undiagnosed in a considerable proportion of patients [25], ultimately to the detriment of the patients.

As in the general population, the prevalence and incidence of depression in women COPD patients are greater than in male patients [24]. This is attributed to differences in brain structure, function, stress, hormones, and social pressures experienced by both genders [26]. Nevertheless, depression remains an issue for both genders with COPD, and it is important not to underestimate its burden on men.

In patients with COPD, depression frequently co-exists with anxiety, with an estimated prevalence between 26% and 43% [27, 28]. Current evidence also suggests that patients with COPD and depression are seven times more prone to clinical anxiety compared to non-depressed patients with COPD. Indeed, the impact of the co-existence of anxiety and depression is significant, as they increase the risk of suicidal ideation and physical disability compared to either disorder alone [7].

The Potential Link between Mental Disability and COPD

The exact mechanisms linking COPD to mental health illness remain uncertain, although several factors have been suggested (Table 1). However, current evidence indicates that mental health-related disorders, particularly depression, have a bidirectional association with COPD [29]. In other words, mental health illness could increase COPD-related outcomes, and COPD heightens the risk of developing mental illness. Findings from a previous study including 60 clinically stable patients showed that more breathlessness and decreased exercise capacity could have mechanistic roles in increased mental health-related disorders [30]. Moreover, a three-year follow-up study of 1,589 patients with COPD demonstrated that patients with moderate-to-severe dyspnea have an increased risk of new depression [31]. In turn, depression is a significant risk factor for dyspnea in patients with COPD [32].

Although smoking is a major risk factor for both mental illness and COPD, the interrelationship between the two remains to be determined. Previous prospective cohort studies reported that depression is likely to contribute to smoking initiation, increased smoking behavior [33], and reduced physical activity [34]. Smoking is also a significant risk factor for COPD and reduced exercise capacity (which is an indicator of a poor COPD prognosis). Therefore, there could be a mechanistic link through these associations.

Table 1. Associations and impacts of mental health on patients with COPD

The link between mental health and COPD	• Systemic inflammation • Female gender • Lower socioeconomic class • Presence of comorbidities • Prolonged hospital stay • Frequent hospital admissions • More severe COPD
Impacts of mental health on COPD	• Reduced physical activity • Reduced exercise capacity • Reduced sexual drive • Reduced cognitive functioning • Loss of self-confidence • Dependence of caregivers

COPD not only contributes to physical disability but can also be emotionally devastating, leading to hopelessness, helplessness, social isolation, and an unhealthy lifestyle, all of which increase the risk of mental health illness. Indeed, it has been demonstrated that a lack of social support might increase the risk of anxiety in COPD patients [35]. Therefore, it is important to ensure high-quality social support to minimize the suffering from anxiety and depression [36].

Current research suggests that the relationship between lung function impairment and depression may be mediated through low-grade chronic inflammation. Previous studies demonstrated that inflammatory markers were elevated in late-stage depression and COPD. For example, a study of older adults (n = 2077) showed that the inflammatory biomarkers interleukin-6 and C-reactive protein mediated the relationship between symptoms of depression and pulmonary obstruction [37].

The association between mental health-related disorders and COPD has also been attributed to patient-related factors, such as gender (female), smoking status, and lower socioeconomic class; all have been linked to a greater prevalence and incidence of mental health illness [16, 38, 39]. The presence of comorbidities, which occur in up 98% of patients [40], and frequent episodes of hospital admissions have also been associated with an increased risk of depression and anxiety in COPD. Further, pain, which is largely overlooked in patients with COPD, has also been linked to increased symptoms related to anxiety and depression. Interestingly, poor sleep quality, impaired quality of life, and reduced physical activity, which occur because of pain, are what drive symptoms related to anxiety and depression [37].

Impact of Mental Health on COPD

Mental health-related disorders have severe impacts on COPD, and current evidence suggests that anxiety and depression heighten the risk of death in COPD patients. In a cohort study, anxiety was the factor most associated to increased mortality risk compared to the other proposed comorbidities [41]. Anxiety and depression are also linked to worse clinical outcomes, such as an increased risk of COPD exacerbation [9, 42], hospitalization [43], re-hospitalization [18], and longer length of stay [44] compared to patients without these mental health disorders. Further, current evidence shows that mental health illness is associated with worse lung function, breathlessness, and respiratory symptoms; all contribute to a significant challenge in COPD management.

The impact of psychological comorbidities is significant even on the natural course of COPD. Anxiety contributes to worse dyspnea at an earlier stage, and patients with anxiety symptoms are more likely to experience their first hospitalization episode earlier than patients without such symptoms [45].

Evidence increasingly suggests that mood disorders are associated with worse patient-centered outcomes. In fact, the current literature demonstrates that anxiety and depression are associated with reduced health-related quality of life (HRQoL), exercise capacity, and poor physical and functional status. A previous systematic review demonstrated that patients with COPD and co-existing psychological disorders at baseline were likely to experience reduced HRQoL after a year of follow-up [1].

Patients with COPD and mental health-related disorders are associated with poor adherence to medication regimens [46, 47], including PR [2, 3], contributing to worse clinical outcomes. Indeed, studies show that nonadherence to therapies is related to an increased risk of COPD exacerbation, higher prevalence of hospital and emergency admissions, and re-hospitalization [48, 49]. Thus, these comorbidities should be targeted and managed accordingly.

Screening and Diagnosis

Underdiagnosed and undertreated psychological disorders, such as anxiety and depression, have adverse effects on the clinical outcomes of patients with COPD. Healthcare providers who are in direct contact with COPD patients should be aware of this and target these disorders accordingly. Screening may play a crucial role in increasing early detection and determining whether further assessment is needed. A number of validated screening tools are suitable for clinical purposes.

Anxiety Screening Tools

Several screening tools for anxiety disorders are available, including the Beck Anxiety Inventory (BAI), Anxiety Inventory for Respiratory (AIR) Disease scale [50], COPD Anxiety Questionnaire (CAF) [51], and Generalized Anxiety Disorder 7-item (GAD-7) scale [52]. There are also tools for assessing global psychological disorders, such as the Hospital Anxiety and Depression Scale (HADS) [53], Hopkins Symptom Check List, and Patient Health Questionnaire (PHQ).

One of the most valuable tools for identifying patients at risk of psychological disorders is the Primary Care Evaluation of Mental Disorders (PRIME-MD) [54], which uses five simple questions (Table 2). However, it is not a diagnostic tool but rather provides scores based on a specified cutoff, which indicates a mental illness concern for which the patient should be referred for further evaluation.

Table 2. Screening questions for anxiety and depression [54]

Depression screening[a]	In the past month, have you been bothered a lot by: 1. Little interest or pleasure in doing things? 2. Feeling down, depressed, or hopeless?
Anxiety screening[b]	In the past month, have you been bothered a lot by: 1. "Nerves," or feeling anxious or on edge? 2. Worrying about a lot of different things? During the last month: 3. Have you had an anxiety attack (suddenly feeling fear or panic)?

[a]PHQ-2 two-item Patient Health Questionnaire
[b]PHQ-3 three-item Patient Health Questionnaire

A specialized physician usually makes a confirmed clinical diagnosis of anxiety disorders. Importantly, symptoms of anxiety and COPD may overlap; thus, a detailed interview assessment should be conducted to make a clear distinction between symptoms due to anxiety and those due to COPD.

Depression Screening Tools

One of the most helpful ways to identify patients with major depression is through screening. There are a number of screening tools that may be implemented in clinical practice, including the Beck Depression Inventory (BDI), Zung Depression Scale, and the Patient Health Questionnaire-2 (PHQ-2) and Patient Health Questionnaire-9 (PHQ-9) [55]; all have reasonable sensitivity and specificity. Again, the five simple questions from the PRIME-MD tool are a good screening tool for depression.

Although screening tools are useful for identifying patients at risk, a physician should confirm the clinical diagnosis of depression. A firm diagnosis is made in an interview based on the Diagnostic and Statistical Manual of Mental Disorders (DSM-V) and International Classification of Disease (ICD 10) criteria.

In addition to the specific and global psychological assessments, there are also more general assessments for patients with COPD, including the COPD Assessment Test (CAT) and the COPD Clinical Questionnaire, which consider symptoms related to mental illness [56].

Mental Health Management for Patients with COPD

Although mental health-related disorders are common in patients with COPD, many patients do not receive effective treatments. Therefore, healthcare workers need to be alert to the symptoms of these comorbidities and intervene accordingly. For optimal COPD management, a multidisciplinary team approach is needed, involving primary care physicians, nurses, pulmonary medicine specialists, mental health specialists, social workers, and physical therapists. This will ensure that psychological disorders are managed alongside the physical illness (COPD). An example of a multidisciplinary approach is pulmonary rehabilitation, which has many beneficial effects; for example, ameliorating anxiety and depressive symptoms [57, 58]. It is also important to optimize medical therapies, such as bronchodilators, corticosteroids, and oxygen therapy, as they have been shown to improve pulmonary function and functional capacity and thereby improve psychological symptoms [26].

Although the prevalence of mental health-related disorders is significantly high, and while the current COPD guidelines recommend identifying these comorbid conditions [57], assessment of such comorbidities is not currently part of standard COPD practice. The identification of mental health illness not only helps in developing an appropriate treatment plan that meets patients' needs but also guides the choice of pharmacological therapies. However, the current COPD guidelines do not offer specific management approaches to these comorbidities and in fact recommend that they should be managed using standard care, as if the patients do not have COPD (Figure 1). This makes managing these comorbidities difficult, especially when pharmacological treatments are needed, as the risk of drug interactions may increase.

Non-Pharmacological Treatment

Non-pharmacological interventions are a preferred approach and have been shown to be as effective as pharmacological therapies (e.g., antidepressants). Indeed, current recommendations for managing patients with mental-health related disorders consider non-pharmacological interventions the first-line approach. Such therapies include cognitive behavioral therapy (CBT), pulmonary rehabilitation, and relaxation therapy [59].

CBT is a form of psychotherapy treatment administered by a psychologist/psychiatrist that aims to address maladaptive coping in patients with COPD and mental-health related disorders. It helps correct the patient's view about living with COPD, as emotional distress magnifies symptoms related to physical illness (COPD) [59]. The key feature of CBT is its focus on changing individuals' thoughts and, consequently, influencing their behavior and emotional state. Not only does CBT aim to raise patients' awareness of their negative thoughts, which could aggravate depression and anxiety symptoms, but more importantly, it tries to change them. CBT can be provided on either an individual or group basis, and both have been shown to be effective. CBT is recommended for a wide range of mental health illnesses. A previous meta-analysis of four studies on CBT demonstrated that CBT improved anxiety and depression in patients with COPD [60]. Furthermore, based on a systematic review of RCT findings, CBT is an effective therapy for resolving anxiety and depressive symptoms, especially when provided in conjunction with exercise and education [61].

Muscle relaxation is another form of non-pharmacological therapy that aims to reduce psychological symptoms by managing physiological changes associated with anxiety. Relaxation therapy includes a wide range of techniques, such as breathing exercises, mindfulness, distraction therapy, and sequential muscle relaxation [62]. Several of these techniques may be offered as part of a PR program or provided in conjunction with CBT. Current evidence on the effect of muscle relaxation therapy on mental health illness is discrepant, with some studies showing positive effects and others showing minimal or no beneficial effects.

Increasing evidence suggests that pulmonary rehabilitation offers multiple benefits for patients with COPD, such as improving dyspnea, exercise tolerance, health status, anxiety, and depressive symptoms and reducing hospital admission for patients recovering from recent COPD exacerbations [57, 58]. Exercise-based PR programs seem to be the most effective intervention in terms of ameliorating mood symptoms. A previous systematic review revealed that PR significantly improved anxiety and depression in COPD patients [63]. However, the long-term effects of pulmonary rehabilitation are not known. PR should be provided with pharmacological and/or psychological therapies, as it has shown to be more beneficial than PR alone. It is worth noting that mental health-related disorders may manifest as physical illness (COPD); thus, a multidisciplinary approach is crucial for identifying and targeting patients' problems.

It is widely known that the most effective treatment for smokers is smoking cessation. Indeed, smoking cessation influences the rapid decline in lung function and alters the natural history of the disease [64]. Patients with COPD and mental health-related disorders may experience greater difficulties when attempting to quit smoking due to nicotine withdrawal. Therefore, clinicians should consider these difficulties in the clinical management of COPD patients and mental illness.

Pharmacological Treatment

Few studies have assessed the impact of pharmacological interventions on treating mental health-related disorders in COPD patients. However, it is important to note that the management of mental illness in patients with COPD should not be different from the management of patients without COPD. Thus, pharmacological intervention may be necessary for an acute and severe episode of anxiety and depression.

Antidepressant agents are categorized based on their mechanism of action. They all have similar effectiveness, although they may differ in their types and side effects. The main classes of antidepressants include selective serotonin reuptake inhibitors (SSRIs), serotonin–noradrenaline reuptake inhibitors (SNRIs), tricyclic antidepressants (TCAs), and monoamine oxidase inhibitors (MAOIs). Studies show that serotonergic antidepressants, either SSRIs or SNRIs, have better safety records than TCAs [65, 66]. In fact, current guidelines for managing moderate-to-severe depression recommend using SSRIs/SSNRIs as the first-line therapy for patients with physical illnesses, including those with COPD. However, research results on the effect of antidepressants are mixed, as some studies show that serotonergic agents improve anxiety and depression in patients with COPD while others do not [67].

When prescribing antidepressants to patients with COPD and poor mental health, certain factors must be taken into consideration, such as the possible adverse effects. It is also important that medications have a short life and do not provoke drug interactions. Indeed, the pharmacological approach used for patients with COPD may increase drug–drug or drug–disease interactions [45], leading to undesired outcomes. Some drugs, such as benzodiazepines (unless used cautiously), cause respiratory depression, especially in individuals with CO_2 retention, and should therefore be avoided. A prospective study found that benzodiazepines and opioids increase the risk of mortality in patients with severe COPD, especially when they are given in higher doses [68]. Generally, antidepressants have small effects on the ventilatory drive, although caution should be taken when prescribing certain drugs (e.g., TCAs and mirtazapine) for hypercapnic patients with COPD. Hence, the selection of medications should be based on minimizing adverse effects while ensuring effectiveness.

While SSRIs/SNRIs are recommended as the first-line pharmacological intervention, they can have several side effects, including dry mouth, headache, upset stomach, and psychomotor activation. Recent evidence suggests that COPD patients who are new recipients of antidepressants (SSRIs/SNRIs) are at an increased risk of morbidity and mortality compared to those who do not use antidepressants, underlining the harmful outcomes associated with the drugs [65]. However, whether the observed associations are due to the actual drug effects or to unmeasured confounding factors remains to be determined.

Data on the efficacy of antidepressants for treating mental health-related disorders in patients with COPD are currently limited and inconclusive. This is because most studies have had methodological issues, such as a small sample size, sample heterogeneity, short or incomplete follow-up duration (as subjects withdraw from the study because of adverse events), and non-controlled designs.

Based on current evidence, medication adherence is poor. Potential side effects, patients' unwillingness to take more medications (in addition to their medication regimens), and the stigma linked to psychiatric medications all contribute to low acceptance and poor adherence. Thus, a comprehensive approach is needed to increase medication compliance. Moreover, healthcare professionals should also monitor patients for their medication adherence. In particular, depressed patients have significantly low adherence to medications compared to subjects without depressive symptoms [69].

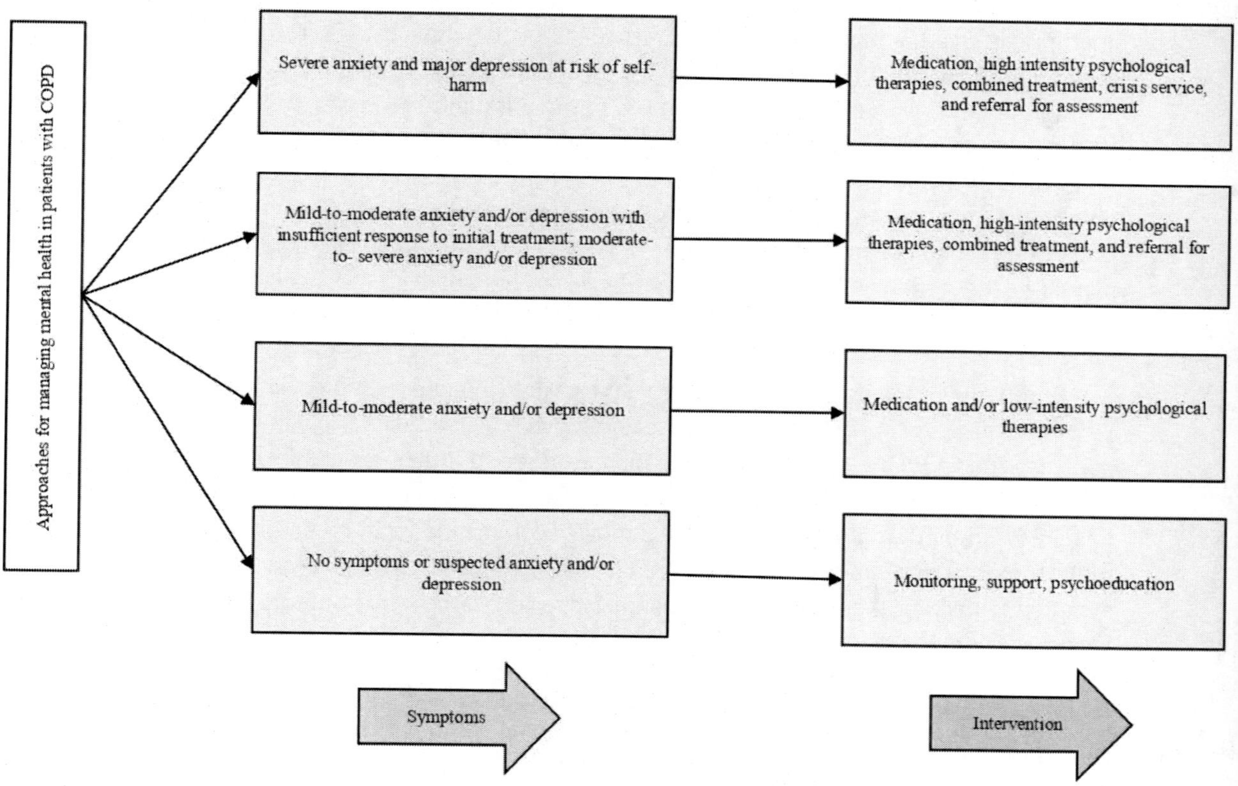

Figure 1. Suggested algorithm for managing mental health (depression and anxiety) in adults based on NICE guidelines.

Since breathlessness is frequently associated with depression and anxiety, it is therefore of clinical significance to target dyspnea in patients with COPD. Several approaches could alleviate dyspnea, such as pulmonary rehabilitation, improving muscle function, and reducing the central neural drive to respiratory muscles (by providing oxygen supplementation or opioids). Bronchodilators may also contribute to ameliorating emotional- and mood-related symptoms, as they have beneficial effects on dyspnea.

Barriers to Treatments

Although mental health-related disorders affect a considerable proportion of patients with COPD, evidence suggests that a significant proportion of these patients do not receive appropriate treatment, contributing to worse clinical outcomes. Therefore, mental health comorbidities should be detected as early as possible and targeted accordingly.

In a review, Maurer et al. discussed the following multi-stage barriers to identifying and treating anxiety and depression in patients with COPD: 1) patient-perceived barrier (e.g., reluctance to disclose symptoms of mental health illness), 2) doctor-perceived barrier (e.g., time constraints for consultation, lack of confidence to disclose a diagnosis, and lack of a standardized diagnostic approach), and 3) system-level barriers (e.g., limited resources for mental health treatment and a lack of coordination/communication between primary care and mental health systems) [70]. These barriers must be overcome in order to optimize clinical outcomes.

Improving practice starts with an early and accurate diagnosis. However, it remains unclear when screening for mental health illness should be done and whether it should be done for all patients with COPD or only for those at increased risk. Further, there are some limitations of the screening tools that are currently used in clinical practice (e.g., they are only valid for patients with chronic illnesses). Even the most recommended and commonly used screening tools for patients with COPD (the HADS, BAI, and BDI) have items including somatic symptoms, making them difficult to decipher due to overlaps in symptoms. Thus, there is a need to design disease-specific tools.

Challenges for Clinical Practice

Reducing the impacts of mental health disabilities starts by recognizing the mental health issues as early as possible. However, routine assessment of mental health in patients with COPD is not currently part of standard practice. In addition, little evidence suggests that routine screening may improve outcomes. Therefore, clinicians managing patients with COPD should play an active role in identifying symptoms and managing them accordingly. This is crucial, as early recognition allows the development of appropriate strategies and guides the choice of antidepressants (if indicated), improving patient outcomes.

Clinicians who are in direct contact with patients should be able to identify existing comorbidities, such as mental health-related disorders, during routine check-ups. Moreover, given the higher prevalence of depression and anxiety, patients should be actively screened. There are many simple screening tools available, including the PHQ-2 and PHQ-3. Current guidelines recommend asking screening questions during patient interviews to determine whether further assessment is needed.

Evidence regarding the effect of antidepressants in patients with COPD is currently limited, as only small trials have been performed. Further well-controlled research is needed to investigate the efficacy of antidepressants. There has also been no strong evidence to show whether antidepressants are cost-effective or reduce healthcare utilization.

It is becoming increasingly evident that pulmonary rehabilitation improves symptoms related to mental health. However, pulmonary rehabilitation programs do not offer specific provisions for patients with COPD and mental health disorders. Therefore, it is important to maximize the benefits of rehabilitation programs. As patients with COPD have a high dropout rate from rehabilitation programs, future studies should focus on understanding the barriers to and facilitators of adherence and completion in patients with coexisting mental health-related disorders. In addition, studies should also seek to determine whether poor adherence and high-dropout rates are related to psychological factors.

Conclusion

Despite the significant impacts of mental health comorbidities, they remain largely overlooked, imposing a substantial burden on patients and the healthcare system. Early identification and management based on an integrated approach are recommended to improve clinical outcomes.

Key Points

- Mental health-related disorders are common in patients with COPD yet are largely overlooked.
- The impacts of mental health comorbidities are significant, leading to increased morbidity and mortality.
- Healthcare professionals should be vigilant to mental health symptoms during the assessment.
- Early identification of these comorbidities allows the development of appropriate treatment plans that meet patients' needs.
- A multidisciplinary team approach for managing such comorbidities is recommended to improve clinical outcomes.

References

[1] Blakemore, A., Dickens, C., Guthrie, E., Bower, P., Kontopantelis, E., Afzal, C., et al. (2014). Depression and anxiety predict health-related quality of life in chronic obstructive pulmonary disease: systematic review and meta-analysis. *Int J Chron Obstruct Pulmon Dis*. 9, 501-12.

[2] Khdour, M. R., Hawwa, A. F., Kidney, J. C., Smyth, B. M., and McElnay, J. C. (2012). Potential risk factors for medication nonadherence in patients with chronic obstructive pulmonary disease (COPD). *European Journal of Clinical Pharmacology*, 68(10), 1365-73.

[3] Keating, A., Lee, A., and Holland, A. E. (2011). What prevents people with chronic obstructive pulmonary disease from attending pulmonary rehabilitation? A systematic review. *Chronic Respiratory Disease.*, 8(2), 89-99.

[4] Xu W., Collet J. P., Shapiro S., Lin Y., Yang T., Platt R. W., et al. (2008). Independent effect of depression and anxiety on chronic obstructive pulmonary disease exacerbations and hospitalizations. *American Journal of Respiratory and Critical Care Medicine.*, 178(9), 913-20.

[5] Laforest L., Roche N., Devouassoux G., Belhassen M., Chouaid C., Ginoux M., et al. (2016). Frequency of comorbidities in chronic obstructive pulmonary disease, and impact on all-cause mortality: A population-based cohort study. *Respir Med.*, 117, 33-9.

[6] Pichot P. (1986). [DSM-III: the 3d edition of the Diagnostic and Statistical Manual of Mental Disorders from the American Psychiatric Association]. *Rev Neurol (Paris).*, 142(5), 489-99.

[7] Willgoss T. G., and Yohannes A. M. (2013). Anxiety disorders in patients with COPD: a systematic review. *Respir Care.*, 58(5), 858-66.

[8] Solano J. P., Gomes B., and Higginson I. J. (2006). A comparison of symptom prevalence in far advanced cancer, AIDS, heart disease, chronic obstructive pulmonary disease and renal disease. *J Pain Symptom Manage.*, 31(1), 58-69.

[9] Eisner M. D., Blanc P. D., Yelin E. H., Katz P. P., Sanchez G., Iribarren C., et al. (2010). Influence of anxiety on health outcomes in COPD. *Thorax.*, 65(3), 229-34.

[10] Dowson C. A., Kuijer R. G., and Mulder R. T. (2004). Anxiety and self-management behaviour in chronic obstructive pulmonary disease: what has been learned? *Chron Respir Dis.*, 1(4), 213-20.

[11] Hynninen K. M., Breitve M. H., Wiborg A. B., Pallesen S., and Nordhus I. H. (2005). Psychological characteristics of patients with chronic obstructive pulmonary disease: a review. *J Psychosom Res.*, 59(6), 429-43.

[12] Livermore N., Sharpe L., and McKenzie D. (2010). Panic attacks and panic disorder in chronic obstructive pulmonary disease: a cognitive behavioral perspective. *Respir Med.*, 104(9), 1246-53.

[13] Kinsman R. A., Yaroush R. A., Fernandez E., Dirks J. F., Schocket M., and Fukuhara J. (1983). Symptoms and experiences in chronic bronchitis and emphysema. *Chest.*, 83(5), 755-61.

[14] Guyatt G. H., Townsend M., Berman L. B., and Pugsley S. O. (1987). Quality of life in patients with chronic airflow limitation. *Br J Dis Chest.*, 81(1), 45-54.

[15] Sirey J. A., Raue P. J., and Alexopoulos G. S. (2007). An intervention to improve depression care in older adults with COPD. *Int J Geriatr Psychiatry.*, 22(2), 154-9.

[16] Matte D. L., Pizzichini M. M., Hoepers A. T., Diaz A. P., Karloh M., Dias M., et al. (2016). Prevalence of depression in COPD: A systematic review and meta-analysis of controlled studies. *Respir Med.*, 117, 154-61.

[17] Yohannes A. M., Willgoss T. G., Baldwin R. C., and Connolly M. J. (2010). Depression and anxiety in chronic heart failure and chronic obstructive pulmonary disease: prevalence, relevance, clinical implications and management principles. *International Journal of Geriatric Psychiatry.*, 25(12), 1209-21.

[18] Lecheler L., Richter M., Franzen D. P., Rampini S. K., Cheetham M., Jenewein J., et al. (2017). The frequent and underrecognized co-occurrence of acute exacerbated COPD and depression warrants screening: a systematic review. *Eur Respir Rev.*, 26(144).

[19] Yohannes A. M., Baldwin R. C., and Connolly M. J. (2003). Prevalence of sub-threshold depression in elderly patients with chronic obstructive pulmonary disease. *Int J Geriatr Psychiatry.*, 18(5), 412-6.

[20] Hanania N. A., Mullerova H., Locantore N. W., Vestbo J., Watkins M. L., Wouters E. F., et al. (2011). Determinants of depression in the ECLIPSE chronic obstructive pulmonary disease cohort. *American Journal of Respiratory and Critical Care Medicine.*, 183(5), 604-11.

[21] van den Bemt L., Schermer T., Bor H., Smink R., van Weel-Baumgarten E., Lucassen P., et al. (2009). The risk for depression comorbidity in patients with COPD. *Chest.*, 135(1), 108-14.

[22] Schneider C., Jick S. S., Bothner U., and Meier C. R. (2010). COPD and the risk of depression. *Chest.*, 137(2), 341-7.

[23] Wagena, E. J., van Amelsvoort, L. G., Kant, I., and Wouters, E. F. (2005). Chronic bronchitis, cigarette smoking, and the subsequent onset of depression and anxiety: results from a prospective population-based cohort study. *Psychosomatic Medicine.*, 67(4), 656-60.

[24] Siraj, R. A., McKeever, T. M., Gibson, J. E., and Bolton, C. E. (2022). Incidence of depression and antidepressant prescription in patients with COPD: A large UK population-based cohort study. *Respir Med.*, 196, 106804.

[25] Dury, R. (2016). COPD and emotional distress: not always noticed and therefore untreated. *British Journal of Community Nursing.*, 21(3), 138-41.

[26] Yohannes, A. M., Kaplan, A., and Hanania, N. A. (2018). Anxiety and Depression in Chronic Obstructive Pulmonary Disease: Recognition and Management. *Cleve Clin J Med.*, 85(2 Suppl 1), S11-s8.

[27] Kunik, M. E., Roundy, K., Veazey, C., Souchek, J., Richardson, P., Wray, N. P., et al. (2005). Surprisingly high prevalence of anxiety and depression in chronic breathing disorders. *Chest.*, 127(4), 1205-11.

[28] Yohannes, A. M., and Alexopoulos, G. S. (2014). Depression and anxiety in patients with COPD. *Eur Respir Rev.*, 23(133), 345-9.

[29] Atlantis, E., Fahey, P., Cochrane, B., and Smith, S. (2013). Bidirectional associations between clinically relevant depression or anxiety and COPD: a systematic review and meta-analysis. *Chest.*, 144(3), 766-77.

[30] Tetikkurt, C., Ozdemir, I., Tetikkurt, S., Yılmaz, N., Ertan, T., and Bayar, N. (2011). Anxiety and depression in COPD patients and correlation with sputum and BAL cytology. *Multidiscip Respir Med.*, 6(4), 226-31.

[31] Yohannes, A. M., Müllerová, H., Hanania, N. A., Lavoie, K., Tal-Singer, R., Vestbo, J., et al. (2016). Long-term Course of Depression Trajectories in Patients With COPD: A 3-Year Follow-up Analysis of the Evaluation of COPD Longitudinally to Identify Predictive Surrogate Endpoints Cohort. *Chest.*, 149(4), 916-26.

[32] Sundh, J., and Ekström, M. (2016). Persistent disabling breathlessness in chronic obstructive pulmonary disease. *Int J Chron Obstruct Pulmon Dis.*, 11, 2805-12.

[33] van Gool, C. H., Kempen, G. I., Penninx, B. W., Deeg, D. J., Beekman, A. T., and van Eijk, J. T. (2003). Relationship between changes in depressive symptoms and unhealthy lifestyles in late middle aged and older persons: results from the Longitudinal Aging Study Amsterdam. *Age Ageing.*, 32(1), 81-7.

[34] Patten, S. B., Williams, J. V., Lavorato, D. H., and Eliasziw, M. A. (2009). longitudinal community study of major depression and physical activity. *Gen Hosp Psychiatry.*, 31(6), 571-5.

[35] Fuller-Thomson, E., and Lacombe-Duncan, A. (2016). Understanding the Association Between Chronic Obstructive Pulmonary Disease and Current Anxiety: A Population-Based Study. *Copd.*, 13(5), 622-31.

[36] Yohannes, A. M. (2013). Is it quality or quantity of social support needed for patients with chronic medical illness? *J Psychosom Res.*, 74(2), 87-8.

[37] Lee, A. L., Harrison, S. L., Goldstein, R. S., and Brooks, D. (2015). Pain and its clinical associations in individuals with COPD: a systematic review. *Chest.*, 147(5), 1246-58.

[38] Martinez Rivera, C., Costan Galicia, J., Alcazar Navarrete, B., Garcia-Polo, C., Ruiz Iturriaga, L. A., Herrejon, A., et al. (2016). Factors Associated with Depression in COPD: A Multicenter Study. *Lung.*, 194(3), 335-43.

[39] Di Marco, F., Verga, M., Reggente, M., Maria Casanova, F., Santus, P., Blasi, F., et al. (2006). Anxiety and depression in COPD patients: The roles of gender and disease severity. *Respir Med.*, 100(10), 1767-74.

[40] Schnell, K., Weiss, C. O., Lee, T., Krishnan, J. A., Leff, B., Wolff, J. L., et al. (2012). The prevalence of clinically-relevant comorbid conditions in patients with physician-diagnosed COPD: a cross-sectional study using data from NHANES 1999-2008. *BMC Pulmonary Medicine.*, 12, 26.

[41] Divo, M. J., Casanova, C., Marin, J. M., Pinto-Plata, V. M., de-Torres, J. P., Zulueta, J. J., et al. (2015). COPD comorbidities network. *The European Respiratory Journal.*, 46(3), 640-50.

[42] Dalal, A. A., Shah, M., Lunacsek, O., and Hanania, N. A. (2011). Clinical and economic burden of depression/anxiety in chronic obstructive pulmonary disease patients within a managed care population. *Copd.*, 8(4), 293-9.

[43] Pooler, A., and Beech, R. (2014). Examining the relationship between anxiety and depression and exacerbations of COPD which result in hospital admission: a systematic review. *Int J Chron Obstruct Pulmon Dis.*, 9, 315-30.

[44] Ng, T. P., Niti, M., Tan, W. C., Cao, Z., Ong, K. C., and Eng, P. (2007). Depressive symptoms and chronic obstructive pulmonary disease: effect on mortality, hospital readmission, symptom burden, functional status, and quality of life. *Arch Intern Med.*, 167(1), 60-7.

[45] Hillas, G., Perlikos, F., Tsiligianni, I., and Tzanakis, N. (2015). Managing comorbidities in COPD. *Int J Chron Obstruct Pulmon Dis.*, 10, 95-109.

[46] Stapleton, R. D., Nielsen, E. L., Engelberg, R. A., Patrick, D. L., and Curtis, J. R. (2005). Association of depression and life-sustaining treatment preferences in patients with COPD. *Chest.*, 127(1), 328-34.

[47] George, J., Kong, D. C., Thoman, R., and Stewart, K. (2005). Factors associated with medication nonadherence in patients with COPD. *Chest.*, 128(5), 3198-204.

[48] Bourbeau, J., and Bartlett, S. J. (2008). Patient adherence in COPD. *Thorax.*, 63(9), 831-8.

[49] van Boven, J. F., Chavannes, N. H., van der Molen, T., Rutten-van Mölken, M. P., Postma, M. J., and Vegter, S. (2014). Clinical and economic impact of non-adherence in COPD: a systematic review. *Respir Med.*, 108(1), 103-13.

[50] Yohannes, A. M., Dryden, S., and Hanania, N. A. (2016). The Responsiveness of the Anxiety Inventory for Respiratory Disease Scale Following Pulmonary Rehabilitation. *Chest.*, 150(1), 188-95.

[51] Kühl, K., Kuhn, C., Kenn, K., and Rief, W. (2011). The COPD-Anxiety-Questionnaire (CAF): a new instrument to assess illness specific anxiety in COPD patients. *Psychother Psychosom Med Psychol.*, 61(1), e1-9.

[52] Spitzer, R. L., Kroenke, K., Williams, J. B., and Löwe, B. (2006). A brief measure for assessing generalized anxiety disorder: the GAD-7. *Arch Intern Med.*, 166(10), 1092-7.

[53] Bratås, O., Grønning, K., and Forbord, T. (2014). Psychometric properties of the Hospital Anxiety and Depression Scale and The General Health Questionnaire-20 in COPD inpatients. *Scand J Caring Sci.*, 28(2), 413-20.

[54] Spitzer, R. L., Williams, J. B., Kroenke, K., Linzer, M., deGruy, F. V., 3rd, Hahn, S. R., et al. (1994). Utility of a new procedure for diagnosing mental disorders in primary care. The PRIME-MD 1000 study. *Jama.*, 272(22), 1749-56.

[55] Kroenke, K., Spitzer, R. L., and Williams, J. B. (2001). The PHQ-9: validity of a brief depression severity measure. *J Gen Intern Med.*, 16(9), 606-13.

[56] Sundh, J., Ställberg, B., Lisspers, K., Kämpe, M., Janson, C., and Montgomery, S. (2016). Comparison of the COPD Assessment Test (CAT) and the Clinical COPD Questionnaire (CCQ) in a Clinical Population. *Copd.*, 13(1), 57-65.

[57] Global Initiative for Chronic Obstructive Lung Disease. the Global Strategy for the Diagnosis, Management and Prevention of COPD 2020 2020 [cited 2020 18 February]. Available from: https://goldcopd.org/wp-content/uploads/2019/11/GOLD-2020-REPORT-ver1.0wms.pdf.

[58] Bolton, C. E., Bevan-Smith, E. F., Blakey, J. D., Crowe, P., Elkin, S. L., Garrod, R., et al. (2013). British Thoracic Society guideline on pulmonary rehabilitation in adults. *Thorax.*, 68 Suppl 2, ii1-30.

[59] Tselebis, A., Pachi, A., Ilias, I., Kosmas, E., Bratis, D., Moussas, G., et al. (2016). Strategies to improve anxiety and depression in patients with COPD: a mental health perspective. *Neuropsychiatr Dis Treat.*, 12, 297-328.

[60] Smith, S. M., Sonego, S., Ketcheson, L., and Larson, J. L. (2014). A review of the effectiveness of psychological interventions used for anxiety and depression in chronic obstructive pulmonary disease. *BMJ Open Respir Res.*, 1(1), e000042.

[61] Coventry, P. A., and Gellatly, J. L. (2008). Improving outcomes for COPD patients with mild-to-moderate anxiety and depression: a systematic review of cognitive behavioural therapy. *Br J Health Psychol.*, 13(Pt 3), 381-400.

[62] Volpato, E., Banfi, P., Rogers, S. M., and Pagnini, F. (2015). Relaxation Techniques for People with Chronic Obstructive Pulmonary Disease: A Systematic Review and a Meta-Analysis. *Evid Based Complement Alternat Med.*, 2015, 628365.

[63] Coventry, P. A., and Hind, D. (2007). Comprehensive pulmonary rehabilitation for anxiety and depression in adults with chronic obstructive pulmonary disease: Systematic review and meta-analysis. *J Psychosom Res.*, 63(5), 551-65.

[64] Anthonisen N. R., Connett J. E., and Murray R. P. (2002). Smoking and lung function of Lung Health Study participants after 11 years. *American Journal of Respiratory and Critical Care Medicine.*, 166(5), 675-9.

[65] Vozoris N. T., Wang X., Austin P. C., Stephenson A. L., O'Donnell D. E., Gershon A. S., et al. (2018). Serotonergic antidepressant use and morbidity and mortality among older adults with COPD. *The European Respiratory Journal.*, 52(1).

[66] von Wolff, A., Holzel, L. P., Westphal, A., Harter, M., and Kriston, L. (2013). Selective serotonin reuptake inhibitors and tricyclic antidepressants in the acute treatment of chronic depression and dysthymia: a systematic review and meta-analysis. *Journal of Affective Disorders.*, 144(1-2), 7-15.

[67] Yohannes, A. M., and Alexopoulos, G. S. (2014). Pharmacological treatment of depression in older patients with chronic obstructive pulmonary disease: impact on the course of the disease and health outcomes. *Drugs Aging.*, 31(7), 483-92.

[68] Ekström, M. P., Bornefalk-Hermansson, A., Abernethy, A. P., and Currow, D. C. (2014). Safety of benzodiazepines and opioids in very severe respiratory disease: national prospective study. *Bmj.*, 348, g445.

[69] Grenard, J. L., Munjas, B. A., Adams, J. L., Suttorp, M., Maglione, M., McGlynn, E. A., et al. (2011). Depression and medication adherence in the treatment of chronic diseases in the United States: a meta-analysis. *J Gen Intern Med.*, 26(10), 1175-82.

[70] Maurer, J., Rebbapragada, V., Borson, S., Goldstein, R., Kunik, M. E., Yohannes, A. M., et al. (2008). Anxiety and depression in COPD: current understanding, unanswered questions, and research needs. *Chest.*, 134(4 Suppl), 43s-56s.

Chapter 6

Spirometry as a Diagnostic Tool in COPD

Noor AlKhathlan*, PhD
Department Respiratory Care,
Imam Abdulrahman bin Faisal University, Saudi Arabia

Abstract

The importance of spirometry as a diagnostic tool in chronic obstructive pulmonary disease (COPD) has been addressed in the clinical practice guideline update from the American College of Physicians, American College of Chest Physicians, American Thoracic Society, and European Respiratory Society. The guideline update recommended that spirometry should be obtained to diagnose airflow obstruction in patients with respiratory symptoms and to screen for airflow obstruction in individuals without respiratory symptoms [1]. Therefore, it is essential that healthcare providers involved in managing COPD understand this physiological test, relevant measurements obtained from it, how to perform good quality tests and their value in diagnosing, monitoring, and assessing the severity of the disease. This chapter is intended to give an overview of all-important aspects related to spirometry.

Keywords: spirometry, FEV_1, FVC, chronic obstructive pulmonary disease (COPD)

Introduction

Chronic obstructive pulmonary disease (COPD) is characterized by incompletely reversible expiratory airflow limitation. The etiology of COPD is chronic lung inflammation which is most commonly caused by smoking. Therefore, the major risk factor for developing COPD is the exposure to cigarette smoke or fumes and occupational or environmental exposures [2]. The prevalence and incidence of COPD worldwide have been steadily rising and still remain a leading cause of morbidity and mortality in the US. Spirometry, among many different tests used to evaluate lung function, is recommended as the "gold standard" for diagnosing and assessing the severity of COPD as well as assessing the response to the bronchodilator regimen [2].

* Corresponding Author's Email: naalkhathlan@iau.edu.sa.

In: Chronic Obstructive Pulmonary Disease
Editor: Jaber S. Alqahtani
ISBN: 979-8-88697-333-4

What Is Spirometry?

Spirometry is a simple test used to assess lung function by measuring the volume of air that can be expired from the lungs after a maximal inspiration. It can be performed using a device called a spirometer. Spirometry parameters: forced vital capacity (FVC), forced expiratory volume in 1 second (FEV_1) and FEV_1/FVC (%) are used to determine the presence and extent of obstruction [3]. It can be obtained from the resultant flow volume loop (Figure 1) and/or volume time curve. In which FEV_1 measure the volume of gas expired in the first second of an FVC maneuver. Whereas FVC is the maximum volume of air that can expired when the subject exhales as forcefully and rapidly as possible after a maximal inspiration. In obstructive pulmonary disease, the changes seen in spirometry are a reduction in FEV_1 with respect to FVC by <0.70.

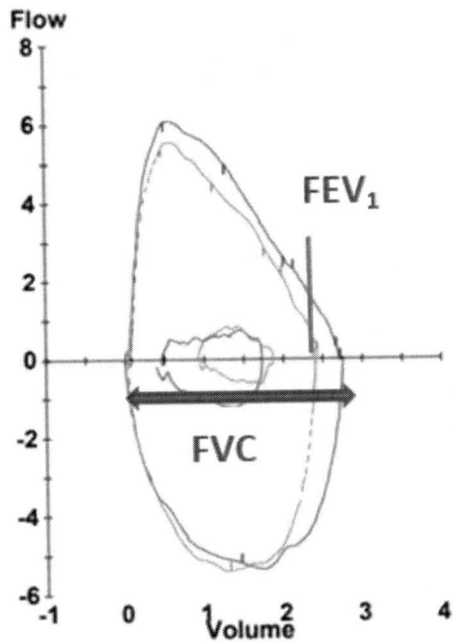

Figure 1. Flow-volume loop

Other measures that can be obtained from spirometry are the forced expiratory flows at low lung volumes (FEF). The reduction in the instantaneous flow measured after 75% of the forced vital capacity (FVC) has been exhaled (FEF_{75}) and/or the reduction in mean expiratory flow between 25% and 75% of FVC have been considered as early signs of small airways obstruction and peripheral lung damage even before FEV_1 becomes abnormal. However, the consensus recommendation from the American Thoracic Society and the European Respiratory Society (ATS/ERS) do not support the use of $FEF_{25\text{-}75}$ and FEF_{75} for determining small airways changes and they stated that "abnormalities in these mid-range flow measurements during a forced exhalation are not specific for small airway disease in individual patients" [4] (p. 953). This is because these parameters may be affected by airflows and volume changes in the larger airways, highly dependent on an accurate FVC maneuver, have a very high variability and poor correlation with measures of air trapping [5].

Reasons for Conducting Spirometry

Patients with dyspnoea, cough, chest tightness, wheezing, and sputum production may benefit from spirometry [6]. A particular pattern of normality or abnormality, such as airway obstruction, lung restriction, or (a combination of obstruction and possible restriction), may be determined from this test's findings. If the spirometry findings are abnormal, the patient may be referred for further pulmonary function testing and assessment. Indication and relative contraindication of spirometry are presented in Table 1.

Table 1. Indication and relative contraindication of spirometry

Indication for Spirometry
1. To detect the presence or absence of lung disease.
2. To quantify the extent of known disease on lung function.
3. It can help in the investigation of certain respiratory symptoms, such as persistent cough or shortness of breath, also known as dyspnea.
4. It is also useful to determine the baseline lung function of an individual, providing a point of reference to compare future results against and notice any changes that occur over time. This is particularly valuable for individuals that work in an environment with a high occupational risk for lung disease.
5. To evaluate the efficacy of the medications used in the treatment.
6. To evaluate the risk of pulmonary complications prior to undertaking some surgical procedures.
7. Evaluate disability or impairment.
Relative Contraindications
• It is recommended that patients should not be tested within 1 month of a myocardial infarction [6].
• Also, patients with any of the following conditions: chest or abdominal pain of any cause, oral or facial pain exacerbated by a mouthpiece, and stress are unlikely to achieve optimal or repeatable results.

Phases of Spirometry Testing

Spirometry testing is recommended to be performed to all patients with respiratory disorders or symptoms, especially long-term conditions as it help to assess the progression of the disease and track changes. However, it needs a high level of patient cooperation. The test procedure consists of four phases in sequential [7].

***Phase one*:** Starts with normal breathing, followed by
***Phase two*:** Inspiration rapidly until completely full, then
***Phase three*:** Expiration with maximal effort until completely empty, and
***Phase four*:** Inspiration with maximal effort until completely full.

Test should be repeated for a minimum of three maneuvers, but usually no more than eight for adults. Therefore, it's important to train the patient to practice the test before the actual measurements and confirm that the patient understands the instructions and is willing to comply, repeat instructions as necessary and be coached vigorously [7]. Performing maneuver usually takes 30 minutes to complete.

Operator and Equipment Quality Assurance

To ensure obtaining valid spirometry test results, equipment quality assurance standards should be strictly followed. The international joint task force, the American Thoracic Society and the European Respiratory Society, have developed such standards [7]. The daily calibration verification for spirometer is performed at low, medium, and high flow with a 3 L syringe.

This procedure is performed to establish a relationship between sensor-determined values of flow or volume and the actual flow or volume with accuracy of ±3% within the calibration limit. If the calibration verification fails, technologists need to check for and remediate problems and repeat calibration verification. Attention to equipment quality control and calibration is an important part of good laboratory practice.

At a minimum, the requirements are as follows:

1. A log of calibration results is maintained.
2. The documentation of repairs or other alterations which return the equipment to acceptable operation.

The dates of computer software and hardware updates or changes; and if equipment is changed or relocated, calibration checks and quality-control procedures must be repeated before further testing begins.

Table 2. Acceptability, repeatability criteria and data reporting for spirometry

The Acceptability Criteria for FEV_1 and FVC Measurements

- Satisfactory start-of-test without hesitation or delay starting (back-extrapolated volume should be <5% or 150 ml whichever is greater).
- There should be no coughing, glottis closure or hesitation during the first second.
- No evidence of obstructed mouthpiece or spirometer.
- No evidence of a leak.
- The tracing should show at least 6 seconds of forced effort.
- An obvious plateau with no volume change (<30 ml) for at least 1 second (children, adolescents, and some restricted patients may plateau in less than 6 seconds, while in severe obstruction, very low flows may be observed at the end of expiration, but has no significant changes in results).
- A minimum of three acceptable efforts should be obtained.
- Test should be discontinued if repeatable values cannot be obtained after 8 attempts.

Repeatability Criteria (Applied to Acceptable FVC and FEV_1, Values)

- The difference between the two largest FVC values must be ≤0.150 L, and the difference between the two largest FEV_1 values must be ≤0.150 L.

Data Reporting

- The largest FVC and the largest FEV_1 should be recorded after examining the data from all of the acceptable curves, even if they do not come from the same curve.
- A single best test should be selected. The test maneuver that has the largest combined sum of its values for FVC and FEV_1 is considered to be the best test.

Acceptability, Repeatability Criteria and Data Reporting

The ATS/ERS joint force have also developed acceptability and repeatability criteria for FEV_1 and FVC measurements [7] (Table 2). These criteria are essential to get a high-quality spirometry data that guide diagnosis of COPD and treatment decisions. To get the "best" test result, the test is repeated three times with a rest between tests.

Therefore, performing spirometry test and interpreting the results should be performed by trained healthcare professionals. NICE guideline has recommended that *"all healthcare professionals managing patients with COPD should be competent in the interpretation of the results of spirometry and all healthcare professionals performing spirometry should have undergone appropriate training and should keep their skills up to date"* [8].

Eligibility for Spirometry

Early assessment of lung function with the use of spirometry is recommended for symptomatic patients present with progressive shortness of breath, wheeze, cough, and sputum production, who have a history of smoking. Also, patients whose occupations may expose them to respiratory irritants, such as fumes and dusts. While it is not recommended for asymptomatic patients, even those with risk factors [9].

Global Initiative for Chronic Obstructive Lung Disease (GOLD) stated that: *"COPD is commonly both overdiagnosed and underdiagnosed because of lack of spirometry testing among symptomatic patients"* [9]. Therefore, it is recommended to perform spirometry to all symptomatic patients. As this will enable early identification of the disease, assist appropriate therapy, delay disease progression and improve quality of life.

COPD is diagnosed when symptomatic patients with risk factors has irreversible airway obstruction indicated by FEV_1/FVC ratio of less than 0.70 [9]. However, this is a point of great controversy. There is an alternative approach to the use of a fixed FEV_1/FVC ratio of less than 0.70 that has been introduced by GOLD using the lower limit of normal value for FEV_1/FVC ratio or z-scores [5]. This method avoids sex and height bias in assessing bronchodilator responsiveness, however, is relatively new to clinicians and difficult to understand which ultimately confirms the use of a fixed FEV_1/FVC ratio of less than 0.70.

Assessing Severity of COPD Using Spirometry

Global Initiative for Chronic Obstructive Lung Disease (GOLD) set criteria for classification of severity of airflow limitation in COPD based on pulmonary function testing [9]. A postbronchodilator FEV_1/FVC ratio of <0.70 is commonly considered diagnostic for COPD.

They categorize airflow limitation into stages. In patients with $FEV_1/FVC < 0.70$:

- GOLD 1 - mild: $FEV_1 \geq 80\%$ predicted
- GOLD 2 - moderate: $50\% \leq FEV_1 < 80\%$ predicted
- GOLD 3 - severe: $30\% \leq FEV_1 < 50\%$ predicted
- GOLD 4 - very severe: $FEV_1 < 30\%$ predicted

Bronchodilator Responsiveness Testing in COPD

Bronchodilator responsiveness testing is considered vital to diagnose COPD and to distinguish COPD from asthma [10]. In the presence of obstructive lung disease, airway resistance increased and therefore airflow into or out of the lungs is reduced. Bronchodilator responsiveness testing determines the degree of improvement of airflow in response to inhalation of a dose of a bronchodilator as measured by changes in FEV_1 and FVC" [10].

COPD is characterized by progressive airflow obstruction that is only partly reversible, whereas asthma is associated with airflow obstruction that is often reversible either spontaneously or with treatment. The ATS/ERS recommendation stated that an increase in FEV_1 and/or FVC $\geq 12\%$ from baseline values, with a minimal absolute change of 200 mL constitutes a positive bronchodilator response [4]. In the absence of a significant increase in FEV_1 and/or FVC, a decrease in lung hyperinflation may indicate a significant response [4].

According to GOLD, postbronchodilator FEV_1/FVC ratio of less than 0.70 is considered one of the 3 features required to diagnose COPD, which "confirms the presence of persistent airflow limitation [11]. The second feature is "appropriate symptoms" including dyspnea, chronic cough, sputum production, or wheezing, and the third is "significant exposure to noxious stimuli" such as a history of smoking cigarettes, or other environmental exposures [9].

Approaches to Spirometry Interpretation

The *classic approach* to interpret spirometry measurements and assess the level of abnormality is the use of % predicted:

% predicted = measured/ predicted x 100

In which the predicted value is calculated using a prediction equation taken from a population of comparable subjects (in terms of their height, weight, age, sex and ethnic group) and using equipment similar to that used for the subject's recording. This method is not supported, either by ATS or by ERS as it leads to *age-related bias*, due to which the severity of airway obstruction will be systematically overestimated in elderly people [5].

Whereas the *new approach* was introduced by an international collaboration of >40 countries and resulted in standardized GLI spirometry reference equations that can be used globally for people aged from 3 to 95 years [5]. From which z-scores can be derived and used to interpret lung function data:

z-score = (measured-predicted)/standard deviation

This method calculates how far the subject's measurements are from their predicted value.

In clinical medicine, the 'normal range' is generally defined as the range of values which encompasses 95% of a healthy population. Therefore, the lower limit of normal (LLN) is the cut-off below which results from only 2.5% of healthy individuals will fall, while the upper limit of normal (ULN) represents the threshold above which results from only 2.5% of healthy individuals will be found [5].

Patterns of Spirometry Impairment

There are three common patterns of spirometry impairment, all of which illustrated in Table 3 with their interpretation guidelines.

Table 3. Patterns of spirometry impairment

Obstructive Pattern 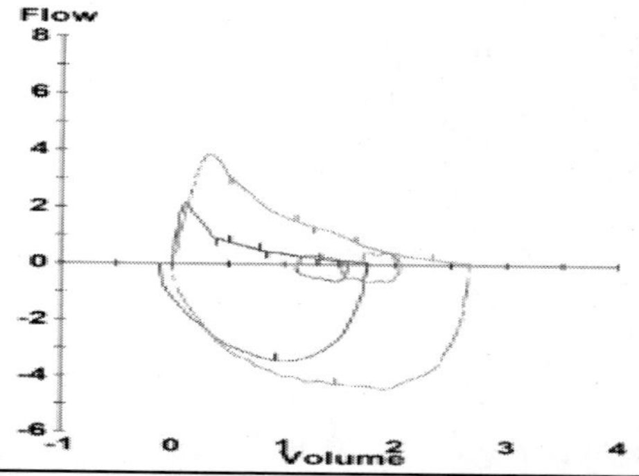	• FEV_1/FVC% is <LLN (ATS criteria) or <70% (GOLD criteria). • Grade severity based on FEV_1 < 80% of predicted.
Restrictive Pattern 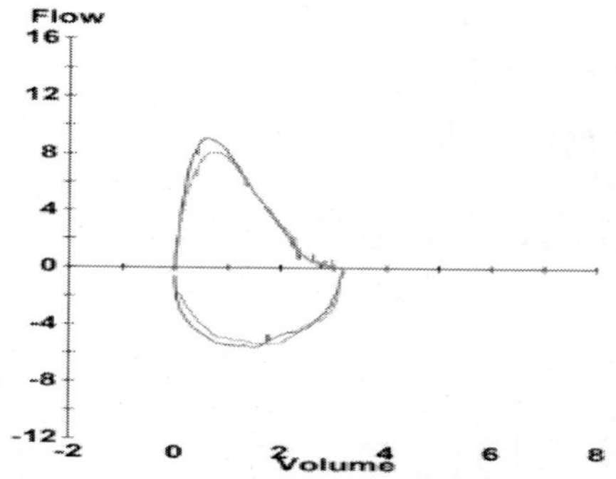	• FEV_1/FVC% is ≥LLN (ATS criteria) or ≥70% (GOLD criteria). • Grade severity based on FVC < 80% of predicted.
***Combined Obstructive and Restrictive (Mixed Pattern)** 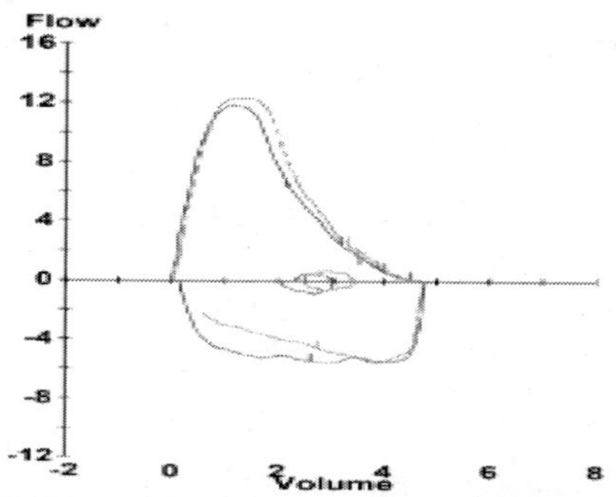	• FEV_1/FVC% is <LLN (ATS criteria) or <70% (GOLD criteria) with FVC < 80% of predicted.

* The causes of mixed pattern were classified as either a pulmonary parenchymal disorder (most commonly COPD) or a combination of pulmonary parenchymal and non-pulmonary diseases [12].

Limitations of Spirometry Testing

One of the biggest limitations of spirometry testing is the need for patient cooperation especially among children and the elderly. Therefore, Impulse Oscillometery (IOS) which is a newer technology that uses small-amplitude pressure oscillations to determine the resistance of the airway was developed to overcome this problem [13]. This technique can be used in infants, the elderly, for neuromuscular disease, sleep apnoea and critical care because it is simple to perform in clinics and needs only normal breathing patterns.

Conclusion

Spirometry is a crucial test to diagnose airflow obstruction in symptomatic patients and to screen for airflow obstruction in individuals without respiratory symptoms. Therefore, all healthcare providers involved in managing COPD should be aware of this physiological test including its outcome measures, their acceptability, reproducibility and value in diagnosing, monitoring, and assessing the severity of the disease.

Key Points

- It is recommended that spirometry be performed on all patients with respiratory symptoms and to screen for airflow obstruction in individuals without respiratory symptoms.
- Quality assurance of the equipment, in parallel with meeting the acceptability and repeatability criteria of testing is crucial to get accurate test results that guide the diagnosis.
- In obstructive lung pattern, a positive bronchodilator response means reversible obstruction (asthma) whereas a negative response means irreversible obstruction (consider differential diagnosis).
- In a mixed lung pattern, an increase in FVC > LLN of predicted; >80% of predicted post bronchodilator therapy is considered pure obstruction with air trapping which is likely to be COPD.
- Using LLN is recommended when interpreting spirometry test results, as it is completely independent of age, height and sex.

References

[1] Qaseem A, Wilt TJ, Weinberger SE, Hanania NA, Criner G, van der Molen T, et al. Diagnosis and Management of Stable Chronic Obstructive Pulmonary Disease: A Clinical Practice Guideline Update from the American College of Physicians, American College of Chest Physicians, American Thoracic Society, and European Respiratory Society. Philadelphia, PA: American College of Physicians; 2011;155(3): 179–192. Available from: http://doi.org/10.7326/0003-4819-155-3-201108020-00008.

[2] Webber EM, Lin JS, Thomas RG. Screening for Chronic Obstructive Pulmonary Disease: Updated Evidence Report and Systematic Review for the US Preventive Services Task Force. *JAMA*. 2022;327(18):1812–1816. http://doi.org/10.1001/jama.2022.4708.

[3] Riley CM, Sciurba FC. Diagnosis and Outpatient Management of Chronic Obstructive Pulmonary Disease: A Review. United States: American Medical Association; 2019;321(8): 786–797. Available from: http://doi.org/10.1001/jama.2019.0131.

[4] Pellegrino R, Viegi G, Jensen R, Johnson Dc, Maclntyre N, McKay R, et al. Interpretative strategies for lung function tests. Leeds: Maney; 2005;26(5): 948–968. Available from: http://doi.org/10.1183/09031936.05.00035205.

[5] Quanjer PH, Stanojevic S, Cole TJ, et al. and the ERS Global Lung Function Initiative. Multi-ethnic reference values for spirometry for the 3-95 years age range: the Global Lung Function 2012 equations. *Eur Respir J* 2012; 40: 1324-1343.

[6] Mottram C. Ruppel's manual of pulmonary function testing. [Online] St. Louis, MO: Elsevier; 2018. Available from: https://bit.ly/3OtwOhR.

[7] Graham BL, Steenbruggen I, Miller MR, Barjaktarevic IZ, Cooper BG, Hall GL, et al. Standardization of Spirometry 2019 Update. An Official American Thoracic Society and European Respiratory Society Technical Statement. United States: American Thoracic Society; 2019;200(8): e70–e88. Available from: http://doi.org/10.1164/rccm.201908-1590ST.

[8] Bellamy D. Spirometry in Practice: *A Practical Guide to Using Spirometry in Primary Care.* Second Edition. London: British Thoracic Society (BTS) COPD Consortium; 2005.

[9] Mirza S, Clay RD, Koslow MA, Scanlon PD. COPD Guidelines: A Review of the 2018 GOLD Report. England: Elsevier Inc; 2018;93(10): 1488–1502. http://doi.org/10.1016/j.mayocp.2018.05.026.

[10] Vigna M, Aiello M, Bertorelli G, Crisafulli E, Chetta A. Flow and volume response to bronchodilator in patients with COPD. Acta Biomed. 2018 Oct 8;89(3):332-336. doi: 10.23750/abm.v89i3.5631. PMID: 30333454; PMCID: PMC6502113.

[11] Delzell JE Jr. Common lung conditions: chronic obstructive pulmonary disease. United States; 2013;409: 23. Available from: https://go.exlibris.link/CZNVtFDN.

[12] Diaz-Guzman E, McCarthy K, Siu A, Stoller JK. Frequency and causes of combined obstruction and restriction identified in pulmonary function tests in adults. *Respir Care.* 2010 Mar;55(3):310-6. PMID: 20196880.

[13] Kaminsky, D. et al. Clinical significance and applications of oscillometry. *European Respiratory Review.* 2022 31: 210208. http://doi.org/10.1183/16000617.0208-2021.

Chapter 7

Alternative Methods of Physiological Lung Function Assessments in COPD

Mohammed A. Almeshari[1,2,*], Abdulrhman S. Alghamdi[1], Sulaiman S. Alsaif[1], Abdulrahman M. Alshehri[1] and Khalid S. Alwadeai[1]

[1]Rehabilitation Health Sciences Department,
College of Applied Medical Sciences,
King Saud University, Riyadh, Saudi Arabia
[2]Institute of Inflammation and Ageing,
University of Birmingham, Birmingham, UK

Abstract

Chronic obstructive pulmonary disease (COPD) is a complex disease with different clinical manifestations. Pulmonary diseases are usually assessed using physiological tests such as forced expiratory maneuver via spirometry. Indeed, spirometry is the most widely used physiological assessment for COPD. It is used in the diagnosis and monitoring of the disease progression or improvement. In clinical practice, the use of spirometry has some limitations, including being an effort-dependent test, and may not be tolerated in advanced disease stages or during exacerbations. Other physiological assessment modalities have been proposed to help in assessing airways diseases such as COPD. Unlike spirometry, body plethysmography is used in assessing lung volumes and airways resistance. Another method, oscillometry, soundwaves are used to obtain the impedance of the airways of which the resistance and reactance are obtained. In multiple and single breath washout tests, the exhaled gases fractions are used in determining lung volumes and ventilation heterogeneity. These modalities require minimal effort and may give more insights into the airways' conditions. In this chapter, the alternative physiological modalities (body plethysmography, oscillometry, and multiple/single breathe washout tests) will be explored and discussed to better understand their utility in clinical practice.

Keywords: oscillation, small airways, physiology, COPD, multiple breath washout, body plethysmography, lung volumes

* Corresponding Author's Email: malmeshari@ksu.edu.sa.

In: Chronic Obstructive Pulmonary Disease
Editor: Jaber S. Alqahtani
ISBN: 979-8-88697-333-4

Introduction

Chronic obstructive pulmonary disease (COPD) is one of the leading causes of death worldwide [1]. The disease primarily affects the airways and the alveoli causing air trapping. The disease is defined as an irreversible airflow limitation [2]. The Global Initiative of COPD (GOLD) confirms COPD diagnosis via spirometry and using the post-bronchodilator ratio of 0.7 of the forced expiratory volume in the first second (FEV_1) over the forced vital capacity (FVC) [2]. Spirometry has also been used to define the stages and severity of airflow limitation in patients with COPD by using the FEV_1 [3]. Although spirometry is a reliable and valid instrument, it remains a patient-dependent test and requires a forceful and unnatural maneuver. Nevertheless, there were some concerns in interpreting and conducting a clinically valid spirometry assessment in primary clinics [4, 5]. Moreover, spirometry only assesses the flow and derives the amount of volume in the vital capacity (VC). Physiologically, COPD causes air trapping and primarily affects the residual volume (RV), the functional reserve capacity (FRC), and the total lung capacity (TLC) [6], however, none of them is measured by spirometry. Nevertheless, spirometry assesses flow rates and derives VC, which is representative of a major region of the lungs and the breathing process. Spirometry assessments are sometimes difficult for patients to perform and require good coaching from the clinician to get a reliable result [7].

Other and more recent physiological pulmonary assessment modalities have been proposed for patients with COPD. Body plethysmography is a test that uses Boyle's law to assess lung volumes. Body plethysmography is mainly used to assess RV, FRC, TLC, and airways resistance, which are all directly related to COPD. Moreover, it does not require a forceful maneuver, therefore considered a patient-independent test. Similarly, oscillometry does not require a forceful maneuver. However, it only assesses the resistance and reactance of the airways at different frequencies. In multiple breath washout (MBW) and single breath washout (SBW) tests, intrinsic or extrinsic gases are used to assess the ventilation heterogeneity and lung volumes and capacities such as RV and FRC. In this chapter, the alternative methods of physiological assessment for COPD are described and discussed to formulate a general understanding of minimally patient-dependent tests. This chapter aims to describe the tests and how they are performed. Also, to evaluate its utility and benefits in assessing COPD patients in clinical practice.

Oscillation Technique

The oscillation technique was first described in 1956 by Dubois [8]. The oscillation technique involves sending sound waves through the airways via the mouth using a loudspeaker. The sound waves are sent at multiple frequencies and respiratory impedance (Zrs) is measured. There are two main types of oscillometry techniques, the forced oscillation technique (FOT) and impulse oscillation (IOS). The FOT uses a single sinusoidal wave at a certain frequency at a time. In IOS, which was first introduced by Michaelson in 1976, a square-shaped wave is sent through the airways at multiple frequencies at the same time.

Oscillometry devices produce oscillating waveforms between 3 and 35 Hz [9], where the lower the frequency waves are the further the waves travel. Higher frequencies are considered as a measure of larger airways as waves travel for a short distance through the airways, whereas lower frequencies are considered as measures of whole airways as oscillations waves travel throughout the airways [10]. Figure 1 (adapted from Almeshari et al. [10]) illustrates how far oscillation waves travel within the airways in relation to frequency (5 and 20 Hz). Therefore, the use of multiple frequencies helps in assessing most of the airways and distinguishing the site of impairment [11].

The oscillation technique is non-invasive and simple to perform by subjects. It does not require the patient to do unnatural breathing or maximal breathing maneuvers. The test requires the patient to put on a nose clip and make a seal with their lips around the mouthpiece of the filter of the oscillometry device while holding their cheeks with their hands and breathing normally [12]. The cheeks are held during the maneuver because the oscillation of the devices causes the cheeks to vibrate, which can affect the reading of the outcomes. The test is conducted in a very short time, with readings obtained in less than 20 seconds. The use of normal breathing makes this type of assessment more practical in subjects with trouble following directions or performing forced maneuvers, such as spirometry [9].

The oscillation technique assesses respiratory impedance (Zrs), defined as the spectral relationship between pressure and volume. Of Zrs, respiratory resistance (Rrs) is derived. The Rrs is the sum of energy needed for the oscillation waves to move through the airways [13]. Furthermore, the respiratory reactance (Xrs) is also derived from the Zrs. The Xrs is defined as the sum of airways recoil against the oscillation, mainly representing the lungs' compliance.

The Rrs is usually reported at two frequencies (5 and 20). The Rrs at 20 Hz (R20) represents the larger airways' resistance as the oscillation waves only travel for a short distance [10]. In the Rrs at 5 Hz (R5), oscillation waves travel throughout the airways, and it is considered the total lung resistance measure. The difference between R20 and R5 (R5-R20) is considered a specific assessment for the smaller airways [14, 15], sometimes referred to as the quiet zone.

In the presence of a physiological increase in airways resistance (i.e., bronchoconstriction), the Rrs readings will increase, which is not specific to COPD alone as it may occur in other lung diseases such as asthma [16]. In COPD, hyperinflation is prevalent and may increase the compliance of the lungs. This is where other parameters, namely Xrs, and specifically at 5 Hz (X5), are known to be specific for assessing chest compliance [17]. Indeed, X5 is decreased in COPD where there is an increase in lung compliance [18].

The oscillation technique has many advantages that promote the utility in its use in clinical practice, mainly as a complementary marker to spirometry or where spirometry is not available or difficult to perform. In cases such as COPD exacerbation, oscillometry should be a feasible test to assess the improvement of patients during hospitalization [19]. Moreover, the oscillation technique was found to be feasible for home testing as it is simple to use and performed by patients with minimal training as it is an effort-independent test [20]. Furthermore, the Oscillation technique was found to be an accurate test of lung function in the older population who may not be able to perform a forceful maneuver such as used in spirometry [21]. The oscillation technique provides multiple indices that help assess physiological lung parameters that pertain directly to the COPD disease process (airways resistance, lung compliance) in different areas of the airways.

Despite being simple to perform, time-efficient, and practical, oscillation techniques have some limitations in clinical practice. 1) Reference ranges are lacking in many ethnic groups limiting their use in such groups [12]. 2) Oscillation devices have been shown to generate different values, limiting their ability to compare outcomes across reports. There are differences in how oscillation devices send the waves and how the devices read them [22]. Indeed, this may also contribute to the practicality of implementing reference ranges as there are variances between the devices.

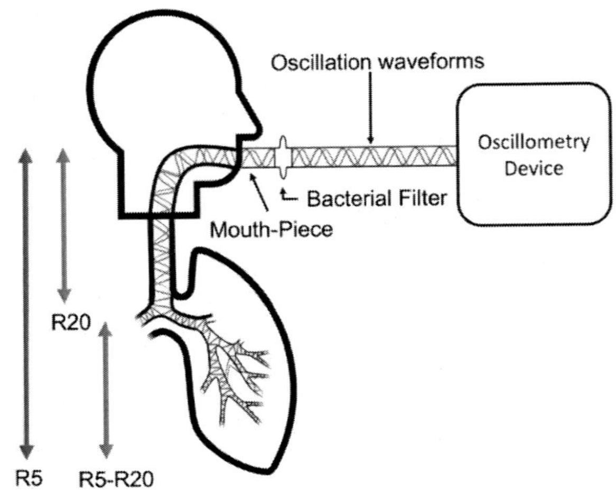

Figure 1. Adapted from [Almeshari et al. (10)], the oscillating wave at 5 Hz (red) travels throughout the airways tree, whereas the wave at 20 Hz (blue) only travels through the larger airways; therefore, the difference between the two is considered as a test of the small airways.

Body Plethysmography

Body plethysmography was first described by DuBois et al. in 1956 to measure the volume of gas within the thoracic cavity [23]. The technique implemented Boyle's law for pressure and gases which states "under isothermal conditions, when gas in a closed container is compressed, its volume decreases while the pressure inside the container increases, such that the product of volume and pressure, at any given moment, is constant." Compared to spirometry, RV, FRC, and TLC measurements are technically more difficult, limiting their application in clinical practice [24]. Although the usefulness of lung volume measures in assessing illness severity, functional impairment, disease course, and responsiveness to treatment has yet to be identified. Nonetheless, in some cases, measures of lung capacity are vital for a precise physiological diagnosis [25].

According to the ATS/ERS task force [24], the following steps should be done when testing subjects using whole-body plethysmography; 1) The equipment should be turned on and sufficient time is given for warming up the machine, and calibration is carried out per the manufacturing guidelines. 2) The subject should be sitting upright with their head in a neutral position. 3) The equipment is adjusted for the patient to sit comfortably in the chamber and in a proper position to reach the mouthpiece without flexing or extending the neck. The subject does not have to remove dentures as removal may introduce leaks at the mouthpiece. 4) The procedure and its purpose should be explained to the subject for better test performance. The patient's cheeks are supported by both hands, and a nose clip is to be used. 5) The box door is closed, and sufficient time is allowed for thermal equilibration before the beginning of the test. 6) The patient is instructed to attach to the mouthpiece and breathe quietly for 3–10 tidal breaths until a stable end-expiratory level is reached. 7) When the patient reaches FRC or near it, the mechanical shutter is closed for 2–3 seconds at end-expiration phase, and the patient is asked to do a series of mild pants at a frequency of 0.5–1.0 Hz. Panting in frequencies of more than 1.5 Hz may cause errors, whereas those with a frequency of less than 0.5 Hz may lead to issues with the leak system of the body plethysmograph. 8) Three to five technically acceptable panting maneuvers should be documented, then the shutter is opened and an ERV maneuver is performed by the patient, and a slow IVC maneuver is followed thereafter. The patient can remove the mouthpiece and relax between TGV/VC procedures if necessary. At least 3 maneuvers that agree within 5% are required to meet the repeatability criteria and the mean value should be reported [24].

The measurement of lung volumes using whole-body plethysmography is widely performed. The changes in Thoracic Gas Volume (TGV) during breathing maneuvers can be obtained using a whole-body plethysmograph by measuring the changes in the pressure while the volume in the chamber is constant, and volume and airflow while the pressure in the chamber is constant [26]. The TGV is the volume of compressible gas within the thorax at the same time as the airflow occlusion occurs during plethysmography measurement [26, 27], which may be higher or lower than the Functional residual capacity (FRC) depending on where airflow occlusion occurs during the breathing maneuvers [3]. The static lung volumes characterized by the FRC, RV, and TLC cannot be measured directly [3, 27]. However, whole-body plethysmography is recognized as a 'gold standard' method for measuring static lung volumes [3].

Whole-body plethysmography is one of the most common methods for measuring airway resistance. The results of plethysmography include, among others, the following parameters: airway resistance (Raw), specific airway resistance (sRaw), and specific airway conductance (sGaw) [28, 29].

The Raw results depend on lung volume; however, the sRaw and sGaw are relatively independent of the changes in lung volume [28]. The Raw is the result of sRaw and TGV measured during breathing maneuvers with a closed shutter [29]. The sRaw is computed from the pressure of the gas and the proportion of the change in TGV to the flow in the mouth [30]. The sRaw does not require the measurement of lung volume using breathing maneuvers against a closed shutter [29]. The sGaw is a sensitive method for the assessment of airways resistance [29]. Specific conductance is used to evaluate the pulmonary system in patients with severe airways obstruction [28, 29].

As hyperinflation is one of the main disease processes in COPD, measuring lung volumes is vital in assessing the response to treatment and disease progression. It was shown that measuring RV/TLC using body plethysmography was a reliable index of hyperinflation in patients with COPD [31], however, its utility as a disease progression index was not evaluated. Moreover, RV/TLC as a marker for hyperinflation was found to be lower in COPD patients that survived within five years versus those who did not survive [32]. Indeed, RV is considered an early marker for obstructive lung diseases [33]. In severe cases of hyperinflation, inspiratory capacity is decreased at rest [34], therefore, it should be considered for disease progression assessment in COPD. Nevertheless, the body plethysmograph has disadvantages compared to other modalities. Claustrophobic people may find it difficult to go into the body plethysmograph chamber. Moreover, unlike spirometry or oscillometry, body plethysmograph devices are not portable and require some space. The body plethysmograph also costs more than other MBW which the FRC, RV, and TLC can also be derived from, although the values are not interchangeable between the two techniques [35].

Inert Gas Washout Tests

Facilitating efficient gas exchange is the main function of the human lung. For decades, conventional spirometry has been used for most chronic lung diseases as a standard diagnostic technique to assess the level of airway obstruction in chronic respiratory diseases such as COPD [36, 37], cystic fibrosis [38], and asthma [39]. However, emerging evidence raises the need for alternative techniques as spirometry may not be a sensitive tool for assessing peripheral airway involvement and ventilation distribution [40]. Over 60 years ago, inert gas washout was introduced by Ward S. Fowler [41], and as a measure of ventilation inhomogeneity (VI), it provides valuable information on small airways function. Inert gas washout is performed over a single vital capacity breath or a series of tidal breaths; this procedure is called SBW or MBW, respectively, and provides complementary information. However, inert gas washout IGW was an undervalued and underutilized test but has been recently revisited [40, 41]. With the advancements in gas analyzers and computers, the MBW technique has been modified to determine ventilation distribution and gas clearance curves during tidal breaths, allowing for its usage for more types of patients including those at very young ages [42, 43].

The SBW and MBW are non-invasive tests used to measure the ventilation inhomogeneity in the lungs, providing insightful information about the function of the small airways. The tests are performed using suitable and safe inert gases that do not participate in the process of gas exchange [44]. These gases can be either endogenous (e.g., nitrogen: N2, and argon) or exogenous (e.g., Sulphur hexafluoride: SF6, helium: He, and methane) [44].

The SBW test involves a VC maneuver at a low constant flow (04-05 liter/s) and is ideally performed while the patient is sitting upright, wearing a nose clip, and using a mouthpiece or a tight facemask to breathe. The test involves the following steps: patient exhales to RV, then inhales 100% oxygen gas to TLC, followed by a 'washout' where the patient exhales from TLC to RV [45]. For the SBW test using an exogenous inert gas, the gas is 'washed in' when the patient inhales from RV to TLC before its 'washout' when exhaling to RV.

The MBW is deemed to be a more informative test that assesses ventilation distribution inhomogeneity through a series of breaths during tidal (normal) breathing from the functional residual capacity (FRC). This makes it a feasible test for all age groups. The test requires minimal cooperation and coordination from the patient than the SBW test but at the expense of being a time-consuming test [44]. Similar to SBW, the use of exogenous inert gas to perform the test requires an initial 'wash in' phase before the 'washout' [44].

The main outcome of an SBW test is an expirogram with 4 distinct phases. The absolute dead space is depicted in phase I, and phase II represents the bronchial (or transitional) phase. Phase III, the alveolar phase, is followed by phase IV, the fast deflection phase at end of expiration [44]. In the classical SBW test, the Phase III slope reflects the ventilation inhomogeneity across the different lung volumes [42], representing a combination of large and small-scale inhomogeneities. While gravity contributes to 30-40% inhomogeneity, the remaining happens among or within the peripheral lung units [46].

The main outcome parameters reported by the MBW are the functional residual capacity (FRC), lung clearance index (LCI), and the slopes of the alveolar phase III (SIII) of the inert gas. The FRC represents the volume of gas remaining in the lungs at the end of exhalation. The LCI is a global measure of ventilation inhomogeneity and is considered the simplest to calculate and easiest to understand by both clinicians and patients [42]. The LCI reflects the cumulative number of FRC turnovers required to wash out the inert gas until it reaches a given fraction of its starting concertation, historically 1/40th [44, 47]. An increased LCI is a result of an increased number of tidal breaths (turnovers) needed to clear the inert gas, representing a higher ventilation inhomogeneity. Additionally, the expirogram of the inert gas, specifically the SIII phase, provides parameters for peripheral lung ventilation. These parameters are useful in distinguishing between ventilation inhomogeneity arising within diffusion-convection-dependent acinar airways (Sacin) and the inhomogeneity arising within convection-dependent conducting airways (Scond) [40, 48].

Table 1. Advantages and disadvantages of alternative physiological lung function assessments

Test	Advantages	Disadvantages/Limitation
Oscillometry	• Easy to perform • Quick assessment • Can be portable	• Limited clinical implementation • Result interpretation barrier • Lack of reference ranges
Body plethysmography	• Easy to perform • Provides information on lung volume and airways dynamics. • Reference ranges available for a wide population	• Not portable • Expensive • May not be suitable for claustrophobic participants
Multiple breath washout	• Easy to perform • Reference ranges available for a wide population • Cost-effective	• Sacin and Scond measuring equipment and software can be expensive • Time-consuming test • Result interpretation barrier

The SBW and MBW both evaluate inhomogeneity of ventilation distribution at different lung volumes. In recent years, MBW implementation has increased and the reasons for this renaissance involve technological and physiological considerations [40]. The approach is sensitive enough to identify early signs of lung function deterioration, which often occurs in small peripheral airways. The MBW provides information that is not given via other lung function testing at the moment [40]. Moreover, MBW examines inert gas clearance over a series of breaths to assess ventilation distribution inhomogeneity during tidal breathing from Functional residual capacity (FRC) [44]. The LCI is a widely used measurement derived from MBW tests, which is shown to distinguish between COPD and healthy patients [49]. LCI raises in the event of airflow obstruction, which is supported by earlier emphysema study results, which show that LCI can distinguish between healthy and COPD participants (50). In addition, LCI also detects small airway damage at the acinar entrance in smokers (≤10 pack-years) compared to spirometry [51].

Additional research indicated that the MBW test might detect small airway alterations in smokers before routine spirometry became abnormal [52]. The MBW test is sometimes used with young patients due to the minimal level of cooperation required for the measurements. Although one of the key disadvantages of MBW is that it is a time-consuming test compared to other lung function test modalities. Moreover, additional validation of MBW tests for non-invasive identification of early abnormalities in peripheral or parenchymal locations is required [53]. SBW has been utilized to assess the involvement of small airways in COPD patients [54]. SBW can be performed during normal tidal breathing or forceful maneuvers [40]. SBW could be more attractive in healthcare settings since its measurements could be performed faster than

MBW [40]. Although the SBW test has been shown to be reproducible in adults [55], it is less reproducible than MBW. Table 1 presents the advantages and disadvantages of alternative physiological lung function assessments.

Conclusion

Spirometry is the most widely used method in assessing COPD patients and is the gold standard in diagnosing it. Other physiological assessments described in this chapter may be used as an alternative to spirometry to assess COPD patients, especially when they are unable to. Unlike spirometry, these modalities are sub-maximal and therefore can be considered effort-independent tests. In cases where it is difficult for patients to make an optimal effort for FVC maneuver (i.e., during exacerbation), these modalities have been deemed feasible. The alternative physiological modalities provide indices that are directly related to COPD hallmarks (hyperinflation and increased airways resistance) which supports its use in clinical practice and in clinical decision making. These modalities can also be used in addition to spirometry to provide an additional dimension of the physiological status of the lungs to confirm the diagnosis and assess deterioration or improvement of the lungs' condition. The use of physiological lung function assessments discussed in this chapter are easy to perform by patients and should be utilized in clinical practice for assessing COPD patients to have a better understanding of the status of the disease.

Key Points

- Although spirometry is the gold standard for diagnosing and assessing COPD, other physiological lung function modalities provide different indices that are related to COPD disease process.
- Oscillometry tests are simple to perform and time efficient and require minimal patient effort, making them ideal for patients who have difficulty following instructions or during exacerbation.
- Body plethysmography is an easily performed test that is mainly used to get a perspective of the lung volumes to assess for hyperinflation.
- Multiple breath washout is a simple test that is easy to perform to get lung volumes and assess hyperinflation, with the main limitation of being a time-consuming test.
- The alternative tests discussed in this chapter face different drawbacks for use in clinical practice mainly due to being only available in specialized centers or clinics and the limitation of interpreting the results.

References

[1] World Health Organization (WHO). *The top 10 causes of death* [2022/05/10]. Available from: https://www.who.int/news-room/fact-sheets/detail/the-top-10-causes-of-death.

[2] Global Initiative for Chronic Obstructive Lung Disease 2022 Report. *Global Initiative for Chronic Obstructive Lung Disease - GOLD.*

[3] Sylvester, KP, Clayton, N, Cliff, I, Hepple, M, Kendrick, A, Kirkby, J, Miller, M, Moore, A, Rafferty, GF, O'Reilly, L, Shakespeare, J, Smith, L, Watts, T, Bucknall, M, & Butterfield, K. ARTP statement on pulmonary function testing 2020. *BMJ Open Respiratory Research*. 2020;7(1):e000575.

[4] Eaton T, Withy S, Garrett JE, Mercer J, Whitlock RM, Rea HH. Spirometry in primary care practice: the importance of quality assurance and the impact of spirometry workshops. *Chest*. 1999;116(2):416-23.

[5] Schermer T, van Schayck O, van Weel C, Folgering H, Bottema B, Jacobs A. The value of spirometry for primary care: asthma and COPD. *Primary Care Respiratory Journal*. 2000;9(3):51-5.

[6] Pellegrino R, Brusasco V. On the causes of lung hyperinflation during bronchoconstriction. *European Respiratory Journal*. 1997;10(2):468.

[7] Melo SMdA, Oliveira LAd, Wanderley JLF, Rocha RDA. Evaluating the extremely elderly at a pulmonary function clinic for the diagnosis of respiratory disease: frequency and technical quality of spirometry. *Jornal brasileiro de pneumologia: publicacao oficial da Sociedade Brasileira de Pneumologia e Tisilogia*. 2019;45(4):e20180232-e.

[8] Dubois AB, Brody AW, Lewis DH, Burgess BF, Jr. Oscillation mechanics of lungs and chest in man. *J Appl Physiol*. 1956;8(6):587-94.

[9] Kuo CR, Jabbal S, Lipworth B. I Say IOS You Say AOS: Comparative Bias in Respiratory Impedance Measurements. *Lung*. 2019;197(4):473-81.

[10] Almeshari MA, Stockley J, Sapey E. The diagnosis of asthma. Can physiological tests of small airways function help? *Chronic Respiratory Disease*. 2021;18:14799731211053332.

[11] Komarow HD, Myles IA, Uzzaman A, Metcalfe DD. Impulse oscillometry in the evaluation of diseases of the airways in children. *Annals of Allergy, Asthma & Immunology*. 2011;106(3):191-9.

[12] King, GG, Bates, J, Berger, KI, Calverley, P, de Melo, PL, Dellacà, RL, Farré, R, Hall, GL, Ioan, I, Irvin, CG, Kaczka, DW, Kaminsky, DA, Kurosawa, H, Lombardi, E, Maksym, GN, Marchal, F, Oppenheimer, BW, Simpson, SJ, Thamrin, C, … Oostveen, E. Technical standards for respiratory oscillometry. *European Respiratory Journal*. 2020;55(2):1900753.

[13] Oostveen E, MacLeod D, Lorino H, Farre R, Hantos Z, Desager K, Marchal, F. The forced oscillation technique in clinical practice: methodology, recommendations and future developments. *European Respiratory Journal*. 2003;22(6):1026-41.

[14] Contoli M, Bellini F, Morandi L, Forini G, Bianchi S, Gnesini G, Marku, B, Rabe, KF, & Papi, A. Assessing small airway impairment in mild-to-moderate smoking asthmatic patients. *European Respiratory Journal*. 2016;47(4):1264.

[15] Foy BH, Soares M, Bordas R, Richardson M, Bell A, Singapuri A, Hargadon, B, Brightling, C, Burrowes, K, Kay, D, Owers-Bradley, J, Siddiqui, S. Lung Computational Models and the Role of the Small Airways in Asthma. *American Journal of Respiratory and Critical Care Medicine*. 2019; 200(8):982-91.

[16] Watts JC, Farah CS, Seccombe LM, Handley BM, Schoeffel RE, Bertolin A, Dame Carroll, J, King, GG, & Thamrin, C. Measurement duration impacts variability but not impedance measured by the forced oscillation technique in healthy, asthma and COPD subjects. *ERJ Open Research*. 2016;2(2):00094-2015.

[17] Yamagami H, Tanaka A, Kishino Y, Mikuni H, Kawahara T, Ohta S, Yamamoto, M, Suzuki, S, Ohnishi, T, Sagara, H. Association between respiratory impedance measured by forced oscillation technique and exacerbations in patients with COPD. *Int J Chron Obstruct Pulmon Dis*. 2018;13:79-89.

[18] Crim C, Celli B, Edwards LD, Wouters E, Coxson HO, Tal-Singer R, Calverley, PMA. Respiratory system impedance with impulse oscillometry in healthy and COPD subjects: ECLIPSE baseline results. *Respiratory Medicine*. 2011;105(7):1069-78.

[19] Alqahtani JS, Al Rajeh AM, Aldhahir AM, Aldabayan YS, Hurst JR, Mandal S. The Clinical Utility of Forced Oscillation Technique (FOT) during Hospitalisation in patients with exacerbation of COPD. *ERJ Open Research*. 2021:00448-2021.

[20] Timmins SC, Diba C, Thamrin C, Berend N, Salome CM, King GG. The feasibility of home monitoring of impedance with the forced oscillation technique in chronic obstructive pulmonary disease subjects. *Physiol Meas*. 2013;34(1):67-81.

[21] Tse HN, Tseng CZS, Wong KY, Yee KS, Ng LY. Accuracy of forced oscillation technique to assess lung function in geriatric COPD population. *International Journal of Chronic Obstructive Pulmonary Disease*. 2016;11:1105-18.

[22] Dandurand RJ, Lavoie J-P, Lands LC, Hantos Z, the Oscillometry Harmonisation Study G. Comparison of oscillometry devices using active mechanical test loads. *ERJ Open Research*. 2019;5(4):00160-2019.

[23] Dubois AB, Botelho SY, Bedell GN, Marshall R, Comroe JH, Jr. A rapid plethysmographic method for measuring thoracic gas volume: a comparison with a nitrogen washout method for measuring functional residual capacity in normal subjects. *The Journal of Clinical Investigation*. 1956;35(3):322-6.

[24] Wanger J, Clausen JL, Coates A, Pedersen OF, Brusasco V, Burgos F, Casaburi, R, Crapo, R, Enright, P, van der Grinten, CPM, Gustafsson, P, Hankinson, J, Jensen, R, Johnson, D, MacIntyre, N, McKay, R, Miller, MR, Navajas, D, Pellegrino, R, & Viegi, G. Standardisation of the measurement of lung volumes. *European Respiratory Journal*. 2005;26(3):511.

[25] Pellegrino R, Viegi G, Brusasco V, Crapo RO, Burgos F, Casaburi R, Coates, A, van der Grinten, CPM, Gustafsson, P, Hankinson, J, Jensen, R, Johnson, DC, Maclntyre, N, McKay, R, Miller, MR, Navajas, D, Pedersen, OF, Wanger, J. Interpretative strategies for lung function tests. *European Respiratory Journal*. 2005;26(5):948.

[26] Coates AL, Peslin R, Rodenstein D, Stocks J. Measurement of lung volumes by plethysmography. *Eur Respir J*. 1997;10(6):1415-27.

[27] Criée CP, Sorichter S, Smith HJ, Kardos P, Merget R, Heise D, Berdel, D, Köhler, D, Magnussen, H, Marek, W, Mitfessel, H, Rasche, K, Rolke, M, Worth, H, & Jörres, RA. Body plethysmography – Its principles and clinical use. *Respiratory Medicine*. 2011;105(7):959-71.

[28] Kaminsky DA. What Does Airway Resistance Tell Us About Lung Function? *Respiratory Care*. 2012;57(1):85.

[29] Urbankowski T, Przybyłowski T. Methods of airway resistance assessment. *Pneumonol Alergol Pol*. 2016;84(2):134-41.

[30] Goldman MD SH, Ulmer WT. *Whole-Body Plethysmography*. UK: European Respiratory Monograph; 2005.

[31] D'Ascanio M, Viccaro F, Calabrò N, Guerrieri G, Salvucci C, Pizzirusso D, Mancini, R, De Vitis, C, Pezzuto, A, Ricci, A. Assessing Static Lung Hyperinflation by Whole-Body Plethysmography, Helium Dilution, and Impulse Oscillometry System (IOS) in Patients with COPD. *Int J Chron Obstruct Pulmon Dis*. 2020;15:2583-9.

[32] Nishimura K, Izumi T, Tsukino M, Oga T. Dyspnea is a better predictor of 5-year survival than airway obstruction in patients with COPD. *Chest*. 2002;121(5):1434-40.

[33] Kakavas S, Kotsiou OS, Perlikos F, Mermiri M, Mavrovounis G, Gourgoulianis K, Pantazopoulos, I. Pulmonary function testing in COPD: looking beyond the curtain of FEV1. *NPJ Primary Care Respiratory Medicine*. 2021;31(1):23.

[34] O'Donnell DE, Laveneziana P, Webb K, Neder JA. Chronic obstructive pulmonary disease: clinical integrative physiology. *Clin Chest Med*. 2014;35(1):51-69.

[35] Hall GL, Filipow N, Ruppel G, Okitika T, Thompson B, Kirkby J, Steenbruggen, I, Cooper, BG, & Stanojevic, S. Official ERS technical standard: Global Lung Function Initiative reference values for static lung volumes in individuals of European ancestry. *European Respiratory Journal*. 2021;57(3):2000289.

[36] Huygen PE, Gültuna I, Ince C, Zwart A, Bogaard JM, Feenstra BW, Bruining, HA. A new ventilation inhomogeneity index from multiple breath indicator gas washout tests in mechanically ventilated patients. *Crit Care Med*. 1993;21(8):1149-58.

[37] Verbanck S, Schuermans D, Van Muylem A, Melot C, Noppen M, Vincken W, Paiva, M. Conductive and acinar lung-zone contributions to ventilation inhomogeneity in COPD. *Am J Respir Crit Care Med*. 1998;157(5 Pt 1):1573-7.

[38] Aurora P, Bush A, Gustafsson P, Oliver C, Wallis C, Price J, Stroobant, J, Carr, S, & Stocks, J. Multiple-breath washout as a marker of lung disease in preschool children with cystic fibrosis. *Am J Respir Crit Care Med*. 2005;171(3):249-56.

[39] Verbanck S, Schuermans D, Vincken W. Inflammation and airway function in the lung periphery of patients with stable asthma. *J Allergy Clin Immunol*. 2010;125(3):611-6.

[40] Usemann J, Yammine S, Singer F, Latzin P. Inert gas washout: background and application in various lung diseases. *Swiss Med Wkly*. 2017;147:w14483.

[41] Fowler WS, Cornish ER, Jr., Kety SS. Lung function studies. VIII. Analysis of alveolar ventilation by pulmonary N2 clearance curves. *J Clin Invest*. 1952;31(1):40-50.

[42] Robinson PD, Goldman MD, Gustafsson PM. Inert Gas Washout: Theoretical Background and Clinical Utility in Respiratory Disease. *Respiration*. 2009;78(3):339-55.

[43] Kraemer R, Meister B. Fast real-time moment-ratio analysis of multibreath nitrogen washout in children. *Journal of Applied Physiology* (Bethesda, Md : 1985). 1985;59(4):1137-44.

[44] Robinson PD, Latzin P, Verbanck S, Hall GL, Horsley A, Gappa M, Thamrin, C, Arets, HGM, Aurora, P, Fuchs, SI, King, GG, Lum, S, Macleod, K, Paiva, M, Pillow, JJ, Ranganathan, S, Ratjen, F, Singer, F, Sonnappa, S, … Gustafsson, PM. Consensus statement for inert gas washout measurement using multiple- and single- breath tests. *Eur Respir J*. 2013;41(3):507-22.

[45] Comroe JH, Fowler WS. Lung function studies: VI. Detection of uneven alveolar ventilation during a single breath of oxygen. *The American Journal of Medicine*. 1951;10(4):408-13.

[46] Dutrieue B, Lauzon A-M, Verbanck S, Elliott AR, West JB, Paiva M, Prisk, G. Helium and sulfur hexafluoride bolus washin in short-term microgravity. *J Appl Physiol*. 1999;86(5):1594-602.

[47] Bouhuys A, Lennep HJv. Effect of body posture on gas distribution in the lungs. *J Appl Physiol*. 1962;17(1):38-42.

[48] Verbanck S, Paiva M. Model simulations of gas mixing and ventilation distribution in the human lung. *Journal of Applied Physiology* (Bethesda, Md : 1985). 1990;69(6):2269-79.

[49] Şerifoğlu İ, Ulubay G. The methods other than spirometry in the early diagnosis of COPD. *Tuberk Toraks*. 2019;67(1):63-70.

[50] von Nieding G, Löllgen H, Smidt U, Linde H. Simultaneous washout of helium and sulfur hexafluoride in healthy subjects and patients with chronic bronchitis, bronchial asthma, and emphysema. *Am Rev Respir Dis*. 1977;116(4):649-60.

[51] Liu B, Zhou Q, He B. [The application of multiple breath nitrogen washout in chronic obstructive pulmonary disease]. *Zhonghua Jie He He Hu Xi Za Zhi*. 2015;38(7):492-6.

[52] Verbanck S, Schuermans D, Paiva M, Meysman M, Vincken W. Small airway function improvement after smoking cessation in smokers without airway obstruction. *Am J Respir Crit Care Med*. 2006; 174(8):853-7.

[53] Brusasco V, Barisione G, Crimi E. Pulmonary physiology: future directions for lung function testing in COPD. *Respirology*. 2015;20(2):209-18.

[54] Mikamo M, Shirai T, Mori K, Shishido Y, Akita T, Morita S, Asada, K, Fujii, M, Tsuchiya, T, & Suda, T. Predictors of phase III slope of nitrogen single-breath washout in COPD. *Respir Physiolo Neurobiol*. 2013;189(1):42-6.

[55] Husemann K, Berg N, Engel J, Port J, Joppek C, Tao Z, Singer, F, Schulz, H, & Kohlhäufl, M. Double tracer gas single-breath washout: reproducibility in healthy subjects and COPD. *Eur Respir J*. 2014; 44(5):1210-22.

Chapter 8

COPD Case-Findings Tools for COPD Diagnosis

Naiara Tais Leonardi, Alessandro Domingues Heubel and Renata Gonçalves Mendes*, PhD
Department of Physical Therapy,
Federal University of São Carlos (UFSCar),
São Carlos, São Paulo, Brazil

Abstract

Chronic obstructive pulmonary disease (COPD) is a leading cause of morbidity and mortality worldwide. Raising awareness of COPD and early detection of the disease are recommended strategies to combat this important public health issue. COPD case-finding tools are promising useful alternatives to identify patients at-risk for COPD and refer to a confirmatory diagnosis and adequate early management favoring better clinical outcomes and prognosis. A simple, safe, feasible and accurate tool may be cost-effective to identify patients who require diagnostic spirometry. Questionnaires, peak expiratory flow (PEF) and a handheld micro-spirometer or a combination of them have emerged as COPD case-finding tools. Thus, the knowledge of these different approaches and their performances in different settings is essential for applications in clinical practice. However, there are some questions that are still unclear about the feasibility, effectiveness and long-term cost-effectiveness of COPD case-finding tools in health outcomes, in the primary care system and in different settings. In this chapter we will explore, in light of science, these alternative approaches and their evidence, challenges and future perspectives.

Keywords: chronic obstructive pulmonary disease, case-finding, early diagnosis, primary health care

Introduction

COPD Case-Finding Tools: What and Why?

According to Global Initiative for Chronic Obstructive Lung Disease (GOLD) recommendations, spirometry is the gold standard assessment for confirming the diagnosis of

* Corresponding Author's Email: renatamendes@ufscar.br.

In: Chronic Obstructive Pulmonary Disease
Editor: Jaber S. Alqahtani
ISBN: 979-8-88697-333-4

COPD [1]. However, studies indicate that 65% to 80% of subjects living with chronic airway obstruction remain undiagnosed [2]. There are some barriers that may be related to this non-diagnosis, such as the difficulty in accessing spirometry, trained technicians and specialized clinicians to interpret the test [2] and lack of awareness of COPD by patients and general practitioners, mainly in low-and-middle income countries (LMIC) [3].

Undiagnosed COPD patients may not receive adequate treatment and may be diagnosed later, increasing possible complications and risk of events, such as exacerbation. Labonté et al., [4], in the CanCOLD study, found that patients with undiagnosed COPD used similar amounts of health services for exacerbation events, such as emergency department visits and hospital admissions, compared to diagnosed COPD patients [4]. Thus, the GOLD Board of Directors has recently highlighted the importance of increasing awareness of COPD at all levels of society, including actions in the earlier diagnosis of COPD aiming to reduce the impact of COPD worldwide [5].

Therefore, some less costly and simpler alternatives to spirometry have emerged to identify patients at-risk for COPD: the case-finding tools. These approaches may include questionnaires, peak expiratory flow (PEF) and/or handheld micro-spirometer and have recently been recommended by the American Thoracic Society Workshop Report [3]. GOLD does not recommend screening spirometry in asymptomatic individuals without any significant exposure to tobacco or other noxious stimuli, but advocates active case-finding, identifying patients with symptoms and/or risk factors to refer to spirometry [1]. It is important to distinguish between screening, which involves testing a large number of individuals, and case-finding, which involves testing target subgroups of individuals at higher risk of airway obstruction [2]. Thus, COPD case-finding tools are an alternative approach to identify patients at-risk for COPD and refer to diagnostic spirometry in order to provide adequate and early assistance to undiagnosed patients and improve clinical outcomes and prognosis.

Alternative Approaches

Considering the need to identify early individuals at risk for COPD in primary care, several COPD case-finding approaches have been developed in high income settings [6-8] and recently in LMIC [9, 10]. These approaches may include questionnaires, peak expiratory flow (PEF) and/or micro-spirometry devices [11]. Case-finding questionnaires are a simple and inexpensive alternative, which consider symptomatic individuals previously exposed to risk factors. These tools may involve questions about exposure, symptoms, age and gender [6-10] associated with PEF [6, 10] or not.

Regarding case-finding questionnaires, questions about exposure to risk factors are generally related to smoking habit [6-9] while CAPTURE (COPD Assessment in Primary Care to Identify Undiagnosed Respiratory Disease and Exacerbation Risk) included second-hand smoke and air pollution [6] and the COLA questionnaire (COPD in LMICs Assessment) included questions related to biomass fuel smoke, such as household use of wood or charcoal as primary fuel for cooking or heating [10]. These differences in relation to the questions are important in choosing the best case-finding tool in different settings, such as LMIC and rural and urban settings.

In resource-constrained settings, where a PEF device is available, case-finding questionnaires plus PEF may be an option. CAPTURE plus PEF (males 350 L/min; females

250 L/min) showed an improved sensitivity and specificity for COPD cases versus no-COPD control subjects (sensitivity (SN) 89.7%; specificity (SP) 93.1%) than CAPTURE alone (SN 95.7%; SP 67.8%) [6]; while in the COLA questionnaire, the inclusion of PEF (value less than 250 L/min) and age improved the prediction in a validation sample (AUC = 0.83, 95% CI 0.78-0.88) compared to the questionnaire alone (AUC = 0.68 95% CI 0.61-0.75) [10]. However, PEF is effort dependent and trained health professionals are required for applications. Therefore, choosing the appropriate COPD case-finding tool depends on available resources, target populations and setting and ability to treat identified patients with COPD.

Micro-spirometers are a simple and cheaper hand-held device that use values of lung function, such as forced expiratory volume in the first second (FEV_1) to forced expiratory volume in the sixth second, to diagnose COPD patients [11]. In a meta-analysis with 17 studies, Schnieders et al., [11] found that the overall area under curve (AUC) of the micro-spirometer (0.84, 95% CI 0.80-0.89) was larger when compared to the case-finding questionnaires in the COPD diagnosis. However, case-finding questionnaires should not be used alone in the COPD diagnosis, but as an adjunct to identify patients who should be referred for diagnosis by spirometry.

What Is the Evidence?

There are a variety of COPD case-finding questionnaires that have been developed over the last two decades in different countries and settings and most of these tools have been developed and validated in high income and urban settings. Some case-finding questionnaires and their characteristics can be seen in Table 1. In addition to those described in this chapter, there are other questionnaires in the literature, such as the CDQ (COPD diagnostic questionnaire) and RHSQ (respiratory health screening questionnaire) (11). In a systematic review with meta-analysis, Schnieders et al., [11] summarized all the alternative case-finding tools that were compared to post-bronchodilator spirometry in studies available up to May, 2020. They found a summary AUC of the COPD-PS of 0.77 (95% confidence interval (CI) of 0.63 to 0.85) and a summary AUC of CDQ of 0.72 (95% CI of 0.64 to 0.78), with approximately equal accuracy in diagnosing COPD [11]. The authors concluded that although case-finding questionnaires were less accurate diagnostic tools than micro-spirometers, they are able to determine symptomatic patients and are easier to implement, which is especially important in resource-limited settings [11].

Considering the high prevalence of undiagnosed COPD cases in LMIC, difficulties in accessing spirometry, lack of guidelines [3], different exposure to risk factors, and the need to better identify and treat subjects with COPD in these settings [5], Siddharthan et al., [12] assessed the discriminative accuracy of 3 COPD case-finding tools (CAPTURE – COPD Assessment in Primary Care to Identify Undiagnosed Respiratory Disease and Exacerbation Risk, LFQ – Lung Function questionnaire and COLA-6 – COPD in LMICs Assessment questionnaire) in 3 diverse LMIC settings (semiurban Bhaktapur, Nepal; urban Lima, Peru; and rural Nakaseke, Uganda). According to a previously established threshold for the case-finding tools to identify people at high risk for airway obstruction (CAPTURE - high risk as a score of 5 or more or an intermediate score (2-5) with low PEF (<250 L/min for females or <350 L/min for males); COLA-6 - score of 4 or more; and LFQ – score of 18 or less), they found the following discriminative performance: AUC ranged from 0.72 (95% CI of 0.68 to 0.77) for

LFQ in Peru to 0.79 (95% CI of 0.77 to 0.81) for COLA-6 in Nepal, and sensitivity ranged from 34.8% (95% CI of 25.3 to 45.2) for COLA-6 in Nepal to 64.2% (95% CI of 60.3% to 67.9%) for CAPTURE in Nepal. They concluded that these three case-finding instruments for COPD were feasible to administer in these 3 LMIC [12].

Case-finding tool performance and the results of the validation studies are described in Table 2, showing a context dependent performance. Thus, knowledge about the local COPD prevalence, severity and mortality is crucial to determine whether the use of any case-finding approach can be justified. In addition, understanding the local population risk factors and the availability of PEF devices at the application setting is important to choose the better COPD case-finding tool. A simple, safe, feasible, reliable and inexpensive questionnaire may be cost-effective in identifying individuals who require diagnostic spirometry test. Thus, knowledge about the case-finding tool structure and performance (Tables 1 and 2), the case-finding objectives and the study methodology may help to make this decision. For example, CAPTURE was developed to identify symptomatic patients with more severe airway obstruction ($FEV_1 <$ 60%) or at risk for exacerbation, [6] while LFQ, COLA, COPD-PS and PUMA were developed to identify individual at-risk for COPD, defined by post-bronchodilator (post-BD) VEF_1/CVF < 70% [7, 9], post-BD lower limit of normal (LLN) for FEV_1/FVC [9], pre-BD $VEF_1/CVF <$ 70% [8] or post-BD FEV_1/FVC ratio Z-score ≤ -1.64 standard deviations and post-BD reversibility as an increase in FEV_1 of 12% or more from baseline or an increase in FVC of 200 mL or more [10].

Regarding COPD case-finding questionnaire performance, it can be observed that it varies across questionnaires (Table 2) and the context [12]. Considering that a perfect combination of sensitivity and specificity (i.e., high sensitivity and high specificity) may be not feasible, the trade-off between the best sensitivity and specificity depends on the purpose of the COPD case-finding tool. If the objective is to identify as many individuals with at-risk for COPD as possible, with less concern about including those who do not have the disease, not missing many cases, a higher sensitivity may be considered [7-9]. However, this may lead to more healthcare costs to confirm all at-risk cases with spirometry. On the other hand, if the objective is a higher level of certainty that all identified individuals have COPD and reduce health system costs from false-positive results to the detriment of not detecting many real COPD patients, a higher specificity may be considered [7, 12]. For example, although the LFQ questionnaire had presented a higher AUC with score of ≤ 16 (AUC 0.69; SN 71,0; SP 66.5; predictive positive value (PPV) 32.5; negative predictive value (NPV) 90.9), the authors selected a cut point score of ≤ 18 (AUC 0.65; SN 82.6; SP 47.8; PPV 26.5; NPV 92.3) to identify patients at risk of airway obstruction, because their aim was not to lose undiagnosed patients and capture early COPD [8]. In contrast, the authors of the COLA questionnaire chose a score ≥ 5 for the highest combination of sensitivity, specificity and positive predictive value, at the expense of a low sensitivity, but a greater specificity, PPV and NPV (SN 19%; SP 99%, PPV 50%; NPV 96%) [10]. It highlights the importance of PPV and NPV in clinical practice and some authors described these results in their validation studies (Table 2).

Another important result to know about the case-finding questionnaires before deciding them and interpret the data is the false-positive and false-negative value. False-positive is expressed as 1-specificity and true-positive as the sensitivity while false-negative is expressed as 1-sensitivity and true-negative as specificity. Siddharthan et al., [12] found in their study with 3 tool (LFQ, CAPTURE and COLA-6) in 3 settings (Uganda, Peru and Nepal) that participants with false-positive were older and more likely to report a history of asthma than true-negative, while false-negatives were more likely to have milder disease and be younger than true-positive. The consequence of false-positive tests is the need for spirometry, and false-negatives are not identifying patients with mild COPD. However, in the first case, another condition may be present and identified with assessment and in the second case, a systematic approach of COPD case-finding may identify these patients in the future.

Finally, it is essential to recognize the limitations of case-finding questionnaires. They should not be used as a diagnostic test, but rather as a case-finding approach to identify patients who should be referred for confirmatory diagnosis by spirometry, according to recommendations [1]. Thus, the case-finding tool should not be used for the decision on initial treatment before the confirmatory test. Another limitation is the discrimination between asthma and COPD, because some symptoms may be shared by both diseases and the ability to define fixed airway obstruction in a case-finding tool needs to be explored, amongst a pragmatic approach of evaluation of these patients in primary care settings. Furthermore, there is a need to test COPD case-finding tools across a range of settings, such as LMIC, primary care and rural area to assess the feasibility and effectiveness as a public health intervention.

Table 1. Characteristics of COPD case-finding questionnaires

Tool	Population/Local	Structure	Score
# CAPTURE COPD Assessment in Primary Care to Identify Undiagnosed Respiratory Disease and Exacerbation Risk [6]	♂ and ♀; ≥40 y/USA	*5 items*: 4: symptoms and habits; 1: event during the past	Score → from 0 (“no” to all) to 6 (“yes” to all questions and at least 2 events past year).
# COPD-PS COPD Population Screener™ COPD-PSTM; Quality Metric Incorporated, Lincoln, Rhode Island, USA) [7]	≥35 y/USA	*5 items*: 3: symptoms; 1: smoking history; 1: age	Score → from 0 (unlikely to have AO) to 10 (likely to have AO). Each item has value of 0-2
# PUMA score Prevalence Study and Regular Practice, Diagnosis and Treatment, Among General Practitioners in Populations at Risk of COPD in Latin America [9]	≥40 y, current or ex-smokers, and/or exposure to biomass smoke; Argentina, Colombia, Venezuela and Uruguay	*7 items*: gender, age, pack-years smoking, dyspnea, sputum, cough and data of previous spirometry.	Score → from 0 to 9 (higher scores indicating higher COPD risk). Each item has value of 0–2
# LFQ Lung Function Questionnaire) [8]	♂ and ♀; ≥40 y/USA – rural (Hazard) and large metropolitan Kentucky area (Lexington)	*5 items*: 1: age; 1: smoking; 3 symptoms	Score → from 5 to 25 points
# COLA COPD in LMICs Assessment [10]	≥35 y and >95 y/Uganda – rural and urban	*3 parts: 7 questions*: respiratory symptoms, functional status, personal exposures; 1 age score; 1 peak expiratory flow score.	Score → from 0 to 10. 1-point for each of the 7 questions, 1-point if age ≥55 y, 1-point if PEF 250 to 399 L/min and 2-points if PEF ≤ 250 L/min

Note: LMICs: low-and-middle income countries; PEF: peak expiratory flow; AO: fixed airway obstruction.

Table 2. Performance of COPD case-finding questionnaires

Tool	Cut-off	AUC	Sensitivity (%)	Specificity (%)	Observation
CAPTURE(6)	CAPTURE alone; score ≥ 2	CAPTURE alone: 0.79	95.7	44.4	Low (0 or 1) or high scores (5 or 6), PEF is not required. Score of 5: high risk of COPD
	CAPTURE (2-5) + PEF ♂ - 350 L/min; ♀ - 250 L/min	CAPTURE + PEF: 0.91	89.7	78.1	
COPD-PS (7)	score ≥ 5	0.73 (screening AO)	84.4 (screening AO)	60.7 (screening AO)	PPV: 56.8% NPV: 86.4%.
PUMA score (9)	score ≥ 5	0.76	74.2	64.8	PPV: 34.7% NPV: 90.9%
LFQ (8)	score ≤ 18	0.65	82.6	47.8	PPV: 26.5% NPV: 92.3%
COLA(10)	score ≥ 5	0.83	19	99	PPV: 50% NPV: 96%.

Note: PEF: peak expiratory flow; AO: fixed-airway obstruction; PPV: positive predictive value; NPV: negative predictive value. *Control group: mild COPD FEV_1 > 60% and non-COPD.

Challenges and Future Perspectives

As mentioned before in other chapters, COPD patients commonly present limiting symptoms, resulting in reduced exercise tolerance, physical activity and health-related quality of life (HRQoL). Besides that, exacerbations and hospitalizations may significantly increase the systemic impairment in these patients, increasing morbidity and mortality risk. Thus, there is a need for COPD awareness to reduce the impact of this pulmonary disease worldwide, making an early diagnosis as soon as possible to ensure that all patients receive effective treatment, preventing development and progression of COPD [5].

It is well-known that COPD treatment may reduce symptoms and thereby improve HRQoL. For example, regarding non-pharmacology treatment, smoking cessation may influence natural history of disease, vaccination may reduce serious illness and death and pulmonary rehabilitation may reduce symptoms, such as dyspnea, anxiety and depression, and improve health status and exercise tolerance [1]. Concerning pharmacological therapy, medication may reduce symptoms, improve FEV_1 and health status and reduce the exacerbation rate. However, there is no sufficient conclusion about the FEV_1 decline and changes in the natural history of disease, in addition to the adverse effects [1]. In this perspective, the question about the COPD case-finding is: What is the effectiveness of COPD case-finding tools in the natural history of disease compared to usual practice? Is the COPD case-finding tool able to reduce impact of disease in COPD patients compared to the usual practice?

Unfortunately, there are few studies on the effectiveness of COPD case-finding tools. In 2015, Haroon et al., [13] conducted a systematic review to summarize and compare the effectiveness of different case-finding approaches. They found only 3 randomized controlled trials (RCT) and 35 uncontrolled studies including questionnaires, handheld flow meters and diagnostic spirometry, with an extensive heterogeneity among studies. Studies varied with respect to target population, recruitment strategies and the clinical definition of COPD. Despite that, their results suggested that targeting COPD patients with a higher risk with questionnaires may increase the yield [13]. Lambe et al., [14] studied long-term cost-effectiveness of a regular case-finding programme in primary care and found inconclusive results about treatment effectiveness, but they did not consider non-pharmacological strategies, such as smoking cessation and pulmonary rehabilitation [14]. Comparing target case-finding for COPD and routine practice, Jordan et al., [15], in a sample of 74,818 patients, found that target case-finding detected more news cases than routine care (4% vs 1%, respectively) and active case-finding group presented higher percentage of new COPD cases than opportunistic case-finding group (5% vs 2%, respectively). In the active case-finding strategy, a questionnaire about symptoms was sent to patients and in the opportunistic case-finding strategy, questionnaires were distributed during some general medical practice visits to flagged patients and in both strategies patients who reported respiratory symptoms in the questionnaire were invited to attend the general practice for confirmatory spirometry [15].

In view of the high prevalence of undiagnosed COPD patients [2] and potential impact in health services [4], there is the need for the COPD case-finding to identify patients at-risk COPD and properly refer the patient to spirometry and early treatment, reducing undiagnosed patients and costs. However, another question that remains is: What is the cost-effectiveness of the COPD case-finding tool in clinical practice compared to usual care?

Jordan et al., [15], in their Target COPD RCT previously cited in this topic, found that active case-finding was more cost-effective than an opportunistic case-finding and routine care in a well-established primary care system. However, they included short-term effects and did not calculate lifetime costs per quality-adjusted life year (QALY) gained as is recommended by the UK's National Institute for Health and Care Excellence [16]. Therefore, in their study using a Markov decision analytic model to evaluate long-term cost-effectiveness of a 3-year systematic case-finding programme, Lambe et al., [14] compared an active case-finding questionnaire with routine practice and calculated the cost per QALY gained. They found that a systematic approach in primary care to active COPD case-finding is likely to be cost-effective in long term. However, as previously mentioned, they did not consider other interventions in their model, such as smoking cessation, pulmonary rehabilitation, and self-management which could improve HRQoL and reduce exacerbation [14]. Thus, although it is thought that these interventions could make a case-finding approach more cost-effective, the question about the cost-effectiveness of these interventions in a case-finding programme remains unclear.

When analyzing some studies on the development and validation of COPD case-finding tools, mainly questionnaires, we notice that the most of them occur in high-income settings, considering smoking as the main risk factor [6-8] (Table 1). Regarding this, the last question about the COPD case-finding tool is: Can we generalize the results about performance, effectiveness and cost-effectiveness to other settings?

Siddharthan et al., [12], recently assessed the performance of three COPD case-finding questionnaires in 3 LMIC settings (Uganda, Peru and Nepal) considering the biomass fuel as a risk factor in the COLA-6 questionnaire. In their study, they found that the performance of the COPD case-finding questionnaire is context dependent and it is necessary to assess instrument performance in other LMIC settings, as well as the acceptability, feasibility and effectiveness in improving clinical outcomes [10, 12]. In an editorial for the Thorax Journal, Van Boven [16] gave his opinion on case-finding costs and the COPD value pyramid, which was introduced by the London Respiratory Network. The COPD's value pyramid shows the value of interventions to diagnosed COPD patients, such as influenza vaccination, smoking cessation and pulmonary rehabilitation in relation to pharmacotherapy and telehealth. Thus, considering the evidence on cost-effectiveness of COPD case-finding and the importance of primary prevention in these patients, the author considered turning COPD's value pyramid into an iceberg and expanding with options for non-diagnosed people at risk for COPD [16].

Conclusion

COPD case finding may favor the early diagnosis and allow an early pharmacological and non-pharmacological intervention with consequent reduction of events and prognosis improvement (Figure 1). There are some alternative approaches, such as questionnaires, PEF and/or micro-spirometer or a combination of them, with good discriminative accuracy to identify patients with airflow obstruction, developed mainly in high income settings and context dependent performance. Therefore, it is essential to know the available COPD case-finding tools and choose the one that best applies to intended context. However, although there are some effectiveness and cost-effectiveness of COPD case-finding tool evidence, mainly questionnaires, high quality RCT with long-term follow-up are necessary to assess the effectiveness of the COPD case-finding in the natural history of disease and impact of disease compared to the usual practice in different settings

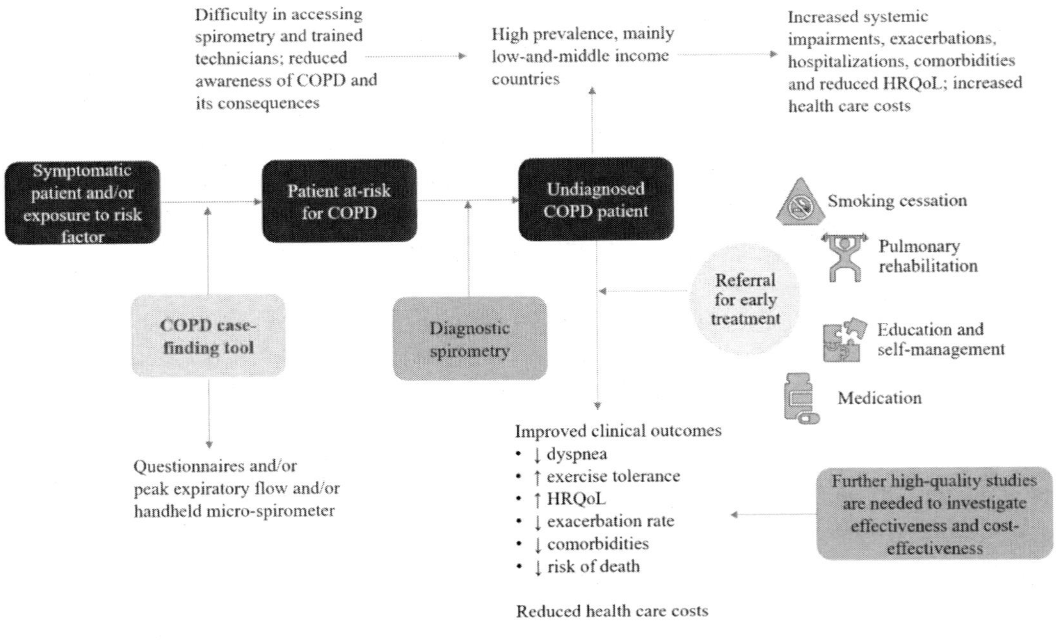

Figure 1. Flowchart on how the COPD case finding tool should work.

Key Points

- COPD case-finding tools are alternative approaches to identify patients at-risk for COPD and refer to diagnostic spirometry, in order to provide adequate early treatment to undiagnosed COPD patients.

- COPD case-finding tool may include questionnaires, peak expiratory flow (PEF) and/or micro-spirometry devices or a combination of them.
- There are several alternative COPD case-finding questionnaires, with or without PEF, focusing on symptoms and risk factors, with sufficient performance showed by discriminative accuracy.
- There are few and heterogenous studies on the effectiveness of COPD case-finding and further high quality RCT are needed to investigate the impact in clinical outcomes compared to usual practice in different settings.
- Although scarce, there is some evidence on the cost-effectiveness of COPD case-finding questionnaire compared to usual care in primary care system.

References

[1] Global Initiative for Chronic Obstructive Lung Disease. *Global Strategy for Prevention, Diagnosis and Management of COPD* [Internet]. 2022. Available from: https://goldcopd.org/2022-gold-reports-2/.

[2] Diab N., Gershon A. S., Sin D. D., Tan W. C., Bourbeau J., Boulet L. P., and Shawn D. Aaron Underdiagnosis and Overdiagnosis of Chronic Obstructive Pulmonary Disease. *Am J Respir Crit Care Med* [Internet]. 2018 Nov;198(9):1130-9.
Available from: https://www.atsjournals.org/doi/10.1164/rccm.201804-0621CI.

[3] Hurst J. R., Buist A. S., Gaga M., Gianella G. E., Kirenga B., Khoo E. M., Renata Gonçalves Mendes, Anant Mohan, Kevin Mortimer, Sarah Rylance, Trishul Siddharthan, Sally J. Singh, Job F. M. van Boven, Siân Williams, Jing Zhang, William Checkley Challenges in the Implementation of Chronic Obstructive Pulmonary Disease Guidelines in Low- and Middle-Income Countries: An Official American Thoracic Society Workshop Report. *Ann Am Thorac Soc* [Internet]. 2021 Aug;18(8):1269-77. Available from: https://www.atsjournals.org/doi/10.1513/AnnalsATS.202103-284ST.

[4] Labonté L. E., Tan W. C., Li P. Z., Mancino P., Aaron S. D., Benedetti A., Kenneth R Chapman, Robert Cowie, J Mark FitzGerald, Paul Hernandez, François Maltais, Darcy D Marciniuk, Dennis O'Donnell, Don Sin, Jean Bourbeau, Canadian Respiratory Research Network; CanCOLD Collaborative Research Group Undiagnosed Chronic Obstructive Pulmonary Disease Contributes to the Burden of Health Care Use. Data from the CanCOLD Study. *Am J Respir Crit Care Med* [Internet]. 2016 Aug;194(3):285-98. Available from: http://www.atsjournals.org/doi/10.1164/rccm.201509-1795OC.

[5] Halpin D. M. G., Celli B. R., Criner G. J., Frith P., López Varela M. V., Salvi S., Claus F Vogelmeier, Ronchang Chen, Kevin Mortimer, Maria Montes de Oca, Zaurbek Aisanov, Daniel Obaseki, Rebecca Decker, Alvar Agusti It is time for the world to take COPD seriously: a statement from the GOLD board of directors. *Eur Respir J* [Internet]. 2019 Jul 4;54(1):1900914.
Available from: http://dx.doi.org/10.1183/13993003.00914-2019.

[6] Martinez F. J., Mannino D., Leidy N. K., Malley K. G., Bacci E. D., Barr R. G., Russ P. Bowler, MeiLan K. Han, Julia F. Houfek, Barry Make, Catherine A. Meldrum, Stephen Rennard, Byron Thomashow, John Walsh, Barbara P. Yawn, High-Risk-COPD Screening Study Group A New Approach for Identifying Patients with Undiagnosed Chronic Obstructive Pulmonary Disease. *Am J Respir Crit Care Med* [Internet]. 2017 Mar 15;195(6):748-56.
Available from: http://www.atsjournals.org/doi/10.1164/rccm.201603-0622OC.

[7] Martinez F. J., Raczek A. E., Seifer F. D., Conoscenti C. S., Curtice T. G., D'Eletto T., Claudia Cote, Clare Hawkins, Amy L Phillips, COPD-PS Clinician Working Group. Development and Initial Validation of a Self-Scored COPD Population Screener Questionnaire (COPD-PS). *COPD J Chronic Obstr Pulm Dis* [Internet]. 2008 Jan 2;5(2):85-95.
Available from: http://www.tandfonline.com/doi/full/10.1080/15412550801940721.

[8] Hanania N. A., Mannino D. M., Yawn B. P., Mapel D. W., Martinez F. J., Donohue J. F., Mark Kosinski, Regina Rendas-Baum, Matthew Mintz, Steven Samuels, Priti Jhingran, Anand A. Dalal. Predicting risk of airflow obstruction in primary care: Validation of the lung function questionnaire (LFQ). *Respir Med* [Internet]. 2010 Aug;104:1160-70. Available from: http://dx.doi.org/10.1016/j.rmed.2010.02.009.

[9] López Varela M. V., Montes de Oca M., Rey A., Casas A., Stirbulov R., Di Boscio V. Development of a simple screening tool for opportunistic COPD case finding in primary care in Latin America: The PUMA study. *Respirology* [Internet]. 2016 Oct;21(7):1227-34.
Available from: https://onlinelibrary.wiley.com/doi/10.1111/resp.12834.

[10] Siddharthan T., Wosu A. C., Pollard S. L., Hossen S., Alupo P., Shade T., Robert Kalyesubula, Shumonta Quaderi, Robert A Wise, John R Hurst, Bruce Kirenga, William Checkley, LiNK Cohort Study Investigators. A Novel Case-Finding Instrument for Chronic Obstructive Pulmonary Disease in Low- and Middle-Income Country Settings. *Int J Chron Obstruct Pulmon Dis* [Internet]. 2020 Nov;15:2769-77.
Available from: https://www.dovepress.com/a-novel-case-finding-instrument-for-chronic-obstructive-pulmonary-dise-peer-reviewed-article-COPD.

[11] Schnieders E, Ünal E, Winkler V, Dambach P, Louis VR, Horstick O, Florian Neuhann, Andreas Deckert. Performance of alternative COPD case-finding tools: a systematic review and meta-analysis. *Eur Respir Rev* [Internet]. 2021 Jun 30;30(160):200350.
Available from: http://dx.doi.org/10.1183/16000617.0350-2020.

[12] Siddharthan T., Pollard S. L., Quaderi S. A., Rykiel N. A., Wosu A. C., Alupo P., Julie A. Barber, Maria Kathia Cárdenas, Ram K. Chandyo, Oscar Flores-Flores, Bruce Kirenga, J. Jaime Miranda, Sakshi Mohan, Federico Ricciardi, Arun K. Sharma, Santa Kumar Das, Laxman Shrestha, Marta O. Soares, William Checkley, John R Hurst, GECo Study Investigators. Discriminative Accuracy of Chronic Obstructive Pulmonary Disease Screening Instruments in 3 Low- and Middle-Income Country Settings. *JAMA* [Internet]. 2022 Jan 11;327(2):151.

[13] Available from: https://jamanetwork.com/journals/jama/fullarticle/2787909.

[14] Haroon S. M., Jordan R. E., O'beirne-Elliman J., Adab P. Effectiveness of case finding strategies for COPD in primary care: A systematic review and meta-analysis. *NPJ Prim Care Respir Med*. 2015;25:1-9.

[15] Lambe T., Adab P., Jordan R. E., Sitch A., Enocson A., Jolly K., Jen Marsh, Richard Riley, Martin Miller, Brendan G. Cooper, Alice Margaret Turner, Jon G. Ayres, Robert Stockley, Sheila Greenfield, Stanley Siebert, Amanda Daley, K. K. Cheng, David Fitzmaurice, Sue Jowett Model-based evaluation of the long-term cost-effectiveness of systematic case-finding for COPD in primary care. *Thorax* [Internet]. 2019 Aug;74:730-9. Available from: https://thorax.bmj.com/lookup/doi/10.1136/thoraxjnl-2018-212148.

[16] Jordan R. E., Adab P., Sitch A., Enocson A., Blissett D., Jowett S., Jen Marsh, Richard D. Riley, Martin R. Miller, Brendan G. Cooper, Alice M. Turner, Kate Jolly, Jon G. Ayres, Shamil Haroon, Robert Stockley, Sheila Greenfield, Stanley Siebert, Amanda J. Daley, K. K. Cheng, David Fitzmaurice. Targeted case finding for chronic obstructive pulmonary disease versus routine practice in primary care (TargetCOPD): a cluster-randomised controlled trial. *Lancet Respir Med* [Internet]. 2016 Sep;4(9):720-30. Available from: https://linkinghub.elsevier.com/retrieve/pii/S2213260016301497.

[17] van Boven J. F. M. Costs of case-finding uncovered: time to revisit COPD's value pyramid? *Thorax* [Internet]. 2019 Aug;74(8):727-9.
Available from: https://thorax.bmj.com/lookup/doi/10.1136/thoraxjnl-2019-213440.

Chapter 9

Smoking Cessation in the Management of Stable COPD

Abdullah M. Alanazi*, **PhD, RRT-NPS**
Department of Respiratory Therapy,
College of Applied Medical Sciences,
King Saud bin Abdulaziz University for Health Sciences
and King Abdullah International Medical Research Center,
Riyadh, Saudi Arabia

Abstract

Tobacco smoking is the most common etiological factor in the development and progression of chronic obstructive pulmonary disease (COPD). Although most smokers with COPD are aware of the harmful effects of smoking, they continue to smoke, and those who quit smoking have a high risk of relapse. Smokers with COPD have a long and intense history of smoking and are highly attached to nicotine's rewarding effects. However, there are effective aids to assist smokers with COPD to quit, including pharmacotherapies and behavioral support. Indeed, smoking cessation was found to be the most effective intervention for slowing disease progression and improving lung function among smokers with COPD. Therefore, this chapter addresses smoking cessation in the management of stable COPD from different perspectives, including assessment, treatment, and prevention.

Introduction

Tobacco smoking is a chronic disorder associated with physical and emotional nicotine dependence. [1, 2] Despite its harmful impact on health, smokers continue to smoke tobacco to experience its rewarding effects. [3, 4] While smoking tobacco, nicotine, an addictive chemical in tobacco, binds to $\alpha4\beta2$ nicotine acetylcholine receptors in the brain, which in turn releases neurotransmitters, primarily dopamine, which produces pleasurable emotional effects and reduces withdrawal symptoms. [2] Abstinence from nicotine lowers its level in the blood, leading to craving, irritability, anxiety, and difficulty concentrating. [5]

Quitting tobacco smoking is challenging and has a high relapse rate, [3, 4] particularly in smokers diagnosed with chronic obstructive pulmonary disease (COPD) because of their chronic use of tobacco, greater nicotine dependence, and weaker self-confidence to quit smoking. [6, 7] In comparison to the general population, smokers with COPD are less likely to

* Corresponding Author's Email: Alanaziab@ksau-hs.edu.sa.

In: Chronic Obstructive Pulmonary Disease
Editor: Jaber S. Alqahtani
ISBN: 979-8-88697-333-4

refrain from smoking, particularly among those with higher consumption of cigarettes per day. [7] Up to 35% of smokers with COPD continue to smoke tobacco after diagnosis, and the prevalence of smoking is 77% in individuals with mild COPD and 51% in individuals with severe COPD. [6, 8] Growing evidence emphasizes the need to optimize smoking cessation among smokers with COPD to decelerate disease progression and prevent smoking-induced complications. [9-11]

Tobacco smoking is the most common cause of COPD and is associated with higher mortality and morbidity. [9, 12, 13] Compared to non-smokers with COPD, greater lung function decline and respiratory exacerbation are observed among smokers with COPD. [9] For instance, among adults with mild to moderate COPD, a two-fold decline in forced expiratory volume in one second was observed among smokers with COPD compared to those who refrained from smoking. [14] However, a famous study by Fletcher and Peto that included working men in London revealed that persistent airway obstruction may slow and stop if smokers quit tobacco smoking (Figure 1). [15] Therefore, smoking cessation using pharmacological and behavioral support treatments is an evidence-based approach that is effective in slowing COPD progression. [16, 17]

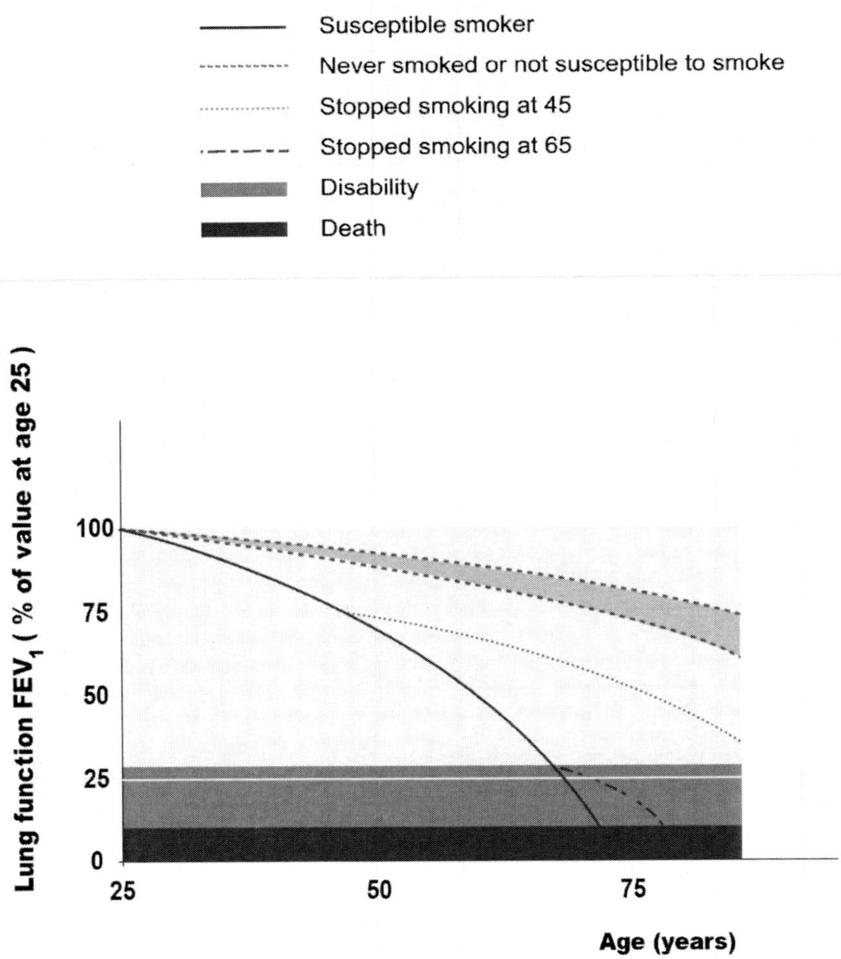

Figure 1. The natural history of chronic airflow obstruction. Adapted from Fletcher & Peto (1977). [15]

Pharmacological and behavioral interventions are most effective when used together for smoking cessation. [18-20] Treatment courses using pharmacological agents help reduce withdrawal symptoms before and after nicotine abstinence, and behavioral interventions help smokers cope with detachment from nicotine addiction. [21] Healthcare providers should utilize teachable moments during smoking-related illness among smokers with COPD to provide effective smoking cessation and increase self-confidence to quit and overcome relapses. [21]

Screening, Assessment, and Enrollment

Healthcare providers are responsible for screening patients for tobacco smoking in every healthcare setting, including outpatient clinics, emergency departments, and inpatient rooms. [21] Considering individuals with COPD, asking about tobacco smoking, advising them to stop smoking, and assisting them in enrolling in smoking cessation are highly warranted. [18, 22] Despite the wide variabilities and challenges to effectively implement such screening, assessment, and enrollment processes for smoking cessation, there are different methods to standardize and ease the process. [23] Among these are the 5As model and the abbreviated 3As model (Figure 2). [24-26]

The 5As model of smoking cessation was first endorsed by the United States Public Health Service in 2008 to briefly deliver smoking cessation services. [27] It provides a systematic direction for healthcare providers to screen, assess, and enroll smokers in smoking cessation. Healthcare providers should 1) *ask* about tobacco use at every patient visit, 2) *advise* those who use tobacco to quit, 3) *assess* their readiness to quit tobacco use, 4) *assist* them to quit by providing pharmacological and behavioral support services, and 5) *arrange* follow-up visits to prevent relapse. [27] Although the 5As model may require additional effort and time, it has been associated with better outcomes in the treatment of tobacco smokers. [27]

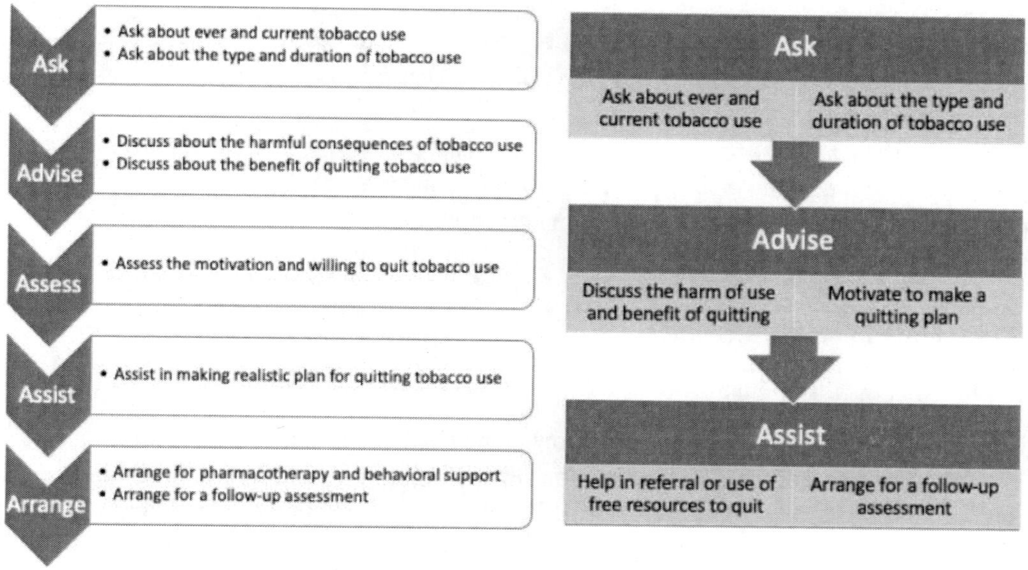

Figure 2. The 5A's and the modified 3A's models for screening, assessment, and enrollment processes in smoking cessation.

The abbreviated 3As model (ask, advise, and assist) has been adapted from the 5As model of smoking cessation to expedite screening, assessment, and enrollment with less work required by healthcare providers. [25, 26] The steps involved are as follows: first, *ask* every patient about any regular or occasional tobacco use during every visit. Second, *advise* those who use tobacco to quit by delivering concise information about the advantages of quitting and available treatment services. Third, *assist* quitting by connecting them with tobacco treatment services provided by the healthcare setting or the national telephone Quitline service that provides pharmacological and/or behavioral support. [25, 26]

The 5As and abbreviated 3As models can be applied via face-to-face, telephone-based, and/or telehealth contact with patients. [21] Screening for tobacco use was optimized by the effective assessment of daily/regular and occasional/recreational tobacco smoking. Those who do not smoke tobacco daily may not be labeled as tobacco smokers. However, intermittent tobacco smoking may cause health-related complications and increase nicotine dependence, especially in individuals with COPD. [1]

Empirical evidence has revealed that a greater degree of nicotine dependence is linked to greater difficulty in refraining from tobacco smoking and requires more intense pharmacological and behavioral interventions. [28] Assessing nicotine dependence can be simplified by asking about the number of cigarettes smoked on a daily basis and whether the first cigarette is smoked within 30 min after waking from sleep. [29] A formal instrument of nicotine dependence can be used to precisely assess the severity of nicotine dependence. The most commonly used instrument is the Fagerström Test for Nicotine Dependence (FTND), a standardized questionnaire for assessing the level of dependence on nicotine. Greater FTND scores suggest the need for more intensive treatment, which can also be integrated into treatment practice to track smokers' progress over time. [30]

Pharmacotherapy for Smoking Cessation

Different types of smoking cessation pharmacotherapies are recommended and effective for adults, including smokers with COPD. Typically, pharmacological agents are started when smokers are ready to quit; however, they are effective when used 2–4 weeks before the quitting date. [31] They are classified as first-line pharmacotherapies (nicotine replacement therapy [NRT], varenicline, and bupropion), which are primarily used (Table 1), and second-line pharmacotherapies (cytisine, clonidine, and nortriptyline).

First-Line Pharmacotherapies

Nicotine Replacement Therapy

NRT delivers nicotine to minimize withdrawal symptoms when smokers refrain from smoking. [8] NRT has been effective in sustaining abstinence from tobacco smoking after smoking cessation. [31] There are different forms of NRT available, such as nicotine gum, lozenge, tablets, spray, inhalers, and patches. [8]

Nicotine gum is chewed as needed every 30 min and can be administered at 2 or 4 mg based on nicotine dependence and intensity of tobacco smoking. [21] To increase its effectiveness, acidic meals and beverages should be avoided for 15 minutes before and after their use. [32, 33] The lung health study reported that the sustained abstinence rate in 1 year among smokers with mild obstructive pulmonary disease who used nicotine gum was 35%, in comparison to 10% in smokers who did not use NRT, and their sustained abstinence rate in 5 years was 22%, in comparison to 5% among smokers who did not use NRT. [34]

Nicotine lozenge is another form of NRT for smokers who do not prefer chewing gum. Nicotine is absorbed through the saliva once placed between the gums and cheek. Nicotine from lozenges is released in greater amounts than nicotine gum after 30 min of use. [33] Nicotine lozenge is available in two doses (2 mg and 4 mg) based on the timing of the smoker's first cigarette after waking, and it is recommended to be used for more than 3 months. [21]

Nicotine sublingual tablets are an oral form of NRT that deliver nicotine equivalent to nicotine lozenges. [8] Among smokers with COPD, those who used nicotine sublingual tablets for smoking cessation had significantly greater sustained abstinence in 1 year (17% vs. 10% in the placebo group). [35]

Nicotine spray and inhalers deliver nicotine via nasal or oral routes. Nicotine spray delivers nicotine through the nasal cavity and is rapidly absorbed into the bloodstream, [31] whereas nicotine inhalers deliver nicotine through the oral cavity (mouth and pharynx). [31] Nicotine spray is available in a 10-ml bottle (200 sprays), and the nicotine inhaler dosage is a 10-mg cartridge (80 puffs). [21]

Transdermal nicotine patches deliver nicotine at a continuously slow-release pace via the skin over 24 h. It is used by smokers without severe nicotine dependence and those who can tolerate nicotine cravings. [21] Transdermal nicotine patch is available in three doses (7, 14, and 21 mg) based on the intensity of cigarette smoking, and it is recommended to be used for more than 3 months. [21] Smokers who experience insomnia while using a transdermal nicotine patch are advised to remove the patch before bedtime. [33] The sustained abstinence rate in 1 year among smokers who used a nicotine transdermal patch was 14% in comparison to 11.3% among smokers who did not use it. [36]

Varenicline

Varenicline stimulates dopamine production by acting on nicotinic acetylcholine receptors of the brain. In addition, varenicline inhibits nicotine binding to $\alpha4\beta2$ nicotine-acetylcholine receptors. All these symptoms reduce withdrawal symptoms from tobacco smoking after abstinence. [8] It is available in two doses (0.5 mg and 1 mg tablets) and is recommended for use for 3–6 months. [21] It should be prescribed with caution to smokers with renal impairment and acute coronary symptoms. It is not recommended for smokers with end-stage renal disease. Varenicline is safe for smokers with stable cardiovascular and psychiatric diseases. [37, 38] Expected side effects of varenicline use are nausea and vivid dreams, which can be minimized by reducing its dose for nausea and avoiding the evening dose for vivid dreams. [39]

Varenicline was safe and effective among smokers with COPD compared to placebo and other smoking cessation treatments. Several studies concluded that varenicline use was a predictor of prolonged sustained abstinence up to 72 weeks. Varenicline can be used even with COPD exacerbations to achieve greater odds of sustained abstinence from tobacco smoking. [17, 40-43]

Table 1. First-line pharmacotherapies for smoking cessation

Drug	Dosing	Administration	Expected adverse effects
Nicotine gum (Nicorette gum; Thrive gum)	2 mg if the first cigarette is smoked >30 min after waking. 4 mg if the first cigarette is smoked ≤30 min after waking.	One piece each hour as needed. No drinking or eating 15 min before use. Chew until mouth tingles, then keep gum inside the cheek. Repeat chewing each time the tingling disappears. Do not use gum for more than 30 minutes.	Mouth irritation, hiccups, nausea; heartburn, and jaw soreness.
Nicotine lozenge (Nicorette lozenge)	2 mg if the first cigarette is smoked >30 min after waking. 4 mg if the first cigarette is smoked ≤30 min after waking.	One piece each hour as needed. No more than 20 pieces a day. No drinking or eating 15 min before use. Keep lozenges between cheek and gum until it melts gradually.	Mouth irritation, hiccups, nausea, and heartburn.
Nicotine sublingual table (Nicorette microtab; Boots NicAssist)	2 mg if the number of cigarettes smoked daily ≤20. 4 mg if the number of cigarettes smoked daily >20.	Place tablet(s) under the tongue until dissolve gradually. One to two tablet(s) based on smoking frequency. Do not exceed dosing instructions.	Headache, throat irritation, hiccups, and feeling sick.
Nicotine spray (Nicotrol NS)	0.5 mg/spray. A bottle contains 200 sprays.	Administer one spray in each nostril every 1–2 h. Do not inhale, swallow, or sniff during spraying.	Nasal discomfort, throat irritation, rhinitis, cough, and sneezing.
Nicotine inhaler (Nicorette; Nicotrol inhalation)	10 mg cartridge (80 puffs)	Inhale one cartridge every 1–2 h. Do not exceed 16 cartridges a day. Do not inhale deep to the lungs. Inhale into mouth and throat. Change cartridge once nicotine taste disappears.	Mouth irritation, throat irritation, and cough.
Transdermal nicotine patch (Nicoderm CQ; Habitrol)	14 mg if the number of cigarettes smoked daily <10. 21 mg if the number of cigarettes smoked daily ≥10. Doses should be tapered gradually to 7 mg after 6 weeks.	Place a new patch on dry skin every morning. Rotate sites every time to avoid skin irritation. Preferred sites are the shoulder or arms.	Skin irritation, sleep disturbance, and vivid dreams.
Varenicline (Chantix; Champix)	0.5 mg once on days 1–3. 0.5 mg twice on days 4–7. 1 mg twice on day 8 and beyond.	Start varenicline 1–4 weeks before the desired quit date.	Headache, nausea, vivid dreams, and insomnia.
Bupropion (Wellbutrin; Zyban)	150 mg once on day 1–3. 150 mg twice on day 4 and beyond.	Start bupropion 1 to 2 weeks before the desired quit date.	Headache, dry mouth, insomnia, and agitation.

Bupropion

Bupropion is an antidepressant that is effective for smoking cessation. It works by minimizing withdrawal symptoms including depression and appetite control. [44] It should be used 2 weeks before the quitting date. Bupropion is used daily at 150 mg of sustained release. The expected side effects are dry mouth, insomnia, agitation, and headaches. [39] It is contraindicated in patients with seizures, epilepsy, brain neoplasms, anorexia nervosa, and pregnant and nursing women. [45] Among smokers with COPD, bupropion showed significantly greater sustained abstinence at 6 months than placebo. [17, 46]

Second-Line Pharmacotherapies

Cytisine is a plant-based substance that is used in smoking cessation because its mechanism of action is similar to that of varenicline. [47] Although no study has assessed cytisine effectiveness among smokers with COPD, it was more effective than NRT in sustaining abstinence, with a low quit-rate among the general population of smokers. [48-50]

Clonidine is an α2-adrenergic receptor agonist that is used as an off-label drug for smoking cessation. It was found to be an effective agent for reducing nicotine withdrawal symptoms, such as craving, anxiety, restlessness, and tension. [24] Expected side effects of clonidine use are hypotension, fatigue, dizziness, dry mouth, and constipation. There are no available data to support clonidine use in COPD; however, clinical trials among general smokers revealed more effective use of oral or transdermal clonidine than placebo to sustain abstinence. [51]

Nortriptyline is an antidepressant that should be used with caution and under supervision for smoking cessation. [52] It is associated with dry mouth, constipation, blurred vision, hypotension, and urinary retention. It is contraindicated in patients with arrhythmias or myocardial infarction. [53] Nortriptyline was more effective in increasing short-term smoking cessation than placebo; however, there was no significant difference in the use of nortriptyline among smokers with COPD. [54]

New Pharmacotherapies

To date, two promising pharmacological agents are being tested for smoking cessation. Acetylcholinesterase inhibitors and N-acetylcysteine (NAC) are in the early stages of clinical trials for the treatment of tobacco smoking in the general population. [55, 56] Neither of these have been assessed among smokers with COPD.

Acetylcholinesterase inhibitors were originally prescribed to manage cognitive decline in patients with Alzheimer's disease. However, acetylcholinesterase inhibitors were efficacious among smokers with nicotine dependence. It is now being investigated in a 12-week randomized placebo-controlled trial. [55] *NAC* is an antioxidant agent being tested to treat tobacco smoking in a 12-week, randomized, double-blind trial. [56] Early results revealed that NAC was effective in reducing daily cigarette use. [56]

Electronic Nicotine Delivery System

Tobacco industry efforts are centered around keeping customers by introducing new products claimed to be less harmful than tobacco cigarettes. There is no strong evidence to support such claims, as some studies were presented and funded by tobacco companies. [57] The most common product is the electronic nicotine delivery system (ENDS), known as electronic cigarettes (e-cigarettes) and JUUL, which has gained popularity in recent years as an alternative tobacco smoking cessation aid, especially for those who are nicotine dependent. [58]

E-cigarettes are battery-powered devices that deliver nicotine through vapor aerosols, without combustion. [59] Adopting ENDS in smoking cessation treatment is debatable, as there is no strong evidence to conclude its long-term safety and effectiveness in helping smokers quit tobacco smoking. [21] A hallmark study in 2021 conducted by a Cochrane group revealed moderate evidence that e-cigarettes containing nicotine were more effective than NRT in helping smokers quit tobacco cigarettes. [60] Among smokers with COPD, it is recommended to direct them to use approved pharmacotherapies to quit tobacco smoking, especially if the ENDS content is not well regulated. For example, commercial and homemade ENDS may contain vitamin E acetate linked to e-cigarette or vaping use-associated lung injury. [61]

Combinations of Different Pharmacotherapies

Combining different first-line smoking cessation agents is a current practice that has been shown to improve sustained abstinence in smokers. [31, 62] A combination of varenicline with bupropion or NRT can be used; however, the only United States Food and Drug Association-approved combination for smoking cessation is bupropion and transdermal nicotine patches. [62] Under physician supervision, any combination can be used if a single agent is not effective in encouraging quitting and/or sustaining abstinence. [62] Combining different agents for smoking cessation is clinically limited, considering the increased cost, side effects, and limited evidence of its efficacy. [21]

Among smokers with COPD, there is limited evidence to support the use of smoking cessation agents to treat tobacco smoking. [8] A combination of nicotine patches and gum was more effective than varenicline in smokers with COPD; however, the recent practice of combining varenicline with other agents is under investigation. [8, 63] Careful inclusion criteria of smokers with COPD and integrations of behavioral support into smoking cessation are highly warranted to effectively assess the combination of different agents into clinical practice. [64]

Behavioral Support for Smoking Cessation

Behavioral support is the recommended practice for smoking cessation. Although its implementation is not well utilized, such interventions have shown promising outcomes in terms of improving the quit rate and sustained abstinence. [65-67] However, combining behavioral support with pharmacotherapies is the most effective approach to increase successful smoking cessation trials. [21] The mode of delivery and intensity of behavioral support varies based on the healthcare settings and smokers' preferences. Behavioral support can be delivered through face-to-face, mobile-based, or web-based interventions. There are several types of behavioral support that differ in intensity; the most recommended are motivational intervention (MI) and cognitive-behavioral therapy (CBT). [18, 21, 65, 68]

Identifying the willingness and readiness of smokers to quit is an important step in designing effective behavioral interventions that fit the smoker's stage. The transtheoretical model (TTM) is a widely used model that assesses behavioral changes in smoking (Figure 3). TTM describes behavior change in five stages, from pre-contemplation, contemplation, preparation, action, maintenance, and relapse. [69] Behavioral interventions by MI, CBT, or both can be tailored to support smokers based on their TTM stage in increasing willingness to quit, adhere to treatment plans, sustain abstinence, and adopt new lifestyle habits. [70]

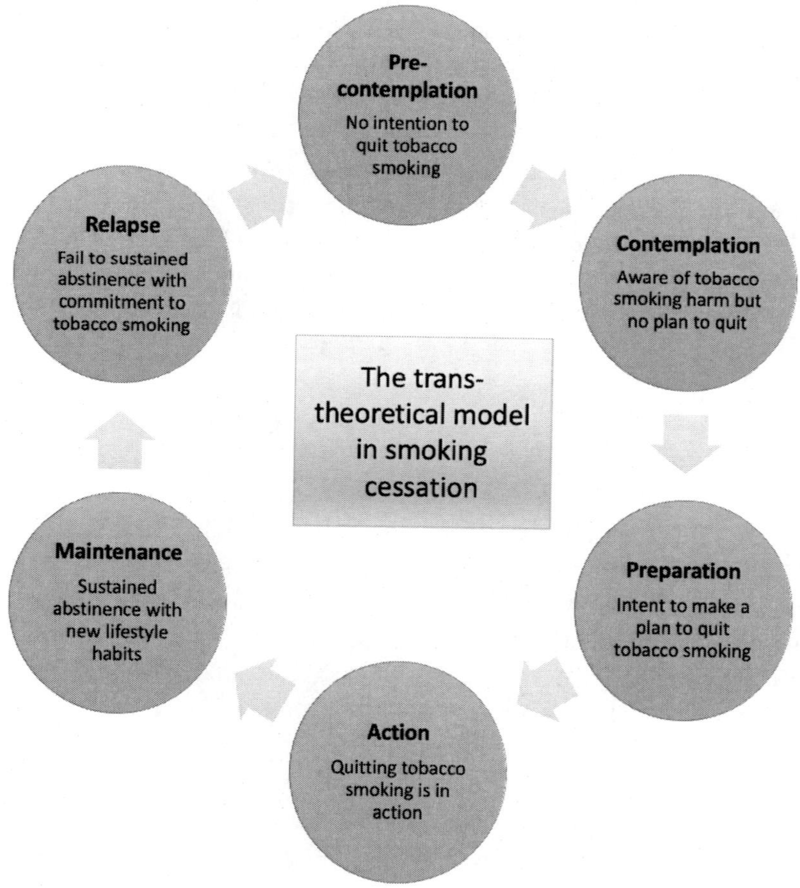

Figure 3. The trans-theoretical model in smoking cessation.

MI is a recommended approach to support smokers with lower motivation by increasing their willingness and commitment to smoking cessation. [70] MI is reciprocal counseling that empowers smokers through active listening and advises them to make a change. [70] Through MI, a counselor should adopt non-confrontational communication and empathize to gain smokers' trust. [70] Discussion related to the barriers and benefits of quitting smoking in the counseling session are highly recommended to set realistic goals for smoking behavior changes. [70]

CBT is another approach to guide motivated smokers in making a change to quit and overcoming their barriers through supervised step-by-step practice. [71] CBT involves intense behavioral training sessions centered on identifying affective, cognitive, and environmental factors that trigger smoking. [70] Smokers with COPD have a long history of smoking tobacco, which makes them highly dependent on nicotine. These individuals usually face obstacles in quitting smoking with multiple failed attempts. CBT has shown effective outcomes in assisting smokers in overcoming craving, withdrawal symptoms, and physical dependence on nicotine. [70, 71]

Behavioral support of any approach should address the cognitive, psychosocial, and environmental factors that trigger smoking and compromise the commitment to smoking cessation. [70] Self-efficacy (an individual's belief in his or her ability to execute or resist behaviors) and outcome expectancies (perceived consequences of a person's behavior) of tobacco smoking are cognitive factors that play a role in resisting and continuing smoking, which can be noted in behavioral support sessions. [72] Psychosocial factors related to mental disorders, social rank, and income are highly associated with smoking status. Therefore, setting realistic expectations in planning a smoking cessation plan is warranted. [70] Finally, smoking behavior is influenced by environmental factors, such as smoking in the workplace, in public places, and with peers and family, which make quitting smoking a challenging task. [70] Directing smokers to quit without social and family isolation is necessary to increase their odds of smoking cessation.

Relapse Prevention

Regardless of the significant efforts to help smokers quit smoking, tobacco smoking remains a public health dilemma. Tobacco smoking is a chronic relapsing behavior that requires long-term planning with several attempts to maintain abstinence from smoking. [21] Smoking cessation is a process that requires continuous support using several techniques to prevent relapse. Most smokers relapse at some time after abstinence from smoking, which necessitates an understanding of the course of smoking abstinence, lapse, relapse, and recovery. [70]

Lapse and relapse are different terms that are commonly misperceived in smoking treatment. Lapse refers to the first episode of smoking after the quit date. However, relapse refers to the failure to maintain smoking abstinence over time with multiple episodes of smoking. [73] A lapse does not indicate relapse unless an individual commits to continue smoking. On the other hand, recovery from smoking is the complete remission of tobacco smoking by overcoming nicotine dependence and commitment to sobriety. [73]

Several intrapersonal and interpersonal factors may mediate relapse in smokers. Intrapersonal factors include emotions, coping issues, willingness to quit, cognitive mechanisms of self-efficacy, outcome expectancies, and craving cues. Interpersonal factors include peers, family, work environment, and social support. [70] All of these can be addressed within a continuous treatment plan to prevent relapse through different clinical interventions, as listed in Table 2.

Table 2. Clinical interventions to prevent relapse in smoking cessation

Assist in understanding between lapse, relapse, and recovery
Assist in identifying high-risk situations and developing coping strategies
Assist in identifying alcohol or other substance issues
Assist in dealing with social pressures
Assist in supporting social networks
Assist in developing coping strategies with negative affect and cognitive issues
Assist in developing a balanced lifestyle
Assist in developing a relapse management plan

Tobacco Control Policies and Tobacco Use Treatment Services

A global movement led by the World Health Organization (WHO) provides a framework of strategies that control tobacco use and support tobacco use treatment services to assist smokers, including vulnerable populations such as smokers with COPD. [74] The WHO Framework Convention on Tobacco Control (WHO-FCTC) guides the country-level implementation of MPOWER measures. The MPOWER consists of six strategies related to tobacco control policies and tobacco use treatment services, as briefly explained below. Adopting such measures varies across countries, based on their legislative power and capacity to implement them. [74]

Monitoring tobacco use. Valid and reliable data on the national prevalence of tobacco use is imperative for the allocation of effective support to control and treat tobacco use. Data should be designed to assess the magnitudes, patterns, determinants, and health consequences of tobacco use. Policymakers and healthcare providers should utilize such data to advocate national tobacco control policies and allocate effective and comprehensive treatment services to smokers. [74, 75]

Protecting people from tobacco smoke. Second-hand smoking is an additional public health issue related to tobacco smoking. Protecting the general population, including newborns, children, and sick people, from exposure to tobacco smoking is a basic human right mandated by WHO. Article 8 of the WHO-FCTC directs countries on methods to protect people from tobacco smoking regardless of the country's income. Primarily, smoke-free legislation prohibits smoking in indoor places, including workplaces, public housing, public transportation, and indoor recreational places. [74, 76]

Offering help to quit smoking. The WHO-FCTC mandates that countries should treat tobacco smoking and increase their capacity to train healthcare providers in smoking cessation. This includes providing pharmacotherapies and behavioral support to smokers. Despite the high global prevalence of tobacco smoking, its trend is decreasing owing to the provision of effective and supportive tobacco treatment services to smokers. [74]

Warning about the dangers of tobacco. Most smokers believe that tobacco smoking is harmful; however, the magnitude and intensity of nicotine dependence makes quitting tobacco smoking an extremely challenging task, apart from the tobacco industry's tactics to advertise tobacco smoking as appealing to use and distract from its devastating health effects. Article 11 of the WHO-FCTC directs policymakers to place health messaging and pictorial warnings representing the health effects of tobacco smoking on tobacco packages. [74, 77]

Enforcing tobacco advertising, promotion, and sponsorship bans. Article 13 of the WHO-FCTC encourages a ban on direct and indirect tobacco advertising, promotion, and sponsorship (TAPS). The tobacco industry implements different strategies to link tobacco use with empowerment, liberty, and success through TAPS, which are significantly associated with tobacco smoking initiation and continuation. Countries are asked to ban such tactics to protect people from TAPS. [74, 78]

Raising taxes on tobacco. Empirical evidence has concluded that tobacco excise taxes and prices are the most effective interventions to prevent and reduce tobacco smoking. This was specifically guided by Article 6 of the WHO-FCTC. Raising taxes works by making purchasing tobacco products less affordable and allocating taxes to support tobacco treatment services. Implementing tobacco taxation is part of the comprehensive strategy led by the WHO to prevent and treat tobacco smoking, in addition to the above-mentioned strategies of the FCTC. [74, 79]

Conclusion

Smokers with COPD constitute a vulnerable group of individuals who are highly addicted to nicotine. Understanding the barriers and motivators to stop smoking is a pivotal component in assisting them with smoking cessation. Smokers with COPD may vary in their willingness to stop smoking, based on their disease symptoms. Those with advanced COPD may be more willing to engage and commit to quitting tobacco smoking.

Smoking cessation plans for smokers with COPD should be tailored in terms of duration and mode of intervention, including pharmacotherapy, behavioral support, and relapse prevention. A combined intervention of pharmacotherapy and behavioral support is highly recommended to increase the effectiveness of smoking cessation. Healthcare providers should utilize the course of illness exacerbation, hospitalizations, and physician visits as teachable moments to encourage smoking cessation among smokers with COPD. Resistance and multiple failures to quit should not discourage healthcare providers from enforcing smoking cessation as it is a proven approach to slow disease progression.

Key Points

- Smoking cessation is the most common intervention to slow disease progression and improve lung function in smokers with COPD.
- Effective screening and assessment of tobacco smoking in healthcare settings are warranted to optimize smoking cessation among smokers with COPD.
- Combining behavioral support with pharmacotherapies for smokers with COPD is the most effective approach to increase successful smoking cessation trials.
- To date, e-cigarettes are not recommended as smoking cessation aids for smokers with COPD.
- A high relapse rate is expected among smokers with COPD, and several attempts to quit smoking should be encouraged.

References

[1] Health UDo, Services H. *The Health Consequences of Smoking—50 Years of Progress: A Report of the Surgeon General.* Atlanta, GA: US Department of Health and Human Services, Centers for Disease; 2014.

[2] Benowitz NL. Nicotine addiction. *New England Journal of Medicine.* 2010;362(24):2295-303.

[3] Chaiton M, Diemert L, Cohen JE, Bondy SJ, Selby P, Philipneri A, et al. Estimating the number of quit attempts it takes to quit smoking successfully in a longitudinal cohort of smokers. *BMJ Open.* 2016;6(6):e011045.

[4] Hughes JR, Solomon LJ, Naud S, Fingar JR, Helzer JE, Callas PW. Natural history of attempts to stop smoking. *Nicotine & Tobacco Research.* 2014;16(9):1190-8.

[5] Piper ME. Withdrawal: expanding a key addiction construct. *Nicotine & Tobacco Research.* 2015;17(12):1405-15.

[6] Tønnesen P. Smoking cessation and COPD. *European Respiratory Review.* 2013;22(127):37-43.

[7] Jiménez-Ruiz CA, Masa F, Miravitlles M, Gabriel R, Viejo JL, Villasante C, et al. Smoking characteristics: differences in attitudes and dependence between healthy smokers and smokers with COPD. *Chest.* 2001;119(5):1365-70.

[8] Antoniu SA, Buculei I, Mihaltan F, Crisan Dabija R, Trofor AC. Pharmacological strategies for smoking cessation in patients with chronic obstructive pulmonary disease: a pragmatic review. *Expert Opinion on Pharmacotherapy.* 2021;22(7):835-47.

[9] Singh D, Agusti A, Anzueto A, Barnes PJ, Bourbeau J, Celli BR, et al. Global strategy for the diagnosis, management, and prevention of chronic obstructive lung disease: the GOLD science committee report 2019. *European Respiratory Journal.* 2019;53(5).

[10] Nizet TA, van den Elshout FJ, Heijdra YF, van de Ven MJ, Mulder PG, Folgering HTM. Survival of chronic hypercapnic COPD patients is predicted by smoking habits, comorbidity, and hypoxemia. *Chest.* 2005;127(6):1904-10.

[11] Trofor AC, Papadakis S, Lotrean L, Buculei-Porosnicu I, Vyzikidou VK, Evangelopoulou V, et al. Tobacco treatment guideline for high risk groups: a pilot study in patients with chronic obstructive pulmonary disease. *Tobacco Induced Diseases.* 2018;16.

[12] Celli BR, MacNee W, Agusti A, Anzueto A, Berg B, Buist AS, et al. Standards for the diagnosis and treatment of patients with COPD: a summary of the ATS/ERS position paper. *European Respiratory Journal.* 2004;23(6):932-46.

[13] Kohansal R, Martinez-Camblor P, Agustí A, Buist AS, Mannino DM, Soriano JB. The natural history of chronic airflow obstruction revisited: an analysis of the Framingham offspring cohort. *American journal of respiratory and critical care medicine.* 2009;180(1):3-10.

[14] Willemse BW, Postma DS, Timens W, ten Hacken NH. The impact of smoking cessation on respiratory symptoms, lung function, airway hyperresponsiveness and inflammation. *European Respiratory Journal.* 2004;23(3):464-76.

[15] Fletcher C, Peto R. The natural history of chronic airflow obstruction. *Br Med J.* 1977;1(6077):1645-8.

[16] Anthonisen NR, Connett JE, Murray RP. Smoking and lung function of Lung Health Study participants after 11 years. *American Journal of Respiratory and Critical Care Medicine.* 2002;166(5):675-9.

[17] van Eerd EA, van der Meer RM, van Schayck OC, Kotz D. Smoking cessation for people with chronic obstructive pulmonary disease. *Cochrane Database of Systematic Reviews.* 2016(8).

[18] Patnode CD, Henderson JT, Coppola EL, Melnikow J, Durbin S, Thomas RG. Interventions for tobacco cessation in adults, including pregnant persons: updated evidence report and systematic review for the US Preventive Services Task Force. *Jama.* 2021;325(3):280-98.

[19] Hartmann-Boyce J, Hong B, Livingstone-Banks J, Wheat H, Fanshawe TR. Additional behavioural support as an adjunct to pharmacotherapy for smoking cessation. *Cochrane Database of Systematic Reviews.* 2019(6).

[20] Stead LF, Koilpillai P, Fanshawe TR, Lancaster T. Combined pharmacotherapy and behavioural interventions for smoking cessation. *Cochrane Database of Systematic Reviews.* 2016(3).

[21] Rigotti NA, Kruse GR, Livingstone-Banks J, Hartmann-Boyce J. Treatment of tobacco smoking: A review. *JAMA*. 2022;327(6):566-77.

[22] Health UDo, Services H. *Smoking Cessation: A Report of the Surgeon General*. Atlanta: US Department of Health and Human Services. 2020.

[23] VanFrank B, Presley-Cantrell L. A comprehensive approach to increase adult tobacco cessation. *JAMA*. 2021;325(3):232-3.

[24] Fiore M, Jaen C, Baker T, Bailey W, Bennett G, Benowitz N. Treati Clinical Practice Guideline. A Clinical Practice Guideline for Treating Tobacco Use and Dependence: 2008 Update-A US Public Health Service report. *American Journal of Preventive Medicine*. 2008;35(2):158-76.

[25] Sherman SE, Takahashi N, Kalra P, Gifford E, Finney JW, Canfield J, et al. Care coordination to increase referrals to smoking cessation telephone counseling: a demonstration project. *The American Journal of Managed Care*. 2008;14(3):141-8.

[26] Vidrine J, Shete S, Cao Y, Greisinger A, Harmonson P, Sharp B, et al. Ask-Advise-Connect: a new approach to smoking treatment delivery in health care settings. *JAMA Intern Med*. 2013; 173 (6): 458–64. Cluster randomized trial that demonstrated than an ask-advise-connect vs an ask-advise-refer strategy resulted in. 2013;13.

[27] Lawson PJ, Flocke SA, Casucci B. Development of an instrument to document the 5A's for smoking cessation. *American Journal of Preventive Medicine*. 2009;37(3):248-54.

[28] Mannino DM. Why won't our patients stop smoking? The power of nicotine addiction. *Diabetes Care*. 2009;32(suppl_2):S426-S8.

[29] Heatherton TF, Kozlowski LT, Frecker RC, Rickert W, Robinson J. Measuring the heaviness of smoking: using self-reported time to the first cigarette of the day and number of cigarettes smoked per day. *British Journal of Addiction*. 1989;84(7):791-800.

[30] Heatherton TF, Kozlowski LT, Frecker RC, Fagerstrom KO. The Fagerström test for nicotine dependence: a revision of the Fagerstrom Tolerance Questionnaire. *British Journal of Addiction*. 1991;86(9):1119-27.

[31] Lindson N, Chepkin SC, Ye W, Fanshawe TR, Bullen C, Hartmann-Boyce J. Different doses, durations and modes of delivery of nicotine replacement therapy for smoking cessation. *Cochrane Database of Systematic Reviews*. 2019(4).

[32] Sachs D, Leone F, Farber H, Bars M, Prezant D, Schane R, et al. *American College of Chest Physicians Tobacco-Dependence Treatment Tool Kit*. American College of Chest Physicians. 2009.

[33] Wadgave U, Nagesh L. Nicotine replacement therapy: an overview. *International Journal of Health Sciences*. 2016;10(3):425.

[34] Anthonisen NR, Connett JE, Kiley JP, Altose MD, Bailey WC, Buist AS, et al. Effects of smoking intervention and the use of an inhaled anticholinergic bronchodilator on the rate of decline of FEV1: the Lung Health Study. *Jama*. 1994;272(19):1497-505.

[35] Tønnesen P, Mikkelsen K, Bremann L. Nurse-conducted smoking cessation in patients with COPD using nicotine sublingual tablets and behavioral support. *Chest*. 2006;130(2):334-42.

[36] Investigators P. Effects on abstinence of nicotine patch treatment before quitting smoking: parallel, two arm, pragmatic randomised trial. *BMJ*. 2018;361.

[37] McClure JB, Swan GE, Catz SL, Jack L, Javitz H, McAfee T, et al. Smoking outcome by psychiatric history after behavioral and varenicline treatment. *Journal of Substance Abuse Treatment*. 2010; 38(4):394-402.

[38] Sterling LH, Windle SB, Filion KB, Touma L, Eisenberg MJ. Varenicline and adverse cardiovascular events: a systematic review and meta-analysis of randomized controlled trials. *Journal of the American Heart Association*. 2016;5(2):e002849.

[39] Giulietti F, Filipponi A, Rosettani G, Giordano P, Iacoacci C, Spannella F, et al. Pharmacological approach to smoking cessation: an updated review for daily clinical practice. *High Blood Pressure & Cardiovascular Prevention*. 2020;27(5):349-62.

[40] Tashkin DP, Rennard S, Hays JT, Ma W, Lawrence D, Lee TC. Effects of varenicline on smoking cessation in patients with mild to moderate COPD: a randomized controlled trial. *Chest*. 2011; 139(3):591-9.

[41] Jiménez Ruiz CA, Ramos Pinedo A, Cicero Guerrero A, Mayayo Ulibarri M, Cristobal Fernández M, Lopez Gonzalez G. Characteristics of COPD smokers and effectiveness and safety of smoking cessation medications. *Nicotine & Tobacco Research.* 2012;14(9):1035-9.

[42] Sansores RH, Ramírez-Venegas A, Arellano-Rocha R, Noé-Díaz V, García-Gómez L, Pérez Bautista O, et al. Use of varenicline for more than 12 months for smoking cessation in heavy chronic obstructive pulmonary disease smokers unmotivated to quit: a pilot study. *Therapeutic Advances in Respiratory Disease.* 2016;10(5):383-90.

[43] Zenteno RJH, Lara DF, Venegas AR, Sansores RH, Pineda JR, Trujillo FF, et al. Varenicline for long term smoking cessation in patients with COPD. *Pulmonary Pharmacology & Therapeutics.* 2018;53: 116-20.

[44] Howes S, Hartmann-Boyce J, Livingstone-Banks J, Hong B, Lindson N. Antidepressants for smoking cessation. *Cochrane Database of Systematic Reviews.* 2020(4).

[45] Benowitz NL, Pipe A, West R, Hays JT, Tonstad S, McRae T, et al. Cardiovascular safety of varenicline, bupropion, and nicotine patch in smokers: a randomized clinical trial. *JAMA Internal Medicine.* 2018;178(5):622-31.

[46] Gonzales D, Rennard SI, Nides M, Oncken C, Azoulay S, Billing CB, et al. Varenicline, an $\alpha 4\beta 2$ nicotinic acetylcholine receptor partial agonist, vs sustained-release bupropion and placebo for smoking cessation: a randomized controlled trial. *Jama.* 2006;296(1):47-55.

[47] Tutka P, Vinnikov D, Courtney RJ, Benowitz NL. Cytisine for nicotine addiction treatment: A review of pharmacology, therapeutics and an update of clinical trial evidence for smoking cessation. *Addiction.* 2019;114(11):1951-69.

[48] Gómez-Coronado N, Walker AJ, Berk M, Dodd S. Current and emerging pharmacotherapies for cessation of tobacco smoking. *Pharmacotherapy: The Journal of Human Pharmacology and Drug Therapy.* 2018;38(2):235-58.

[49] Walker N, Howe C, Glover M, McRobbie H, Barnes J, Nosa V, et al. Cytisine versus nicotine for smoking cessation. *New England Journal of Medicine.* 2014;371(25):2353-62.

[50] West R, Zatonski W, Cedzynska M, Lewandowska D, Pazik J, Aveyard P, et al. Placebo-controlled trial of cytisine for smoking cessation. *New England Journal of Medicine.* 2011;365(13):1193-200.

[51] Gourlay SG, Stead LF, Benowitz N. Clonidine for smoking cessation. *Cochrane Database of Systematic Reviews.* 1999(1).

[52] Prochazka AV, Weaver MJ, Keller RT, Fryer GE, Licari PA, Lofaso D. A randomized trial of nortriptyline for smoking cessation. *Archives of Internal Medicine.* 1998;158(18):2035-9.

[53] Herman AI, Sofuoglu M. Comparison of available treatments for tobacco addiction. *Current Psychiatry Reports.* 2010;12(5):433-40.

[54] Kotz D, Wesseling G, Huibers MJ, van Schayck OC. Efficacy of confronting smokers with airflow limitation for smoking cessation. *European Respiratory Journal.* 2009;33(4):754-62.

[55] Nagano T, Katsurada M, Yasuda Y, Kobayashi K, Nishimura Y. Current pharmacologic treatments for smoking cessation and new agents undergoing clinical trials. *Therapeutic Advances in Respiratory Disease.* 2019;13:1753466619875925.

[56] Prado E, Maes M, Piccoli LG, Baracat M, Barbosa DS, Franco O, et al. N-acetylcysteine for therapy-resistant tobacco use disorder: a pilot study. *Redox Report.* 2015;20(5):215-22.

[57] Pisinger C, Godtfredsen N, Bender AM. A conflict of interest is strongly associated with tobacco industry–favourable results, indicating no harm of e-cigarettes. *Preventive Medicine.* 2019;119:124-31.

[58] Fadus MC, Smith TT, Squeglia LM. The rise of e-cigarettes, pod mod devices, and JUUL among youth: factors influencing use, health implications, and downstream effects. *Drug and Alcohol Dependence.* 2019;201:85-93.

[59] National Academies of Sciences E, Medicine, Health, Medicine D, Board on Population H, Public Health P, et al. In: Eaton DL, Kwan LY, Stratton K, editors. *Public Health Consequences of E-Cigarettes.* Washington (DC): National Academies Press (US) Copyright 2018 by the National Academy of Sciences. All rights reserved.; 2018.

[60] Hartmann-Boyce J, McRobbie H, Butler AR, Lindson N, Bullen C, Begh R, et al. Electronic cigarettes for smoking cessation. *Cochrane Database of Systematic Reviews.* 2021(9).

[61] Matsumoto S, Traber MG, Leonard SW, Choi J, Fang X, Maishan M, et al. Aerosolized Vitamin E Acetate Causes Oxidative Injury in Mice and in Alveolar Macrophages. *American Journal of Physiology-Lung Cellular and Molecular Physiology*. 2022.

[62] Strassmann R, Bausch B, Spaar A, Kleijnen J, Braendli O, Puhan MA. Smoking cessation interventions in COPD: a network meta-analysis of randomised trials. *European Respiratory Journal*. 2009;34(3):634-40.

[63] Jimenez-Ruiz C, Fagerstrom K. Smoking cessation treatment for COPD smokers: the role of pharmacological interventions. *Monaldi Arch Chest Dis*. 2013;79(1):27-32.

[64] Hilberink SR, Jacobs JE, Breteler MH, de Vries H, Grol RP. General practice counseling for patients with chronic obstructive pulmonary disease to quit smoking: impact after 1 year of two complex interventions. *Patient Education and Counseling*. 2011;83(1):120-4.

[65] Hartmann-Boyce J, Livingstone-Banks J, Ordóñez-Mena JM, Fanshawe TR, Lindson N, Freeman SC, et al. Behavioural interventions for smoking cessation: an overview and network meta-analysis. *Cochrane Database of Systematic Reviews*. 2021(1).

[66] Stead LF, Buitrago D, Preciado N, Sanchez G, Hartmann-Boyce J, Lancaster T. *Physician Advice for Smoking Cessation. Cochrane Database of Systematic Reviews. 2013*(5).

[67] Lancaster T, Stead LF. Individual behavioural counselling for smoking cessation. *Cochrane Database of Systematic Reviews*. 2017(3).

[68] Baker TB, McCarthy DE. Smoking treatment: A report card on progress and challenges. *Annual Review of Clinical Psychology*. 2021;17:1-30.

[69] DiClemente CC, Prochaska JO, Fairhurst SK, Velicer WF, Velasquez MM, Rossi JS. The process of smoking cessation: an analysis of precontemplation, contemplation, and preparation stages of change. *Journal of Consulting and Clinical Psychology*. 1991;59(2):295.

[70] Lowinson JH. *Lowinson and Ruiz's Substance Abuse: A Comprehensive Textbook:* Lippincott Williams & Wilkins; 2011.

[71] Patten CA, Martin JE, Myers MG, Calfas KJ, Williams CD. Effectiveness of cognitive-behavioral therapy for smokers with histories of alcohol dependence and depression. *Journal of Studies on Alcohol*. 1998;59(3):327-35.

[72] Bandura A. The Explanatory and Predictive Scope of Self-Efficacy Theory. *Journal of Social and Clinical Psychology*. 1986;4(3):359-73.

[73] Daley DC, Marlatt GA. *Overcoming Your Alcohol or Drug Problem: Effective Recovery Strategies:* Oxford University Press; 2006.

[74] Organization WH. *WHO Framework Convention on Tobacco Control*. WHO Regional Office for South-East Asia; 2004.

[75] Arora S, Gupta S. Monitoring tobacco use and prevention policies: perspective of WHO report on the global tobacco epidemic, 2017. *J Nurs Sci Pract*. 2019;9:39-45.

[76] Edwards R, Thomson G, Wilson N, Waa A, Bullen C, O'dea D, et al. After the smoke has cleared: evaluation of the impact of a new national smoke-free law in New Zealand. *Tobacco Control*. 2008;17(1):e2-e.

[77] Hammond D. Tobacco packaging and labeling policies under the US Tobacco Control Act: research needs and priorities. *Nicotine & Tobacco Research*. 2011;14(1):62-74.

[78] Organization WH. *WHO Report on the Global Tobacco Epidemic, 2013: Enforcing Bans on Tobacco Advertising, Promotion and Sponsorship:* World Health Organization; 2013.

[79] Van Walbeek C, Filby S. Analysis of Article 6 (tax and price measures to reduce the demand for tobacco products) of the WHO Framework Convention on Tobacco Control. *Tobacco Control*. 2019;28(Suppl 2):s97-s103.

Chapter 10

Vaccinations in the Management of Stable COPD

Yaser A. Al Naam*
Clinical Laboratory Sciences Department,
Prince Sultan Military College of Health Sciences,
Dhahran, Saudi Arabia

Abstract

Pneumococcal vaccines have demonstrated substantial advancements in the treatment and prevention of invasive pneumococcal diseases. Both 13-valent pneumococcal conjugate vaccine and pneumococcal polysaccharide vaccine promote active immunization against the serotypes of pneumococcal bacteria. Inactivated influenza vaccines and live attenuated influenza vaccines are produced to protect against three different seasonal influenza viruses. The composition of both influenza vaccines is updated annually. Studies on the vaccine efficacy and effectiveness in COPD have revealed varied results. Since the beginning of the SARS-CoV-2 pandemic, different technologies were used for the development of SARS-CoV-2 vaccines that included weakened and inactive viruses, viral vectors, nucleic acids, and proteins. The efficacy and effectiveness of the various types of SARS-CoV-2 vaccines against infection are still under investigation which might largely depend on age, vaccine type, variants of the virus, and geographic region. The effectiveness and safety concerns for the related COPD vaccinations are discussed in this chapter.

Keywords: COPD, pneumococcal vaccine, influenza vaccine, SARS-CoV-2 vaccines, vaccine efficacy

Introduction

Chronic obstructive pulmonary disease (COPD) is a significant public health concern and is one of the main causes of substantial morbidity and mortality worldwide. Yet COPD is a treatable, preventable, and partially reversible disease characterized by progressive airflow obstruction and associated with an abnormal inflammatory response of the lungs to noxious particles or gases [1]. Both flu and pneumonia can impair lung function and put individuals with COPD at higher risk of complications. COPD patients are more likely to develop

* Corresponding Author's Email: yaser@psmchs.edu.sa.

In: Chronic Obstructive Pulmonary Disease
Editor: Jaber S. Alqahtani
ISBN: 979-8-88697-333-4

pneumonia and other respiratory diseases after a flu infection. Therefore, individuals with COPD are recommended to be immunized against conditions that may affect the lungs. While there is no specific vaccine for COPD, vaccination against *Streptococcus pneumonia* and viral influenza provides secondary prevention or minimizes the severity of COPD exacerbations caused by respiratory infections [2].

Pneumococcal Vaccines

Streptococcus pneumoniae can cause serious illness, including sepsis, meningitis, and pneumonia with or without bacteremia. Pneumococcal vaccines are vaccines that give protection against *Streptococcus pneumoniae* bacteria. These vaccines are developed in two formulations, polysaccharide vaccine, and conjugate vaccine. The advent of pneumococcal vaccines has proven to be a significant advancement in the treatment and prevention of a widespread and sometimes deadly disease process.

Currently available vaccines are the 13-valent pneumococcal conjugate vaccine (PCV13) and the Pneumococcal polysaccharide vaccine (PPSV23). Both vaccines promote active immunization against the serotype's pneumococcal bacteria. Immunity develops approximately two to three weeks after vaccination and lasts for five years [3].

Pneumococcal Conjugate Vaccine (PCV13)

This vaccine formulation demonstrates improved antibody response compared to the pneumococcal polysaccharide vaccine because it contains purified capsular polysaccharides of pneumococcal serotypes conjugated to a carrier protein. PCV 13 actively immunizes against invasive disease caused by *S. pneumoniae* capsular serotypes 1, 3, 4, 5, 6A, 6B, 7F, 9V, 14, 18C, 19A, 19F, and 23F [4]. All of the serotypes are individually conjugated to a CRM197 protein.

PCV13 is recommended differently depending on the patient population. In patients six weeks old through nine years of age, PCV13 is recommended for active immunization for the prevention of diseases considered invasive and caused by Streptococcus pneumoniae serotypes 1, 3, 4, 5, 6A, 6B, 7F, 9V, 14, 18C, 19A, 19F, and 23F [5]. It is also recommended for the prevention and active immunization of otitis media caused by S. pneumoniae serotypes 4, 6B, 9V, 14, 18C, 19F, and 23F. In patients aged 7 to 17 years old, it is recommended to prevent invasive disease in the subtypes mentioned above. In patients 18 years and older, it is indicated for active immunization and prevention of pneumococcal pneumonia, caused by the subtypes of S. pneumoniae, as listed above [5].

Adverse Effects

There are several reports of the most common adverse effects in the different age groups.

The most commonly reported reactions among infants and toddlers are irritability, injection site tenderness, decreased appetite, decreased sleep, increased sleep, fever, injection site redness, and injection site swelling [5]. The most commonly reported reactions among children aged 5 to 17 years old included injection site tenderness, injection site redness, injection site swelling, irritability, decreased appetite, increased sleep, fever, and decreased sleep. The most commonly reported adverse reactions among adults of 18 years and older included pain at the injection site, fatigue, headache, muscle pain, joint pain, decreased appetite, injection site redness, injection site swelling, limitation of arm movement, vomiting, fever, chills, and rash.

Effectiveness

Regarding PCV13 effectiveness and safety, before the 2014 recommendation, a randomized placebo-controlled Community-Acquired Pneumonia Immunization Trial in Adults (CAPiTA) conducted in the Netherlands demonstrated 75% (95% confidence interval [CI] = 41%–91%) efficacy against PCV13-type IPD and 45% (CI = 14%–65%) efficacy against noninvasive PCV13-type pneumonia among adults aged ≥65 years [6].

Pneumococcal Polysaccharide Vaccine (PPSV23)

PPSV23 is the first pneumococcal vaccine formulated from a capsular polysaccharide. PPSV 23 contains 23 capsular polysaccharides types of *S. pneumoniae*, representing at least 85% to 90% of pneumococcal disease isolates in the United States. It has shown a 50% to 80% efficacy in preventing invasive pneumococcal disease in adults [7].

PPSV23 is indicated for all adults 65 years of age and older, as well as younger patients with conditions that increase the risk of developing pneumococcal pneumonia or invasive pneumococcal disease. Conditions that would indicate PPSV23 in patients younger than 65 years of age included chronic heart and lung diseases, diabetes mellitus, cerebrospinal fluid leak, cochlear implant, alcohol use disorder, chronic liver disease, cigarette smoking, hemoglobinopathy, asplenia, immunodeficiency, nephrotic syndrome, leukemia, lymphoma, Hodgkin's disease, generalized malignancy, patients receiving immunosuppressive medications, solid organ transplant, and multiple myeloma [8].

Adverse Reaction

Common Reactions to PPSV23 included injection site pain (60%), injection site induration/swelling (20.3%), headache (17.6%), injection site erythema (16.4%), fatigue (13.2%) and myalgia (11.9%) [9].

Influenza Vaccines

Influenza is caused by negative-stranded, segmented RNA viruses of the family Orthomyxoviridae and includes three distinct types based on their significant antigenic differences in two of their internal proteins, nucleoprotein (NP) and matrix protein (M) [10].

Influenza A, influenza B, and influenza C. Seasonal influenza epidemics caused by influenza A and B viruses result in 3 to 5 million severe cases and thousands of deaths worldwide every year [11].

Occasionally, influenza pandemics occur caused by the influenza A virus because of its ability to spread from migrating birds, pigs, horses, and humans. Pandemics are responsible for increased morbidity and mortality compared with seasonal influenza. Influenza B causes only human-to-human spread [12].

The three types of viruses also differ in their pathogenicity and genome organization. Type A is found in a wide variety of warm-blooded animals (birds and mammals), whereas types B and C are predominantly human pathogens. Influenza A and B viruses are the two types that most commonly cause human disease [13].

Influenza A viruses are further subdivided into subtypes according to the surface glycoproteins hemagglutinin and neuraminidase. However, influenza B viruses have no subtypes. Hemagglutinin and surface protein NA are the most important surface proteins for antigenic stimulus. Currently, 18 subtypes of HA (H1–H18) and nine subtypes of NA (N1–N9) have been found in influenza A viruses, and all subtypes are found in aquatic birds [14].

Both A and B viruses undergo continual antigenic drift by the built-up of point mutations in viral RNA during the virus' replication process, leading to a new virus strain [15]. This continual antigenic drift in these surface proteins complicates the vaccine's development and effectiveness. Therefore, this drift also necessitates the frequent review and change of vaccine strains.

Two types of influenza vaccine are currently available: inactivated influenza vaccines (IIV) and live attenuated influenza vaccines (LAIV) [16]. Generally, both influenza vaccines are produced to protect against three different seasonal influenza viruses, hence called trivalent vaccines. This remains the case in most countries and the current trivalent vaccines contain influenza A(H3N2), pandemic A(H1N1), and one of the two influenza B lineage viruses. Nevertheless, quadrivalent vaccines, which protect against four different viruses including both influenza B lineage viruses, were recently produced in some countries [17].

The annual intake of the inactivated influenza vaccine is necessitated by the continuous emergence of new strains leading to a continuous change in the vaccine architecture and the waning immunity [18].

Influenza A (H3N2) and influenza A (H1N1) viruses represent the two spreading subtypes of human influenza A. Antibody production for one subtype of influenza A provides little or no protection against other subtypes. However, antibody cross-protection against related strains may occur following the vaccination with a relevant strain.

Although influenza B viruses are not subtyped, two distinct lineages of influenza B are currently known worldwide, namely, B/Yamagata-like and B/Victoria-like viruses (CDC 2007). Similarly, immunity to viruses of one lineage provides little or no immunity against the other [19].

Annual Selection of Viruses

The composition of both influenza vaccines is updated annually by the World Health Organization according to the information gathered from the Global Influenza Surveillance and Response System (GISRS), a partnership of 141 national influenza centers in 111 countries

[20]. Influenza virus samples from different parts of the world are gathered and analyzed systematically. Subsequently, one or more components of the vaccine designated for the coming influenza season in the northern and/or southern hemisphere might be modified to reflect the most frequent and recent circulating influenza A and B viruses.

Vaccine administration to individuals at greatest risk of influenza-related complications has been the concern of most influenza programs throughout the globe. Vaccination of persons of close contact with the high-risk groups, including the healthcare workers and the household contacts of the high-risk individuals, is also recommended [21-22]. In the USA, the influenza vaccine has been recommended for all children six months through 18 years old, adults 50–64 years of age, as well as household contacts or persons less than 5 years old or more than 49 years old [23].

Inactivated Influenza Vaccine

The main immunogen in inactivated influenza vaccines is hemagglutinin and the amount of HA administered is correlated with the immunogenicity of the vaccine [24]. During the vaccine processing, some vaccine manufacturers include Aminoglycoside antibiotics to reduce bacterial growth in eggs, which has been reduced to an undetectable amount during the purification process [25].

Inactivated Influenza Vaccination Immune Response

Influenza vaccination essentially induces antibodies to the major surface glycoproteins HA and NA. HA antibodies are the most important for immunity against illness, while NA antibodies may reduce the severity of disease [24]. The immune response to inactivated vaccines is age dependent, with fewer responses among the higher age groups, in addition to the immune competence of the recipient [26]. Moreover, individuals with no antibodies from past influenza infections or previous vaccination may need to get two doses of vaccine to obtain the best response. The immune response peaks at 2–4 weeks after vaccination with one dose among primed individuals [27].

Several studies have demonstrated that only one dose of vaccine received by unvaccinated children less than five years old has resulted in a substantial reduction in morbidity [28-30].

Protection against influenza is usually proportional to the serum HI antibody. Although HI titers of 1:32 to 1:40 are often used as a reference for an adequate immune response to inactivated influenza vaccine, some persons who achieve such titers or higher can remain susceptible to influenza infection [31].

Inactivated influenza virus vaccines are intramuscularly administered. The recommended dose of inactivated influenza vaccines for individuals three years of age and older is 15 mg of HA for each vaccine strain. While 7.5 mg of HA is recommended for children 6–35 months for each vaccine strain. Unimmunized children less than nine years of age require two doses of vaccine for their first time with the doses separated by four or more weeks [32].

Studies on immunogenicity and vaccine effectiveness have shown that unimmunized children require two doses to improve the immune response and thus obtain the best clinical outcomes of the inactivated influenza vaccine.

It has been demonstrated that very low or no clinical effectiveness has been detected after only one dose among children less than five years of age [33]. The ACIP recommends two doses the following year for children aged six months to eight years who received only one dose in their first year of vaccination because the immune response will be better if the child first received two doses with the same antigen [34].

Efficacy and Effectiveness of Inactivated Influenza Vaccine

The age and immune competence of the recipient as well as the antigenic relevance of vaccine strains are among the essential factors relating to the effectiveness of the inactivated influenza vaccine. Although the vaccine still can provide substantial benefit at most ages, especially against more severe outcomes, in years with a suboptimal strain relevance, the vaccine benefit is likely to be suboptimal [35-37].

Studies on vaccine efficacy and effectiveness have revealed varied results because of the lack of standardized outcome measures and the varied influenza case definition [38]. Many different study designs, populations, and outcome measures have been used to assess inactivated influenza vaccine effectiveness. Vaccine efficacy of 86% against serologically confirmed influenza illness, 34% against febrile respiratory illness, and 10% against upper respiratory infection at the same time and population has been reported [39]. Influenza morbidity rates can also vary considerably from one year to another, and during low rates years. The ability of smaller studies to detect a difference in vaccine effectiveness may be compromised, even when using a laboratory-confirmed illness [40-41]. Some meta-analyses have been done, although the differences in study designs and study outcomes provide great challenges while conducting and also when interpreting meta-analyses of vaccine effectiveness. Another major constraint in estimating influenza vaccine outcomes in nonrandomized studies is the biases resulting from the selection of the vaccine recipients. These issues are even more difficult in nonrandomized studies that use non-laboratory-confirmed outcomes, as is the case with most studies on the elderly [42]. It has been found during a season with drifted viruses, severe influenza-associated illness among adults was reduced by 32% [43]. Vaccine effectiveness was high among young adults [43].

Adverse Events

Local reactions include sore arms and redness at the injection site [30]. Systemic reactions occur much less frequently, which include fever, myalgia, arthralgia, and headache [44]. These are more likely to occur in very young children and in those having the vaccine for the first time. Guillain–Barré Syndrome (GBS), a rare neurological syndrome caused by immune system damage to the peripheral nervous system and characterized by ascending paralysis, paresthesia, and dysesthesia, has been associated with the receipt of the 1976 swine influenza vaccine [45]. Subsequent studies did not find similar increases in GBS cases among inactivated vaccine recipients [46]. However, other studies have estimated an incidence of approximately one GBS case per million recipients of inactivated influenza vaccine among adults [46]. Eventually, the Advisory Committee on Immunization Practices stated that the potential benefits of the influenza vaccine in preventing serious illness, hospitalization, and death certainly outweigh the possible risks of developing vaccine-associated GBS [47].

The risk of influenza vaccine-related anaphylaxis has been estimated at one in four million recipients. It is recommended that individuals having a history of anaphylactic hypersensitivity to eggs or previous influenza vaccination should take the inactivated influenza vaccine only under physician assessment [48]. In addition, thimerosal preservative allergic reactions may also occur which are characterized by a delayed hypersensitivity that most often results in a local inflamed lesion [49]. Thimerosal-free influenza vaccines are available. Although few studies of inactivated influenza vaccine safety have been conducted among pregnant women, the vaccine has been used in the USA among pregnant women for many years [50]. Thus, the influenza vaccine is recommended for pregnant women based on their increased risk of hospitalization during seasonal influenza outbreaks and their increased risk of death and fetal loss during pandemics [50].

Live Attenuated Influenza Vaccines

The development of live attenuated influenza virus vaccines (LAIV), also referred to as cold-adapted, live-attenuated influenza vaccine-trivalent (CAIV-T) was considered to be an important scientific achievement. LAIV is developed based on two cold-adapted master donor viruses, A/Ann Arbor/ 6/60 (H2N2) for influenza A vaccines (MDV-A) and B/Ann Arbor/1/66 for influenza B vaccines (MDV-B) [51].

Each donor virus donates the cold-adapted, temperature-sensitive, and attenuated phenotype to the 6:2 reassortant vaccine viruses that contain six internal protein gene segments of MDV and the HA and NA surface proteins of the wild-type influenza virus [52].

Both Influenza A/Ann Arbor/6/60 and Influenza B/ Ann/Arbor/1/66 were subjected to serial in vitro passage at a gradually reduced temperature in primary chicken kidney cells that include plaquing and amplification in embryonated chicken eggs [53].

During the cold passage, the MDV-A and MDV-B acquired several genetic changes in multiple gene segments, which confer the cold adaptive, temperature sensitive, and attenuated phenotypes that can be imparted to 6:2 reassortant vaccine strains [54].

The vaccine viruses infect and replicate in cells lining the nasopharynx of the recipient to induce immunity, but they are not able to replicate in the lower respiratory tract due to their temperature-sensitive and attenuated phenotypes.

Efficacy

The efficacy and effectiveness of an influenza vaccine is usually evaluated by either comparing culture-positive influenza infection rates, especially among children, a 4-fold antibody increase from baseline levels, or observations of acute respiratory illness. The culture-positive rates are the most specific because antibody increase may be biased by natural infections and which is a less specific endpoint [55]. LAIV efficacy trials in the pediatric population consist of nine controlled studies comprising over 20,000 infants and toddlers, children, and adolescents, during seven influenza seasons.

Cold-adapted Ann Arbor-based live attenuated influenza vaccine (LAIV) has been available in the USA since 2003. The vaccine is efficacious against influenza infection. Features of LAIV include easy administration suitable for mass immunization, cross-reactivity to drifted strains for broader coverage, and establishment of herd immunity for control of influenza spread. Annual seasonal LAIV now contains four strains against influenza A H1N1, H3N2, influenza B-Victoria, and B-Yamagata lineages that are co-circulating in humans. LAIV played a significant role in protecting the public from the 2009 H1N1 pandemic and has been evaluated for pandemic preparedness [56].

The most common adverse reactions include runny nose or nasal congestion, fever, and sore throat. Headache and tiredness incidence in LAIV recipients is higher than in a placebo control group but is similar to TIV recipients. One study showed that LAIV was associated with an increased rate of all-cause hospitalization among children aged 6–11 months and an increased rate of medically attended wheezing in children aged 6–23 months [57].

SARS-CoV-2 Vaccines

Since December 2019, there has been an outbreak of SARS-CoV-2, a novel beta-Coronavirus in Wuhan, China. The World Health Organization declared COVID-19 as a pandemic on March 11, 2020. Since then, clinical trial research assessing the efficacy and safety of COVID-19 vaccines have been emerging at an unprecedented rate. Initially, more than a hundred vaccines against SARS-CoV-2 were identified [58]. The technologies used include weakened and inactive viruses, viral vectors, nucleic acids, and proteins. However, a few of these have been approved in some countries. Despite efforts invested in developing SARS-CoV-2 vaccines, more research is still required.

Vaccine Development and Types

Different technologies were put under research and development to create an effective vaccine against COVID-19. Most of these are focused on the coronavirus spike protein (S protein) and its variants as the primary antigen of COVID-19 infection. This is because the S protein triggers strong B-cell and T-cell immune responses [57]. Other SARS-CoV-2 proteins considered for vaccine development were the nucleocapsid as they induce a robust T-cell response and their genes are more conserved and recombine less frequently [58].

Currently, platforms developed for the SARS-CoV-2 vaccine involved nucleic acid technologies (nucleoside-modified messenger RNA and DNA), non-replicating viral vectors, peptides, recombinant proteins, live attenuated viruses, and inactivated viruses.

Unlike influenza, vaccines developed for COVID-19 have used the sing "next-generation technologies for targeting of COVID-19 infection mechanisms precisely.

Several synthetic vaccines use a two prolines mutation for stabilizing the perfusion form of spike proteins, thus stimulating an adaptive immune response to the virus before it attaches to a human cell [59].

Current COVID-19 Vaccines

Recent advances in genomics, bioprocess technology, and immunopathology have greatly contributed to the speedy development of the COVID-19 vaccine. Investigators have used accumulative knowledge from previous vaccine research, and thus the vaccines were made available shortly after the emergence of COVID-19. The different types of COVID-19 vaccine strategies currently available include inactivated, mRNA, viral vector, and nanoparticle-based peptide vaccines.

Inactivated Vaccine

Inactivated vaccines are developed by inactivating virulent particles of viruses chemically. Inactivating chemicals include formaldehyde, β-propiolactone, ethylenimine, phenol, ascorbic acid, β-aminophenylketone, and diethylpyrocarbonate [60]. Such vaccines are safer than attenuated ones even when administered at larger doses. They induce inefficient cellular and humoral immune responses, showing minimal or no long-term memory response. To improve the efficacy of these vaccines, killed virus particles and adjuvants such as aluminum hydroxide are added to the vaccine formulation. These types of vaccines have been developed during the previous coronavirus pandemics.

mRNA Vaccine

mRNA vaccine normally consists of the necessary elements for the encoded protein to be expressed. For this technology, 1-methyl-pseudouridine modification is incorporated in mRNA molecules, enhancing mRNA translation in the body [61]. The antigen is initially identified from the target pathogen. After sequencing and synthesizing, the gene is usually cloned into a plasmid. The mRNA is transcribed in vitro. Before being delivered to the host. After it's administered to the body, it uses the host cellular machinery to translate the mRNA into the target antigen. Both humoral and cellular immunity are activated as the mRNA vaccine mimics the initial viral infection [61]. They elicit adaptive solid immune responses by releasing TNF-α, IFN-α, and other chemokines, by immune cells. Innate immunity is also generated as chemokines and cytokines (i.e., IL-12, TNF) are produced at the injection site. The mRNA vaccine has the advantages of being more stable, easily translatable, rapidly producible, and usually economical [61].

Moderna and Pfizer/BioNTech formulated the mRNA COVID-19 vaccines by implementing nanotechnology, which improves nucleic acid delivery and conformation stabilized subunit vaccines to lymph nodes. It triggers cellular and humoral immunity, preventing viral infection and disease severity.

The human body has ribonuclease enzymes present in every tissue and ready to destroy scattered RNA. Ribonuclease creates a restricted environment for foreign RNA. Lipid nanoparticles can be created to encapsulate RNA and shield it from ribonuclease.

Viral Vector-Based Vaccine

In this technology, a gene/cDNA coding for a pathogen-derived antigen is incorporated into a non-pathogenic or attenuated viral species. These non-pathogenic species serve as a vector. The recombinant vector immunizes against the pathogen while the gene product is expressed on its surface. For this purpose, a few sites are removed from the vector genome where the targeted pathogen's foreign DNA can be integrated. After injecting, foreign DNA can replicate within the host and express the following pathogen's gene product, eliciting cell-mediated and humoral immunity. Many viruses such as adenovirus, vaccinia virus, canarypox virus, and attenuated poliovirus, act as viral vectors. The Adenoviral vector combined with DNA and poxviral vector to induce immunogenicity showed cellular and humoral response enhancement.

The Oxford/AstraZeneca vaccine contains a homologous adenoviral vector that could mitigate the efficiency of the second dose due to anti-vector immunity. The chimpanzee adenovirus was an excellent vector for vaccine formulation from previous vaccine preparations against MERS-CoV [62]. The Oxford/AstraZeneca vaccine is an adenoviral vector-based vaccine comprising DNA that encodes surface glycoprotein protein embedded in a capsid from a modified chimpanzee adenovirus.

Nanoparticle-Based Peptide Vaccine

Nanotechnology has played an important role in vaccine development with variations based on nanoparticles' different compositions, shapes, sizes, and surface properties. Nanoparticles, being smaller in size, can quickly enter living cells through endocytosis. The use of peptide antigens for vaccination has advantages such as purity and low risk of adverse effects. However, such weak immunogenicity necessitates administration with an adjuvant.

Different types of nanoparticles are being used in vaccine development, including polymeric nanoparticles, inorganic nanoparticles, liposomes, immune-stimulating complex (ISCOM), virus-like particles, self-assembled proteins, and emulsions.

Nanoparticles are most commonly used as immunostimulants or delivery materials. In vaccine formulation, the association between nanoparticles and antigens is essential. Nanoparticles act as a temporary carrier and protector of the antigen, which is needed to reach the desired location. By interacting with the antigen, nanoparticles enhance immunogenicity and antigen processing, which activate immune-responsive pathways. Nanotechnology-based vaccine mechanisms are highly efficient, whereas solid nanocarriers transport the core antigen portion of vaccines into the gut-associated lymphoid tissues and mucosa-associated lymphoid tissues, ensuring proper delivery through oral or mucosal routes.

Several studies reported that the current COVID-19 vaccines are highly protective against severe illness, hospitalization, and death due to COVID-19 [63]. In comparison with fully vaccinated people, the CDC reported that unvaccinated people were 10 times more likely to be hospitalized and 11 times more likely to die. One study found that having two doses of a COVID-19 vaccine halved the odds of long COVID. For the two-dose regimens of messenger RNA (mRNA) vaccines BNT162b2 and mRNA-1273, vaccine effectiveness against Covid-19 was 94.5% and 95.9%, respectively, two months after the first dose and decreased to 66.6% and 80.3%, respectively, at seven months [64].

Evidence of Effectiveness of Vaccines in COPD Exacerbations

Human Rhinovirus, Respiratory Syncytial Virus, and Influenza Virus are the most frequent human respiratory viruses linked with COPD exacerbations [2]. Influenza and pneumococcal vaccinations are recommended by international guidelines for COPD patients. The Centers for Disease Control and Prevention in the United States recommends pneumococcal immunization for people suffering from chronic medical conditions such as COPD. Vaccination against infectious exacerbations might increase patient survival and quality of life. According to a comprehensive literature review on the effectiveness of influenza vaccinations in diverse patient categories, the rate of acute respiratory exacerbations may be reduced by influenza vaccinations. However, research on COPD patients is limited and hence inconsistent [65]. A recent Cochrane review found that COPD patients who received an inactivated influenza vaccination had fewer exacerbations [66]. Additional research findings are required to better understand the immunological response of people living with COPD to diverse vaccine formulations, adjuvants, delivery methods, and other innovative techniques. Although vaccinations are the most efficient means of preventing infectious illnesses, the existing approved vaccines for COPD patients are limited.

Conclusion

COPD is a chronic condition with significant morbidity and mortality. Infections are common causes of COPD. Pneumococcal and influenza vaccinations can help reduce infections and exacerbations. Vaccination against pneumococcus reduces community-acquired pneumonia in COPD patients. Overall, vaccination has been shown to reduce the risk of COPD exacerbation, and therefore it is recommended in COPD patients with moderate quality of evidence.

Key Points

- Appropriate pneumococcal vaccination is recommended for all COPD patients. Annual influenza vaccine is recommended for all individuals, particularly those with COPD risk.
- Influenza vaccination reduces the number of exacerbations and influenza-related hospitalization.
- Both pneumococcal vaccine 13 (PCV13) and pneumococcal polysaccharide vaccine 23 (PPSV23) are recommended for all patients ages 65 or older. Studies for comparing the efficacy of the two vaccines were insufficient.
- Influenza vaccination is the most effective strategy to prevent influenza infections, reduce the severity of illness, and save lives during seasonal outbreaks and pandemics. However, the notable disparity remains in vaccine effectiveness, production, acceptance, and coverage.
- Vaccination against COVID-19 reduces the risk of hospitalizations and severe infections. COVID-19 vaccination with appropriate boosters should be recommended for all patients with COPD.

References

[1] Murray CJ, Vos T, Lozano R, Disability-adjusted life years (DALYs) for 291 diseases and injuries in 21 regions, 1990-2010: a systematic analysis for the Global Burden of Disease Study 2010. *Lancet* 2012; 380: 2197 – 223.

[2] Fekete M, Pako J, Nemeth AN, Tarantini S, Varga JT. Prevalence of influenza and pneumococcal vaccination in chronic obstructive pulmonary disease patients in association with the occurrence of acute exacerbations. *J Thorac Dis*. 2020 Aug;12(8):4233-4242. https://doi.org/10.21037/jtd-20-814. PMID: 32944335; PMCID: PMC7475525.

[3] Hsiao A, Hansen J, Timbol J, Lewis N, Isturiz R, Alexander-Parrish R, McLaughlin JM, Gessner BD, Klein NP. Incidence and Estimated Vaccine Effectiveness against Hospitalizations for All-Cause Pneumonia among Older US Adults Who Were Vaccinated and Not Vaccinated With 13-Valent Pneumococcal Conjugate Vaccine. *JAMA Netw Open*. 2022 Mar 1;5(3):e221111. https://doi.org/10.1001/jamanetworkopen.2022.1111. PMID: 35302634; PMCID: PMC8933738.

[4] Berical AC, Harris D, Dela Cruz CS, Possick JD. Pneumococcal Vaccination Strategies. An Update and Perspective. *Ann Am Thorac Soc*. 2016 Jun;13(6):933-44. doi: 10.1513/AnnalsATS.201511-778FR. PMID: 27088424; PMCID: PMC5461988.

[5] Tereziu S, Minter DA. Pneumococcal Vaccine. [Updated 2022 Jan 21]. In: *StatPearls* [Internet]. Treasure Island (FL): StatPearls Publishing; 2022 Jan-. Available from: https://www.ncbi.nlm.nih.gov/books/NBK507794/.

[6] Marra F, Vadlamudi NK. Efficacy and Safety of the Pneumococcal Conjugate-13 Valent Vaccine in Adults. *Aging Dis*. 2019 Apr 1;10(2):404-418. https://doi.org/10.14336/AD.2018.0512. PMID: 31011485; PMCID: PMC6457056.

[7] Cannon K, Elder C, Young M, Scott DA, Scully IL, Baugher G, Peng Y, Jansen KU, Gruber WC, Watson W. A trial to evaluate the safety and immunogenicity of a 20-valent pneumococcal conjugate vaccine in populations of adults ≥65 years of age with different prior pneumococcal vaccination. *Vaccine*. 2021 Dec 17;39(51):7494-7502. [PubMed] [Reference list].

[8] Cannon K, Elder C, Young M, Scott DA, Scully IL, Baugher G, Peng Y, Jansen KU, Gruber WC, Watson W. A trial to evaluate the safety and immunogenicity of a 20-valent pneumococcal conjugate vaccine in populations of adults ≥65 years of age with different prior pneumococcal vaccination. *Vaccine*. 2021 Dec 17;39(51):7494-7502. [PubMed].

[9] Adult immunization. *Med Lett Drugs Ther*. 2018 May 07;60(1546):73-82. [PubMed].

[10] Bouvier NM, Palese P. The biology of influenza viruses. *Vaccine*. 2008;26 Suppl 4(Suppl 4):D49-D53. https://doi.org/10.1016/j.vaccine.2008.07.039.

[11] Ghebrehewet S, MacPherson P, Ho A. Influenza. *BMJ*. 2016; 355:i6258. Published 2016 Dec 7. doi:10.1136/bmj.i6258.

[12] Kilbourne ED. Influenza pandemics of the 20th century. *Emerg Infect Dis*. 2006;12(1):9-14. https://doi.org/10. 3201/eid1201.051254.

[13] Kalarikkal SM, Jaishankar GB. Influenza Vaccine. [Updated 2022 Jan 20]. In: *StatPearls* [Internet]. Treasure Island (FL): StatPearls Publishing; 2022 Jan-. Available from: https://www.ncbi.nlm.nih.gov/books/NBK537197/.

[14] Luo, S., Xie, Z., Huang, J., Xie, Z., Xie, L., Zhang, M., Li, M., Wang, S., Li, D., Zeng, T., Zhang, Y., Fan, Q., & Deng, X. (2019). Simultaneous Differentiation of the N1 to N9 Neuraminidase Subtypes of Avian Influenza Virus by a GeXP Analyzer-Based Multiplex Reverse Transcription PCR Assay. *Frontiers in Microbiology*, 10, 1271. https://doi.org/10.3389/fmicb.2019.01271.

[15] Shao W, Li X, Goraya MU, Wang S, Chen JL. Evolution of Influenza A Virus by Mutation and Re-Assortment. *Int J Mol Sci*. 2017 Aug 7;18(8):1650. https://doi.org/10.3390/ijms18081650. PMID: 28783091; PMCID: PMC5578040.

[16] Ilyushina NA, Haynes BC, Hoen AG, Khalenkov AM, Housman ML, Brown EP, Ackerman ME, Treanor JJ, Luke CJ, Subbarao K, Wright PF. Live attenuated and inactivated influenza vaccines in children. *J Infect Dis*. 2015 Feb 1;211(3):352-60. https://doi.org/10.1093/infdis/jiu458. Epub 2014 Aug 26. PMID: 25165161; PMCID: PMC4296173.

[17] Tisa V, Barberis I, Faccio V, Paganino C, Trucchi C, Martini M, Ansaldi F. Quadrivalent influenza vaccine: a new opportunity to reduce the influenza burden. *J Prev Med Hyg*. 2016;57(1):E28-33. PMID: 27346937; PMCID: PMC4910440.

[18] Weir JP, Gruber MF. An overview of the regulation of influenza vaccines in the United States. *Influenza Other Respir Viruses*. 2016 Sep;10(5):354-60. https://doi.org/10.1111/irv.12383. Epub 2016 Mar 24. PMID: 27426005; PMCID: PMC4947948.

[19] Nakauchi M, Takayama I, Takahashi H, Oba K, Kubo H, Kaida A, Tashiro M, Kageyama T. Real-time RT-PCR assays for discriminating influenza B virus Yamagata and Victoria lineages. *J Virol Methods*. 2014 Sep 1;205:110-5. https://doi.org/10.1016/j.jviromet.2014.04.016. Epub 2014 May 4. PMID: 24797457; PMCID: PMC7172331.

[20] Jester B, Uyeki T, Jernigan D. Readiness for Responding to a Severe Pandemic 100 Years After 1918. *Am J Epidemiol*. 2018 Dec 1;187(12):2596-2602. https://doi.org/10.1093/aje/kwy165. PMID: 30102376; PMCID: PMC7314205.

[21] Grohskopf LA, Alyanak E, Ferdinands JM, Broder KR, Blanton LH, Talbot HK, Fry AM. Prevention and Control of Seasonal Influenza with Vaccines: Recommendations of the Advisory Committee on Immunization Practices, United States, 2021-22 Influenza Season. *MMWR Recomm Rep*. 2021 Aug 27;70(5):1-28. https://doi.org/10.15585/mmwr.rr7005a1. PMID: 34448800; PMCID: PMC8407757.

[22] Kam K, McConnell A. Influenza vaccination among household contacts of children with cystic fibrosis and healthy children. *Paediatr Child Health*. 2013 Nov;18(9):e55-8. PMID: 24426812; PMCID: PMC3885107.

[23] Nowak GJ, Sheedy K, Bursey K, Smith TM, Basket M. Promoting influenza vaccination: insights from a qualitative meta-analysis of 14 years of influenza-related communications research by U.S. Centers for Disease Control and Prevention (CDC). *Vaccine*. 2015 Jun 4;33(24):2741-56. https://doi.org/10.1016/j.vaccine.2015.04.064. Epub 2015 Apr 28. PMID: 25936726; PMCID: PMC5856146.

[24] Gomez Lorenzo MM, Fenton MJ. Immunobiology of influenza vaccines. *Chest*. 2013 Feb 1;143(2):502-510. https://doi.org/10.1378/chest.12-1711. PMID: 23381315; PMCID: PMC3619640.

[25] Krause KM, Serio AW, Kane TR, Connolly LE. Aminoglycosides: An Overview. *Cold Spring Harb Perspect Med*. 2016 Jun 1;6(6):a027029. https://doi.org/10.1101/cshperspect.a027029. PMID: 27252397; PMCID: PMC4888811.

[26] Lord JM. The effect of ageing of the immune system on vaccination responses. *Hum Vaccin Immunother*. 2013 Jun;9(6):1364-7. https://doi.org/10.4161/hv.24696. Epub 2013 Apr 12. PMID: 23584248; PMCID: PMC3901832.

[27] Rudenko L, Naykhin A, Donina S, Korenkov D, Petukhova G, Isakova-Sivak I, Losev I, Stukova M, Erofeeva M, Nikiforova A, Power M, Flores J. Assessment of immune responses to H5N1 inactivated influenza vaccine among individuals previously primed with H5N2 live attenuated influenza vaccine. *Hum Vaccin Immunother*. 2015;11(12):2839-48. https://doi.org/10.1080/21645515.2015.1069931. PMID: 26697973; PMCID: PMC5054797.

[28] Principi N, Esposito S. Pediatric influenza prevention and control. *Emerg Infect Dis*. 2004 Apr;10(4):574-80. https://doi.org/10.3201/eid1004.030398. PMID: 15200844; PMCID: PMC3323102.

[29] Moriarty LF, Omer SB. Infants and the seasonal influenza vaccine. A global perspective on safety, effectiveness, and alternate forms of protection. *Hum Vaccin Immunother*. 2014;10(9):2721-8. https://doi.org/10.4161/hv.29669. PMID: 25483664; PMCID: PMC5283389.

[30] Trombetta CM, Gianchecchi E, Montomoli E. Influenza vaccines: Evaluation of the safety profile. *Hum Vaccin Immunother*. 2018 Mar 4;14(3):657-670. https://doi.org/10.1080/21645515.2017.1423153. Epub 2018 Jan 30. PMID: 29297746; PMCID: PMC5861790.

[31] Cox RJ. Correlates of protection to influenza virus, where do we go from here? *Hum Vaccin Immunother*. 2013 Feb;9(2):405-8. https://doi.org/10.4161/hv.22908. Epub 2013 Jan 4. PMID: 23291930; PMCID: PMC3859764.

[32] Jain VK, Domachowske JB, Wang L, Ofori-Anyinam O, Rodríguez-Weber MA, Leonardi ML, Klein NP, Schlichter G, Jeanfreau R, Haney BL, Chu L, Harris JS, Sarpong KO, Micucio AC, Soni J, Chandrasekaran V, Li P, Innis BL. Time to Change Dosing of Inactivated Quadrivalent Influenza Vaccine in Young Children: Evidence From a Phase III, Randomized, Controlled Trial. *J Pediatric*

Infect Dis Soc. 2017 Mar 1;6(1):9-19. https://doi.org/10.1093/jpids/piw068. PMID: 28062552; PMCID: PMC5907868.

[33] Chung JR, Flannery B, Gaglani M, Smith ME, Reis EC, Hickey RW, Jackson ML, Jackson LA, Belongia EA, McLean HQ, Martin ET, Segaloff HE, Kim SS, Patel MM. Patterns of Influenza Vaccination and Vaccine Effectiveness Among Young US Children Who Receive Outpatient Care for Acute Respiratory Tract Illness. *JAMA Pediatr*. 2020 Jul 1;174(7):705-713. https://doi.org/10.1001/jamapediatrics.2020.0372. PMID: 32364599; PMCID: PMC7199168.

[34] Ventola CL. *Immunization in the United States: Recommendations, Barriers, and Measures to Improve Compliance: Part 1: Childhood Vaccinations*. P T. 2016 Jul;41(7):426-36. PMID: 27408519; PMCID: PMC4927017.

[35] Osterhaus A, Fouchier R, Rimmelzwaan G. Towards universal influenza vaccines? *Philos Trans R Soc Lond B Biol Sci*. 2011 Oct 12;366(1579):2766-73. https://doi.org/10.1098/rstb.2011.0102. PMID: 21893539; PMCID: PMC3146782.

[36] Krammer F, Palese P. Advances in the development of influenza virus vaccines. Nat Rev Drug Discov. 2015 Mar;14(3):167-82. https://doi.org/10.1038/nrd4529. *Erratum in: Nat Rev Drug Discov*. 2015 Apr;14(4):294. PMID: 25722244.

[37] Krammer F, García-Sastre A, Palese P. Is it Possible to Develop a "Universal" Influenza Virus Vaccine? Potential Target Antigens and Critical Aspects for a Universal Influenza Vaccine. *Cold Spring Harb Perspect Biol.* 2018 Jul 2;10(7):a028845. https://doi.org/10.1101/cshperspect.a028845. PMID: 28663209; PMCID: PMC6028071.

[38] Osterholm MT, Kelley NS, Sommer A, Belongia EA. Efficacy and effectiveness of influenza vaccines: a systematic review and meta-analysis. *Lancet Infect Dis*. 2012 Jan;12(1):36-44. https://doi.org/10.1016/S1473-3099(11)70295-X. Epub 2011 Oct 25. Erratum in: Lancet Infect Dis. 2012 Sep;12(9):655. PMID: 22032844.

[39] Nunes MC, Madhi SA. Influenza vaccination during pregnancy for prevention of influenza confirmed illness in the infants: A systematic review and meta-analysis. *Hum Vaccin Immunother.* 2018 Mar 4;14(3):758-766. https://doi.org/10.1080/21645515.2017.1345385. Epub 2017 Oct 18. PMID: 28708952; PMCID: PMC5861794.

[40] Ainslie KEC, Haber M, Orenstein WA. Challenges in estimating influenza vaccine effectiveness. *Expert Rev Vaccines*. 2019 Jun;18(6):615-628. https://doi.org/10.1080/14760584.2019.1622419. Epub 2019 May 31. PMID: 31116070; PMCID: PMC6594904.

[41] Shi M, An Q, Ainslie KEC, Haber M, Orenstein WA. A comparison of the test-negative and the traditional case-control study designs for estimation of influenza vaccine effectiveness under nonrandom vaccination. *BMC Infect Dis*. 2017 Dec 8;17(1):757. https://doi.org/10.1186/s12879-0172838-2. PMID: 29216845; PMCID: PMC5721721.

[42] Shi M, An Q, Ainslie KEC, Haber M, Orenstein WA. A comparison of the test-negative and the traditional case-control study designs for estimation of influenza vaccine effectiveness under nonrandom vaccination. *BMC Infect Dis*. 2017 Dec 8;17(1):757. https://doi.org/10.1186/s12879-0172838-2. PMID: 29216845; PMCID: PMC5721721.

[43] Grijalva CG, Feldstein LR, Talbot HK, Aboodi M, Baughman AH, Brown SM, Casey JD, Erickson HL, Exline MC, Files DC, Gibbs KW, Ginde AA, Gong MN, Halasa N, Khan A, Lindsell CJ, Nwosu SK, Peltan ID, Prekker ME, Rice TW, Shapiro NI, Steingrub JS, Stubblefield WB, Tenforde MW, Patel MM, Self WH; Influenza and Other Viruses in the Acutely Ill (IVY) Network. Influenza Vaccine Effectiveness for Prevention of Severe Influenza-Associated Illness Among Adults in the United States, 2019-2020: A Test-Negative Study. *Clin Infect Dis.* 2021 Oct 20;73(8):1459-1468. https://doi.org/10.1093/cid/ciab462. PMID: 34014274; PMCID: PMC8682606.

[44] Lopes MH, Mascheretti M, Franco MM, Vasconcelos R, Gutierrez EB. Occurrence of early adverse events after vaccination against influenza at a Brazilian reference center. *Clinics* (Sao Paulo). 2008 Feb;63(1):21-6. https://doi.org/10.1590/s1807-59322008000100005. PMID: 18305872; PMCID: PMC-2664188.

[45] Nguyen TP, Taylor RS. Guillain Barre Syndrome. [Updated 2022 May 2]. In: *StatPearls* [Internet]. Treasure Island (FL): StatPearls Publishing; 2022 Jan-. Available from: https://www.ncbi.nlm.nih.gov/books/NBK532254/.

[46] Wang F, Wang D, Wang Y, Li C, Zheng Y, Guo Z, Liu P, Zhang Y, Wang W, Wang Y, Hou H. Population-Based Incidence of Guillain-Barré Syndrome During Mass Immunization With Viral Vaccines: A Pooled Analysis. *Front Immunol*. 2022 Feb 3;13:782198. https://doi.org/10.3389/fimmu.2022.782198. PMID: 35185881; PMCID: PMC8850251.

[47] Institute of Medicine (US) Immunization Safety Review Committee; Stratton K, Alamario DA, Wizemann T, et al., editors. Immunization Safety Review: Influenza Vaccines and Neurological Complications. Washington (DC): National Academies Press (US); 2004. *Immunization Safety Review: Influenza Vaccines and Neurological Complications*. Available from: https://www.ncbi.nlm.nih.gov/books/NBK222009/.

[48] McNeil MM. Vaccine-Associated Anaphylaxis. *Curr Treat Options Allergy*. 2019 Sep;6(3):297-308. https://doi.org/10.1007/s40521-019-00215-0. Epub 2019 Jul 16. PMID: 31815089; PMCID: PMC6896995.

[49] Compans RW, Orenstein WA. Vaccines for pandemic influenza. Preface *Curr Top Microbiol Immunol*. 2009;333:v-viii. PMID: 19787865.

[50] Benowitz I, Esposito DB, Gracey KD, Shapiro ED, Vázquez M. Influenza vaccine given to pregnant women reduces hospitalization due to influenza in their infants. *Clin Infect Dis*. 2010 Dec 15;51(12):1355-61. https://doi.org/10.1086/657309. Epub 2010 Nov 8. PMID: 21058908; PMCID: PMC3106242.

[51] White CL, Chiem K, Perez DR, Santos J, Cardenas Garcia S, Nogales A, Martínez-Sobrido L. A New Master Donor Virus for the Development of Live-Attenuated Influenza B Virus Vaccines. *Viruses*. 2021 Jun 30;13(7):1278. https://doi.org/10.3390/v13071278. PMID: 34208979; PMCID: PMC8310163.

[52] Kiseleva I, Larionova N, Fedorova E, Bazhenova E, Dubrovina I, Isakova-Sivak I, Rudenko L. Contribution of neuraminidase of influenza viruses to the sensitivity to sera inhibitors and reassortment efficiency. *Open Microbiol J*. 2014 Jul 11;8:59-70. https://doi.org/10.2174/1874285801408010059. PMID: 25132869; PMCID: PMC4133923.

[53] Zhou B, Meliopoulos VA, Wang W, Lin X, Stucker KM, Halpin RA, Stockwell TB, Schultz-Cherry S, Wentworth DE. Reversion of Cold-Adapted Live Attenuated Influenza Vaccine into a Pathogenic Virus. *J Virol*. 2016 Sep 12;90(19):8454-63. https://doi.org/10.1128/JVI.00163-16. PMID: 27440882; PMCID: PMC5021423.

[54] Hoffmann E, Mahmood K, Chen Z, Yang CF, Spaete J, Greenberg HB, Herlocher ML, Jin H, Kemble G. Multiple gene segments control the temperature sensitivity and attenuation phenotypes of ca B/Ann Arbor/1/66. *J Virol*. 2005 Sep;79(17):11014-21. https://doi.org/10.1128/JVI.79.17.11014-11021.2005. PMID: 16103152; PMCID: PMC1193632.

[55] Talaat KR, Karron RA, Callahan KA, Luke CJ, DiLorenzo SC, Chen GL, Lamirande EW, Jin H, Coelingh KL, Murphy BR, Kemble G, Subbarao K. A live attenuated H7N3 influenza virus vaccine is well tolerated and immunogenic in a Phase I trial in healthy adults. *Vaccine*. 2009 Jun 8;27(28):3744-53. https://doi.org/10.1016/j.vaccine.2009.03.082. Epub 2009 Apr 17. PMID: 19464558; PMCID: PMC2771405.

[56] Jin H, Subbarao K. Live attenuated influenza vaccine. *Curr Top Microbiol Immunol*. 2015;386:181-204. https://doi.org/10.1007/82_2014_410. PMID: 25059893.

[57] Belshe RB, Edwards KM, Vesikari T, Black SV, Walker RE, Hultquist M, Kemble G, Connor EM; CAIV-T Comparative Efficacy Study Group. Live attenuated versus inactivated influenza vaccine in infants and young children. *N Engl J Med*. 2007 Feb 15;356(7):685-96. https://doi.org/10.1056/NEJMoa065368. Erratum in: N Engl J Med. 2007 Mar 22;356(12):1283. PMID: 17301299.

[58] Azizi A, Aucoin S, Tadesse H, Frost R, Ghorbani M, Soare C, Naas T, Diaz-Mitoma F. A combined nucleocapsid vaccine induces vigorous SARS-CD8+ T-cell immune responses. *Genet Vaccines Ther*. 2005 Aug 22;3:7. https://doi.org/10.1186/1479-0556-3-7. PMID: 16115319; PMCID: PMC1249587.

[59] Rockman S, Laurie KL, Parkes S, Wheatley A, Barr IG. New Technologies for Influenza Vaccines. *Microorganisms*. 2020 Nov 6;8(11):1745. https://doi.org/10.3390/microorganisms8111745. PMID: 33172191; PMCID: PMC7694987.

[60] Sanders B, Koldijk M, Schuitemaker H. Inactivated Viral Vaccines. *Vaccine Analysis: Strategies, Principles, and Control*. 2014 Nov 28:45–80. https://doi.org/10.1007/978-3-662-45024-6_2. PMCID: PMC7189890.

[61] Park JW, Lagniton PNP, Liu Y, Xu RH. mRNA vaccines for COVID-19: what, why and how. *Int J Biol Sci*. 2021 Apr 10;17(6):1446-1460. https://doi.org/10.7150/ijbs.59233. PMID: 33907508; PMCID: PMC8071766.

[62] Vanaparthy R, Mohan G, Vasireddy D, Atluri P. Review of COVID-19 viral vector-based vaccines and COVID-19 variants. *Infez Med*. 2021 Sep 10;29(3):328-338. https://doi.org/10.53854/liim-2903-3. PMID: 35146337; PMCID: PMC8805485.

[63] Varahachalam SP, Lahooti B, Chamaneh M, Bagchi S, Chhibber T, Morris K, Bolanos JF, Kim NY, Kaushik A. Nanomedicine for the SARS-CoV-2: State-of-the-Art and Future Prospects. *Int J Nanomedicine*. 2021 Jan 22;16:539-560. https://doi.org/10.2147/IJN.S283686. PMID: 33519200; PMCID: PMC7837559.

[64] Lin DY, Gu Y, Wheeler B, Young H, Holloway S, Sunny SK, Moore Z, Zeng D. Effectiveness of Covid-19 Vaccines over a 9-Month Period in North Carolina. *N Engl J Med*. 2022 Mar 10;386(10):933-941. https://doi.org/10.1056/NEJMoa2117128. Epub 2022 Jan 12. PMID: 35020982; PMCID: PMC-8781317.

[65] Michiels B, Govaerts F, Remmen R, Vermeire E, Coenen S. A systematic review of the evidence on the effectiveness and risks of inactivated influenza vaccines in different target groups. *Vaccine* 2011; 29(49): 9159-70.

[66] Kopsais Z, Wood-Baker R, Poole P. Influenza vaccine for chronic obstructive pulmonary disease (COPD). *Cochrane Database of Systematic Reviews* 2018, Issue 6. Art. No.: CD002733. https://doi.org/10.1002/14651858.CD002733.pub3.

Chapter 11

Pulmonary Rehabilitation (PR) in the Management of Stable COPD

Yousef S. Aldabayan*, PhD
Respiratory Care Department,
College of Applied Medical Sciences,
King Faisal University,
Al-Hasa, Saudi Arabia.

Abstract

Pulmonary rehabilitation (PR) is a multidisciplinary, patient-focused supplementary program for the treatment of patients with chronic obstructive pulmonary disease (COPD). This program is most suitable for patients with COPD because it involves thorough exercise training to strengthen their lungs and improve their breathing. A 4–12-week PR program with 2–3 supervised visits is effective in controlling dyspnea, tolerating exercise, improving mental health, achieving better Health-related quality of life (HRQOL), facilitating greater independence, reducing hospitalizations, and its consequent economic burden. Supplementation of the two major rehabilitation components—exercise and education—provides an added advantage by improving mental support.

Keywords: pulmonary rehabilitation (PR), COPD, dyspnea, exacerbation, stable COPD, exercise training, education

Introduction

Pulmonary rehabilitation (PR) is a patient-focused, individually tailored, multidisciplinary therapeutic approach consisting of exercise training and education that serves as a supplementary program to avoid pharmacological treatment [1, 2, 3]. It also consists of a pre-rehab assessment and additional patient support that helps in the management of breathing problems and the reduction of breathlessness [4]. The main aim of PR is to improve patients' physical performance and autonomy. Its core components, which include supervised sessions, progressive aerobic and resistance training exercises, and well-defined, proper breathing techniques, enhance performance [2, 3].

---

* Corresponding Author's Email: rt.yousef1@hotmail.com.

In: Chronic Obstructive Pulmonary Disease
Editor: Jaber S. Alqahtani
ISBN: 979-8-88697-333-4

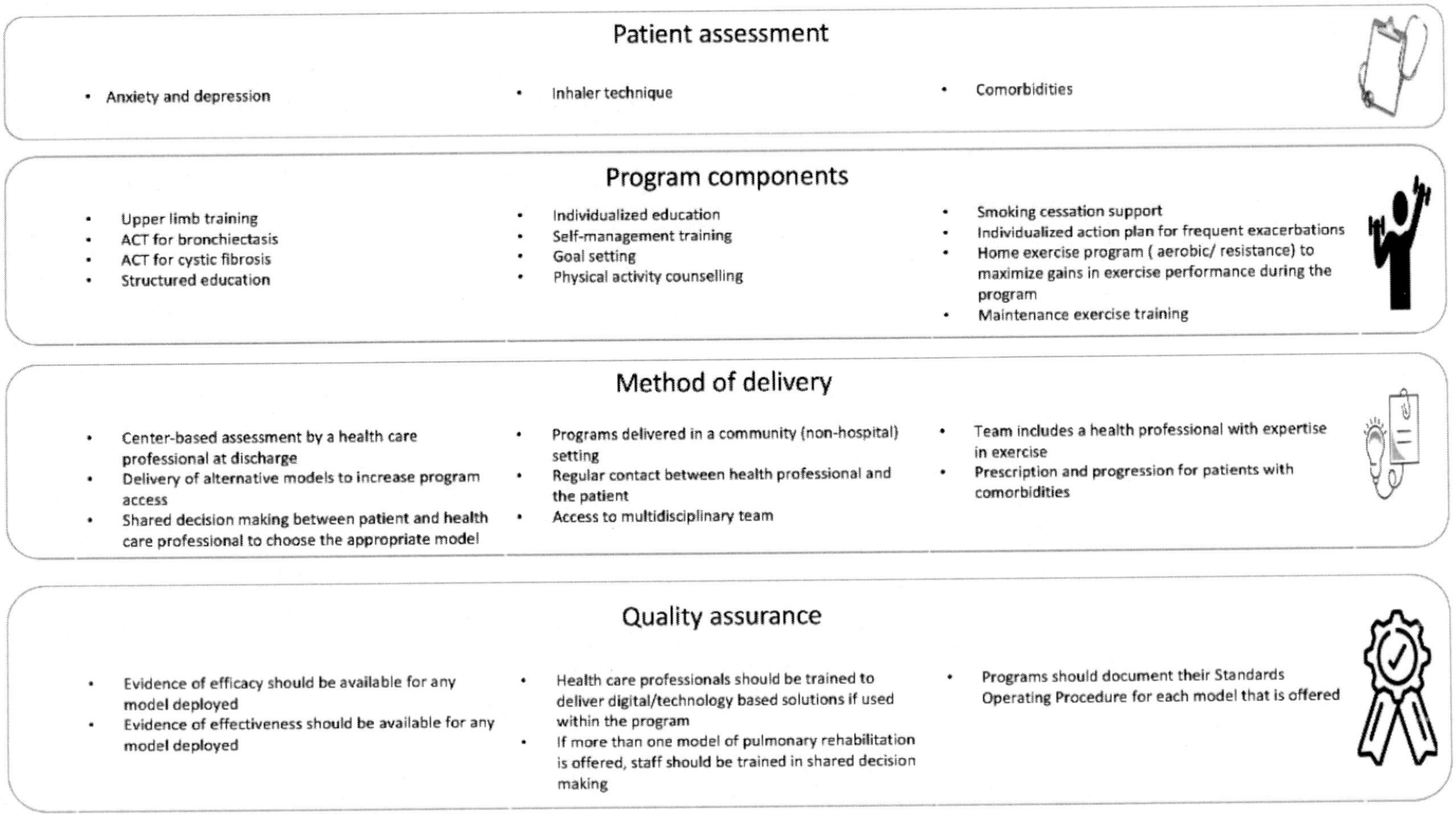

Figure 1. Desirable components of pulmonary rehabilitation.

According to the American Thoracic Society (ATS) Delphi process, pulmonary rehabilitation should include the following components:

(i) Patient assessment, including physical, respiratory, and psychosocial elements;
(ii) Program components, such as exercise, and education sessions;
(iii) Method of delivery, such as models and deliverables; and
(iv) Quality assurance, such as efficacy, and effectiveness (Figure 1) [4].

To achieve better PR outcomes, it is essential to understand what the optimal is regarding: a) program duration, b) program setting, and c) patient referral.

Program Duration

A typical program should last from 4 to 12 weeks (up to 72 weeks if the patient is inclined) with 2 to 3 meetings of supervised training per week [2, 5]. During this time, the program's staff monitors the patient's progress with collateral increase in sustainable training load [3].

Program Setting

PR programs must be undertaken according to times and locations. Therefore, it could be completed conveniently while maintaining environmental safety [2]. It can be organized at home, in healthcare settings, over the phone, online, or in other locations with the right conditions [1, 4]. Moreover, the programs might be available within a reasonable time after referral [2]. The patient's family may also undergo special education and training regarding COPD treatment and other necessary management-related information [1].

Program Referral

Indications

PR is usually most beneficial to patients who have COPD, restrictive lung disease, pulmonary hypertension, heart failure, and musculoskeletal conditions. Moreover, its early induction has shown better recovery outcomes [6]. The modified Medical Research Council breathlessness (mMRC) score is used in this program for evaluation (Table 1) [7, 8]. The mMRC score denotes the patient's disability level due to dyspnea. Scores from 0–4 determine the degree of breathlessness that affects a patient's mobility (0 is the best and 4 is the worst score) [8, 7]. Hence, patients with mMRC scores ≤ 2 (greater or equal to 2) should be referred to a PR program [6] and no change is noticeable for scores between 0 and 1 [9]. The other indices for referral are poor functional state, chronic fatigue, frequent hospitalizations, and waitlisted patients for lung volume reduction surgery [6, 10]. Furthermore, PR is applicable to patients with stable and exacerbated COPD [11].

Table 1. The modified Medical Research Council Breathlessness (mMRC) Scores and Signs

Level of Breathlessness	Descriptions
0	No shortness of breath except when doing a strenuous exercise.
1	Short of breath when walking on an inclined surface.
2	Walking slowly on level ground due to shortness of breath or, when walking at own pace, stopping due to breathlessness.
3	Stopping to catch breath after a few minutes when walking (at least 100 meters) on level ground.
4	Too short of breath to leave the house, or short of breath when dressing and undressing.

Contraindications

The patient's healthcare provider evaluates whether patients qualify for PR. In this evaluation process, the patient's current state of health is scrutinized by examining lung function test results, physical activity levels, and willingness to attend sessions [3]. Admission to PR programs can be selective because the program requires close supervision, and professional staff are few [3]. Non-referral to PR rests solely on the patient's inability to commit to the program physically and mentally. As such, there are only a few contraindications for referral to a program. These include patients with (i) unstable cardiovascular condition; (ii) orthopedic illness, which prevents them from exercising; (iii) severe arthritis or any peripheral vascular disease that prevents safe exercise; (iv) uncontrolled diabetes; (v) psychiatric or cognitive illness, which prevents them from following directions; and (vi) lack of motivation [8, 7].

Nonadherence

The exercise and education sessions are the pre-requisite criteria for this program and its success. Studies have shown that there are relatively higher percentages (20–30%) of patients dropping out of the program due to non-compliance [6]. Most of these patients are: (a) smokers, who are likely to exhibit poor adherence; (b) depressed or socially isolated; (c) having poor quadriceps strength; (d) COPD patients having higher mMRC scores and exacerbations; (e) problems of transportations and (f) financial burden [12-15].

Clinical Impacts

PR is a reliable solution for improving health conditions (i.e., physical, psychosocial, and decreased economic burden). However, in patients with COPD, PR offers more than the usual benefits, such as controlling dyspnea, tolerating exercise, and achieving improved overall health [1, 3, 6].

Controlling Symptoms

In previous studies, PR programs have been found to be effective in diminishing patients' fatigue and dyspnea-related symptoms and improving emotional strength and sense of control [16]. Fatigue can be reduced further if the program incorporates self-management education, optimal nutritional management, and mind–body interventions [17]. However, for patients in palliative care, end of life, and hospice care, the use of opiates, neuromuscular electrical stimulation (NMES), oxygen, and fast-blowing air onto the face can significantly decrease breathlessness [17]. Muscular discomfort in the legs is a major concern for patients with COPD. However, the program also improves the strength of limb muscles and stamina of patients and allows them to perform more rigorous physical tasks without help [18]. Recently, a study conducted by the British Medical Research Council (MRC) using the questionnaire, transitional dyspnea index, modified Borg score during exercise, and Chronic Respiratory Questionnaires among 2,150 stable COPD patients showed that PR improved dyspnea and related symptoms [19]. Overall, this PR program improves the physiological outcome and well-being of patients.

Tolerating Exercise

As patients participate in graduated exercise sessions, there is an expectation of increased physical capacity. As a result, patients become more encouraged to keep exercising, increasing the exercise load when possible, and allowing for more physical activity [1, 20-22]. As per the Global Initiative for Chronic Obstructive Lung Disease (GOLD), exercise tolerance is a very notable change among COPD patients after undergoing the program. [17] Higashimoto et al. showed that PR programs significantly increase the exercise capacity in patients with stable COPD after induction of improved 6-minute walking distance (6MWD), peak workload, and peak VO2 [19]. Furthermore, the Randomized controlled trials (RCT) study also showed significant differences in post-treatment improvement of 6MWD in patients with stable COPD, as revealed by a significant direct relationship with the baseline forced expiratory volume in 1s/forced vital capacity, PaO2, and baseline 6MWD [23]. Similar results were found by Ragaselvi et al. in the 6MWD test and in identifying forced expiratory volume in 1 s/forced vital capacity as a predictor of program efficiency [24]. PR is most appropriate for patients with COPD, as heightened functional exercise capacities have been observed at all levels of COPD severity, although the best outcomes were noted in patients with moderate to severe disease [25].

Improving Mental Health

It is a fact that patients with COPD have difficulties in social activities, and impaired mental health. The benefit of this PR program is determined by improvements in psychosocial and health conditions [18]. Tselebis et al. showed that patients with psychosocial morbidity due to COPD reversed their misfortunes after attending a PR program [26]. Another study by Spruit et al. showed that a PR program improved the psychological conditions of patients, while their physical capacity improved [27]. In a similar study, it was found that the program could better reduce anxiety and depression than standard care [28].

Surviving COPD and Achieving Better Health-Related Quality of Life (HRQOL)

The literature showed that cessation of smoking improved the health conditions of patients with COPD. Studies have also found a link between PR and survival, particularly with the completion of a program [29]. According to GOLD, a successful complete program can greatly improve the health status of patients [17]. Moreover, malnourished patients who receive nutritional supplementation as they participate in the program achieved a better overall health status [17]. Spruit et al. noted that this program helps patients develop long-term adherence to health-enhancing behaviors [27]. Samah et al. showed in their [23] randomized, controlled clinical study of patients with stable COPD that HRQOL using the Saint George Respiratory Questionnaire (SGRQ) revealed a significant difference in the post-treatment improvement in three components of the SGRQ's score and in the total SGRQ score. The above studies show that surviving COPD through PR as a supplement is tantamount to better health outcomes, showing how HRQOL is improved by the program [19].

Facilitating Greater Independence

The goal of PR is to ensure that patients have greater control over their lives. It also helps patients achieve greater independence, as their overall health improves during and after the program [1]. This is a natural phenomenon, as patients are now physically fitter and more mobile. However, patients with severe COPD will take a longer time (i.e., a minimum of 3 months) to be more independent and improve quality of life. However, stable COPD patients require less time to achieve significant benefits [1, 6].

Reducing Hospitalizations and Healthcare Visits

This program made patients more confident and stronger, thus significantly decreasing the number of hospitalizations and/or hospital visits and the economic burden. It also significantly reduced unscheduled hospitalization due to sudden heart attacks in patients with COPD. The economic burden is significantly reduced by reducing diagnostic tests, medicines, and care interventions. It has been noted that if this program is immediately implemented following an exacerbation episode, the incidence of hospitalization also decreases [30, 31].

Reaping the Economic Benefits

It is a fact that PR programs decrease the frequency of hospital visits and lower medical costs due to better overall improvement of the health status of patients with COPD [18]. Therefore, health economic benefits become more favorable as patients regain their strength and limit the need for extra physical support. Therefore, more sincerity toward the program (i.e., zero delays or absences) has a better outcome.

Pulmonary Rehabilitation Models for Stable COPD

Apart from traditional PR programs performed within a healthcare setting, particularly for patients with severe COPD or recuperating from surgery and/or lung- and heart-related diseases, several new models have been developed in recent years as healthcare services have become more flexible, mobile, and accessible. However, the ATS categorized them into 7 different types based on suitability and less involvement of healthcare professionals for patients with stable COPD [4].

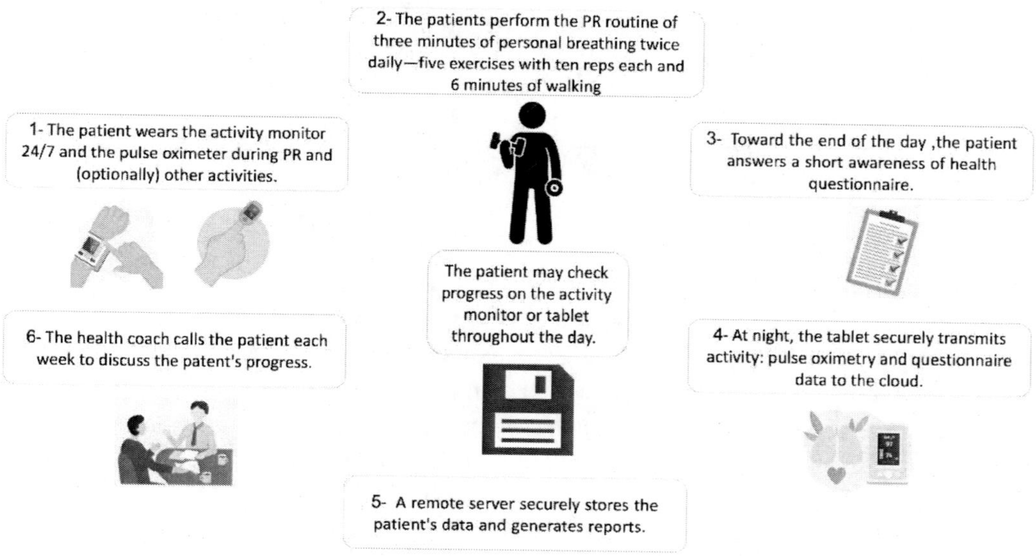

Figure 2. Elements of home-based pulmonary rehabilitation.

1. *Home-based PR*
   This is based on PR programs. (Figure 2). It may include staff visiting patients at home and telephone support. However, it may or may not require the use of specific equipment, such as cycle ergometers.
2. *Telerehabilitation*
   This PR program utilizes modern technologies, such as text messaging, video communication, and social media platforms, in offering rehabilitation. This service might be offered in any place at home, in a healthcare facility, or in community settings.
3. *Web-based Rehabilitation*
   With the advancement of technology, web-based rehabilitation provides a suitable platform for patients to work independently and in a cost-effective manner. So many advanced modules are available, and participants can complete the programs that suit them.
4. *Community PR*
   This program consists of supervised group exercise and/or education undertaken in community-based settings (i.e., non-healthcare and non-residential).
5. *Primary care PR*
   This program is delivered by professional staff within the primary care setting.
6. *PR Using Minimal Equipment*
   This is a self-directed exercise or practical program in which minimal equipment is used. It also requires less routine supervision.

7. *Breathlessness Rehabilitation*
   This PR model aims to manage the symptom-based needs of patients, which might include exercise and nonexercise interventions.

Standard Pulmonary Rehabilitation Program Designed for Stable COPD Patients

The PR program for stable COPD is mainly based on the framework developed by Girdhar et al., as per the guidelines of ATS. (Figure 1) [4, 6].

Pre-Rehabilitation Assessment

Pre-evaluation of the patient is a mandatory requirement for this program. Pulmonologists generally refer the patient to the program after complete examination of the patient's symptoms and laboratory-based diagnosis. A pharmacological supplementary treatment is also provided, and a post-treatment assessment is completed by the pulmonologist at the end of the program [6]. COPD patients might also have to be assessed for their symptomatology, mMRC score, and other information, such as smoking history, oxygen supplementation, comorbidities (e.g., diabetes, obesity, or hypertension), anxiety, and depression levels [4, 6, 8]. A complete pre-rehab assessment is critical, and helps physical therapists design individualized treatment plans to set goals by minimizing potential adverse effects [6].

The physical exam is focused on measuring the functional status of the participant and their ability to take additional physical stress or tolerance (i.e., they will be assessed for muscle wasting, joint mobility, and postural deformities), and a nutritional assessment (weight, height, and BMI, etc.) to determine lung capacity [6]. There is also a need for pertinent respiratory examination for COPD patients to assess their ability to clear respiratory secretions, use of accessory muscles, breathing patterns, and adventitious sounds on auscultation, such as wheezing [6]. Due to the physical deconditioning brought about by COPD, patients suffer from poor nutrition, inflammation, cardiovascular comorbidities, and postural deformities [33]. Questionnaires that will help to determine a patient's baseline functionality include the Functional Independence Measure (FIM), the Assessment of Motor and Process Skills (AMPS), and the Functional Capacity Evaluation (FCE) [34].

Exercise tests also help staff to measure functional capacity. These include a field walking test, a bicycle ergometer, and a treadmill [6]. Simple walk tests like the 6MWD and incremental shuttle walk tests are found to be very effective in clinical settings [6]. The 6MWD test, which measures oxygen desaturation and the development of dyspnea, consists of back and forth walking for a 30-m distance where patients walk at their own pace for 6 minutes [35]. The incremental shuttle walk test measures symptoms with limited maximal exercise capacity. It includes paced continuous walking for 20 minutes on a 10-m marked course or until dyspnea occurs, whichever comes first [8].

Table 2. Suggested Model for a Comprehensive Assessment Scheme Prior to PR Enrollment

Essential Components of Assessment	Other Considerations
• Exercise capacity • Quality of life • Dyspnea • Nutritional status • Occupational status	• Activities of daily living • Advanced care planning needs • Airway clearance requirements • Anxiety and panic • Cognitive status • Comorbidities: impact and management • Coping skills • Depression • Educational needs • Exacerbation management skills • Fall history • Fatigue • Financial needs • Frailty • Goals and priorities • Housing needs • Inhaled medication device technique • Inspiratory muscle strength and endurance • Medication adherence and side effects • Mobility • Musculoskeletal limitations • Oxygen needs, use of oxygen devices • Palliative care needs • Peripheral muscle strength and endurance • Physical activity in daily life • Safety of the home environment • Safety of specific exercise modalities • Self-efficacy • Sleep disturbance • Social support • Speech and swallowing • Smoking status

Therefore, a detailed assessment should be performed before enrollment in the program. A patient-oriented policy (behavior of rehabilitation staff and facilities) might be implemented for maximum outcome in accordance with the ATS assessment model. (Table 2).

Exercise Component

After a successful pre-rehab assessment, the patient is enrolled in the program. Exercise sessions are the core component of the rehab program. The main aim is to help COPD patients by increasing their performance of daily activities independently by reducing dyspnea and fatigue [6]. Exercise training usually begins with a warm-up, which helps in building stamina [3]. The key goal of this program is to strengthen both the upper and lower extremities, according to the advice of the ATS. Such strategies would strengthen the upper limbs and lungs to better cope with physical activity [4].

Endurance Training

Endurance training is a type of athletic training that increases the body's cardiovascular and muscular durability. It helps to develop the body's respiratory capabilities and muscular strength to sustain physical activity for extended periods with lower injury risks. It has also been found to be effective in improving dyspnea among stable COPD patients [19, 23]. This training is delivered in two ways: (i) continuous high-intensity aerobic endurance training and (ii) intermittent training (alternating high-intensity aerobics and low-intensity exercises) [36]. Continuous high-intensity aerobic training (70–80% peak work rate) could be performed with a constant or gradual increase of load. It is found to be most effective in improving oxygen consumption and delaying the anaerobic threshold [33, 37]. In contrast, intermittent training is recommended for patients with advanced COPD and/or more persistent dyspnea. It is best performed with short bouts of high-intensity aerobic training for 30–180 seconds followed by low-intensity exercises or rest [38- 40]. Therefore, interval training results in reduced pulmonary hyperinflation, helping patients exercise longer while having fewer occurrences of dyspnea [6].

Endurance training is provided in several ways, such as walking (treadmill or ground), cycling, rowing, swimming, and aerobic dancing. It could be fulfilled 3–5 times/week with an intensity of 4–6 Borg Dyspnea score (moderate level) [6, 10, 41]. Many programs use initial exercises that target arms and legs (i.e., slow walking for a few minutes) using either a treadmill or an unloaded cycling with an ergometer [1]. Sessions last between 0.5 and 2 hours, including at least half an hour of continuous aerobic activity [42, 43]. The frequency is recommended at two supervised sessions weekly plus a third unsupervised session [44, 45]. To achieve a significant improvement in fitness, at least 12 sessions (4 weeks) are recommended, which could be increased to a maximum of 72 weeks [5, 46]. A longer program (about 8 weeks) is found to be more beneficial as patient physiology and behavior achieve marked changes [47]. During the training period, oxygen levels are also monitored with supplemental oxygen provided as needed [1].

Strength Training

This program helps to increase the muscle strength of the participants. Muscle health helps individuals to improve their gait, limit the risk of falls, and become more independent [48]. Strength training significantly increases physical endurance, longer 6MWD, and higher oxygen consumption [3, 49, 50]. It is most effective for muscles used in daily living, such as the upper and lower extremities, including the trunk muscles [6, 4]. The lower extremities, in particular, suffer the most damage from muscular dystrophy in patients with COPD. It also contributes to maintaining bone mineral density [8]. Hence, to improve lower extremity strength, resistance training with 2–4 sets of 10–15 repetitions in each exercise is recommended for 2–3 days in a week through walking, cycling, and stair climbing, swimming, or using weight machines [6]. Weight increments are prescribed as soon as the patient completes all sets of exercise at a given weight [8].

The targeted approach to upper extremity exercises for COPD patients is beneficial in PR. Upper extremity exercises, such as lifting of arms as well as movements of some parts of the upper extremities (i.e., accessory muscles of respiration), increase metabolic activity in COPD patients. [4, 51-53]. Specific exercise of the upper extremities is critical. However, graded exercise is used to ameliorate skeletal muscle deconditioning, so general aerobic conditioning is better than specific respiratory exercises. Upper extremity resistance training helps patients to complete daily tasks like bathing or cleaning [1]. The upper extremity exercises directly impact the weakest part of the patient's body while employing its deconditioned muscles to complete a set. The exercise might start from low resistance (lightweights) with high frequency and gradually increase to high resistance (heavier load) [44].

Flexibility Training

Flexibility training helps improve patient mobility and posture. Due to hyperinflation, muscle hypertrophy, and inactivity, COPD patients end up having a rather modified chest structure, which affects their posture and movement [6]. Flexibility training can increase the patient's range of movement, reduce stiffness of joints, and regain posture [8]. Whole-body stretching exercises accompanied by proper breathing are best for COPD patients [3, 54, 55]. Stretching of the upper and lower extremity muscles for 2–3 days/week is the minimum required to gain benefits [56]. However, flexibility exercises prepare muscles for more stringent strength and endurance exercises [3].

The staff will teach patients breathing techniques while under stress and while active, and ways to better take medications and use inhalers [3]. Patients undergoing the program will have varying needs for oxygen. The program will conduct tests to measure oxygen levels at rest or during exercise to identify patients who need supplemental oxygen [1, 3]. Patients who smoke will also be provided with appropriate support, guiding them toward a smoking-free lifestyle [3].

Home Exercise Program and Maintenance Exercise Training

To better achieve the gains of endurance, strength, and flexibility training sessions, a home exercise program and maintenance training schedule is necessary [4]. A home exercise program designed by the rehab staff guarantees an improvement in performance and the benefits thereof [4]. Therefore, 3–4 times/week maintenance exercise should be performed to maintain the patient's fitness levels [1].

Education Component

The complete core component of PR is patient education and continuous exercise simultaneously. The education part of the program teaches patients to take control of their breathing, understand more about their illness, and implement behavioral, lifestyle, and dietary changes. A structured learning approach under the supervision of the rehabilitation staff will help patients learn how to breathe properly and take their medications [1, 3, 4]. Patients also have a chance to benefit from occupational therapy and nutritional strategies [6]. This learning could be tailored to a patient's needs and done in classroom settings [3].

COPD Education

Studies have shown that COPD patients with more knowledge are better at the management and treatment of their own conditions [57]. Having more knowledge about their disease gives patients more power/confidence to recognize their symptoms and change their behaviors and lifestyle, which helps them to manage their illnesses proactively [6].

During the pre-rehab assessment, PR staff assist patients in connecting with their educational needs and help them identify what they will need throughout the program [6]. This patient-centerd teaching approach ensures that participants make a significant change in their behaviors [2, 8]. The collaborative nature of the program prepares patients to identify an exacerbation, allows staff to modify their treatment regimen when needed, and creates a communication loop between patients and staff [58, 4]. Exacerbations lead to more hospitalization and hinder patient's physical capacity. Therefore, instituting PR earlier during admission or within a month of discharge is more beneficial than enrolling later [7, 59]. The education aspect of PR informs patients to manage the risks of exacerbations. To better control exacerbations, an individualized action plan for frequent exacerbators can be added to the education component of PR [4]. Smoking cessation support is also recommended for patients trying to live a smoke-free lifestyle [3, 4].

Occupational Therapy

PR, along with occupational therapy, is a more effective program [60, 61]. In occupational therapy, COPD patients are taught to spend their energy efficiently for better outcomes [62, 1]. When patients conserve more energy, they tend to understand managing their breathlessness better, are smarter in performing daily tasks, have more sense of control, and engage with people more effectively [60-63]. The job of occupational therapists is to teach patients to use occupational equipment and technologies (wheeled walking aids) that improve autonomy, ventilatory capacity, and walking efficiency [64, 65].

Nutrition

COPD has more adverse effects on patients' bodies due to obesity and muscle wasting, which is a common phenomenon [66, 67]. The mortality rate is higher in underweight COPD patients [68]. Due to their lower fat-free mass, these patients have less exercise tolerance compared to persons with normal weights [69, 70]. Nutritional screening in pre-rehab assessment is key in identifying the nutritional status of COPD patients. This becomes the nutrition education's basis for the teaching sessions. Nutritional interventions include the addition of nutritional supplements to the patient's diet, especially protein intake, dietary counseling, and positive reinforcement [6, 71, 24].

Mental Health Support

COPD patients undergo a long process of social and psychological battle for being unable to perform their usual daily tasks, and, most specially, the inability to socialize. From the time the patient begins experiencing symptoms and exacerbations, and even toward a more stable and controlled period, the frustration and helplessness pile up. That is why many patients entering PR are in the middle of depression and anxiety [4, 8, 72]. Studies show that almost half of patients are depressive, and about a third have anxiety, whether their COPD is moderate or advanced [73-75]. Hence, it is important to check for the mood and social habits of patients early, at best during the pre-rehab assessment, to determine the breadth of support needed by patients from their family, friends, and even rehab staff [4]. The work of psychologists and psychiatrists has become valuable in these instances. Psychosocial support strategies that boost patient mental health should be available, since desired behavioral changes will not be achieved if a patient is stressed, depressed, or anxious during the life of the program.

Conclusion

Pulmonary rehabilitation is an effective non-pharmacological intervention in patients with stable COPD. It is suitable for people with mild, moderate, or severe chronic lung disease who are limited by breathlessness. Thus, it improves lung function, reduces symptom severity, and improves quality of life. Early initiation of PR is recommended to improve clinical outcomes.

Key Points

- Pulmonary rehabilitation (PR) improves lung function, reduces symptom severity, and improves the quality of life in patients with chronic obstructive pulmonary disease (COPD).
- The delivered education via PR increases the knowledge of the patients, which makes them better at the management and treatment of their own conditions.
- The earlier PR referral would improve the clinical outcomes, especially after acute exacerbations in patients with COPD.
- The objectives of PR are to enhance patients' self-efficiency and to encourage behavioral transformations towards a more significant amount of physical activity in daily life.

References

[1] Wise, RA. *Treatment of Stable COPD*. Merck Manual (Professional Version) July 2020. https://www.merckmanuals.com/professional/pulmonary-disorders/chronic-obstructive-pulmonary-disease-and-related-disorders/treatment-of-stable-copd#:~:text=Treatment%20of%20chronic%20stable%20COPD%20aims%20to%20prevent%20exacerbations%20and,%3D%22disableDrug%22.

[2] NICE. Chronic obstructive pulmonary disease in adults: Quality Standards (QS10). NICE UK 2011. https://www.nice.org.uk/guidance/qs10/chapter/quality-statement-4-pulmonary-rehabilitation-for-stable-copd-and-exercise-limitation.

[3] Lareau SC, Fahy B. Pulmonary Rehabilitation. *Am J Respir Crit Care Med* 2018;198: P19-P20.

[4] Holland, AE, Cox NS, Houchen-Wolloff L, Rochester CL, Garvey C, ZuWallack R, Nici L, Limberg T, Lareau SC, Yawn BP, Galwicki M, Troosters T, Steiner M, Casaburi R, Clini E, Goldstein RS, Singh SJ. Defining Modern Pulmonary Rehabilitation. An Official American Thoracic Society Workshop Report. *Annals of the American Thoracic Society* 2021;18(5). https://doi.org/10.1513/AnnalsATS.202102-146ST.

[5] Ries AL, Bauldoff GS, Carlin BW, et al. Pulmonary rehabilitation: Joint ACCP/AACVPR evidence-based clinical practice guidelines. *Chest.* 2007;131:4-42.

[6] Girdhar, A, Agarwal, P, Singh A. Pulmonary Rehabilitation in Chronic Obstructive Pulmonary Disease. *IntechOpen Book Series* 2018. https://www.intechopen.com/chapters/64166.

[7] Bolton CE et al. British Thoracic Society guideline on pulmonary rehabilitation in adults. *Thorax.* 2013;68:ii1-ii30.

[8] Spruit MA et al. An official American Thoracic Society/European Respiratory Society statement: Key concepts and advances in pulmonary rehabilitation. *American Journal of Respiratory and Critical Care Medicine*. 2013;188:e13-e64.

[9] Evans RA et al. Pulmonary rehabilitation is successful for COPD irrespective of MRC dyspnoea grade. *Respiratory Medicine*. 2009;103:1070-1075.

[10] Ries AL, Make BJ, Lee SM, National Emphysema Treatment Trial Research Group, et al. The effects of pulmonary rehabilitation in the national emphysema treatment trial. *Chest*. 2005;128:3799-3809.

[11] Puhan MA, Scharplatz M, Troosters T, Steurer J. Respiratory rehabilitation after acute exacerbation of COPD may reduce risk for readmission and mortality – A systematic review. *Respiratory Research*. 2005;6:54.

[12] Garrod R, Marshall J, Barley E, Jones PW. Predictors of success and failure in pulmonary rehabilitation. *The European Respiratory Journal*. 2006;27:788-794.

[13] Sabit R, Griffiths TL, Watkins AJ, et al. Predictors of poor attendance at an outpatient pulmonary rehabilitation programme. *Respiratory Medicine*. 2008;102:819-824.

[14] Keating A, Lee A, Holland AE. What prevents people with chronic obstructive pulmonary disease from attending pulmonary rehabilitation? A systematic review. *Chronic Respiratory Disease*. 2011;8:89-99.

[15] Young P, Dewse M, Fergusson W, Kolbe J. Respiratory rehabilitation in chronic obstructive pulmonary disease: Predictors of nonadherence. *The European Respiratory Journal*. 1999;13:855-859.

[16] Lacasse Y, Goldstein R, Lasserson Toby J, et al. Pulmonary rehabilitation for chronic obstructive pulmonary disease. *Cochrane Database of Systematic Reviews*. 2006;4:CD0037993. http://doi.org/10.1002/14651858.CD003793.pub2.

[17] Global Initiative for Chronic obstructive Lung Disease (GOLD). *Pocket Guide to COPD Diagnosis, Management, and Prevention: A Guide for Health Care Professionals,* 2018 Report. GOLD 2018. https://goldcopd.org/wp-content/uploads/2018/02/WMS-GOLD-2018-Feb-Final-to-print-v2.pdf.

[18] Rochester, CL, Vogiatzis, I, Holland, AE, Lareau, SC, Marciniuk, DD, Puhan, MA, Spruit, MA, Masefield, S, Casaburi, R, Clini, EM, Crouch, R, Garcia-Aymerich, J, Garvey, C, Goldstein, RS, Hill, K, Morgan, M, Nici, L, Pitta, F, Ries, AL, ZuWallack, RL. An official ATS/ERS policy statement: Enhancing implementation, use and delivery of pulmonary rehabilitation. *American Journal of Respiratory and Critical Care Medicine*. 2015;192:1373-1386.

[19] Higashimoto Y, Ando M, Sano A, Saeki S, Nishikawa Y, Fukuda K, Tohda Y. Effect of pulmonary rehabilitation programs including lower limb endurance training on dyspnea in stable COPD: A systematic review and meta-analysis. *Respiratory Investigation* 2020;58(5): 355-366.

[20] Garcia-Aymerich, J, Lange, P, Benet, M, Schnohr, P, & Anto, JM. Regular physical activity reduces hospital admission and mortality in chronic obstructive pulmonary disease: A population based cohort study. *Thorax*. 2006;61:772-778.

[21] Griffiths, T, Burr, M, Campbell, I, Lewis-Jenkins, V, Mullins, J, Shiels, K, Turner-Lawlor, P, Payne, N, Newcombe, R, Lonescu, A, Thomas, J, & Tunbridge, J. Results at 1 year of outpatient multidisciplinary pulmonary rehabilitation: A randomised controlled trial. *Lancet*. 2000;355:362-368.

[22] Singh, SJ, Jones, PW, Evans, R, & Morgan, MDL. Minimum clinically important improvement for the incremental shuttle walking test. Thorax. 2008;63:775-777.

[23] Samah M. Shehata MD, Refky, MM, Al gabry MM, Nafae RM. Outcome of pulmonary rehabilitation in patients with stable chronic obstructive pulmonary disease at Chest Department, Zagazig University Hospitals (2014–2016). *Egyptian Journal of Bronchology* 2018;12: 279–287.

[24] Ragaselvi S, Janmeja AK, Aggarwal D, Sidana A, Sood P. Predictors of response to pulmonary rehabilitation in stable chronic obstructive pulmonary disease patients: A prospective cohort study. *Journal of Postgraduate Medicine* 2019;65(2): 101-106.

[25] Vogelmeier, CF, Criner, GJ, Martinez, FJ, Anzueto, A, Barnes, PJ, Bourbeau, J, Celli, BR, Chen, R, Decramer, M, Fabbri, LM, Frith, P, Halpin, DMG, López Varela, MV, Nishimura, M, Roche, N, Rodriguez-Roisin, R, Sin, DD, Singh, D, Stockley, R, Agustí, A. Global strategy for the diagnosis, management, and prevention of chronic obstructive lung disease 2017 report. GOLD executive summary. *American Journal of Respiratory and Critical Care Medicine*. 2017;195(5):557-582.

[26] Tselebis, A, Bratis, D, Pachi, A, Moussas, G, Ilias, I, Harikiopoulou, M, Theodorakopoulou, E, Dumitru, S, Kosmas, E, Vgontzas, A, Siafakas, N, & Tzanakis, N. A pulmonary rehabilitation program reduces levels of anxiety and depression in COPD patients. Multidisciplinary *Respiratory Medicine*. 2013;8:41.

[27] Martijn A Spruit, Sally J Singh, Chris Garvey, Richard ZuWallack, Linda Nici, Carolyn Rochester, Kylie Hill, Anne E Holland, Suzanne C Lareau, William DC Man, Fabio Pitta, Louise Sewell, Jonathan Raskin, Jean Bourbeau, Rebecca Crouch, Frits ME Franssen, Richard Casaburi, Jan H Vercoulen, Ioannis Vogiatzis, Rik Gosselink, Enrico M Clini, Tanja W Effing, François Maltais, Job van der Palen, Thierry Troosters, Daisy JA Janssen, Eileen Collins, Judith Garcia-Aymerich, Dina Brooks, Bonnie F Fahy, Milo A Puhan, Martine Hoogendoorn, Rachel Garrod, Annemie MWJ Schols, Brian Carlin, Roberto Benzo, Paula Meek, Mike Morgan, Maureen PMH Rutten-van Mölken, Andrew L Ries, Barry Make, Roger S Goldstein, Claire A Dowson, Jan L Brozek, Claudio F Donner, Emiel FM Wouters, ATS/ERS Task Force on Pulmonary RehabilitationATS/ERS task force on pulmonary rehabilitation. An official American Thoracic Society/European Respiratory Society statement: Key concepts and advances in pulmonary rehabilitation. *American Journal of Respiratory and Critical Care Medicine*. 2013;188:e13-e64.

[28] Coventry PA, Hind D. Comprehensive pulmonary rehabilitation for anxiety and depression in adults with chronic obstructive pulmonary disease: Systematic review and meta-analysis. *Journal of Psychosomatic Research*. 2007;63:551-565.

[29] Ries AL, Kaplan RM, Limberg TM, Prewitt, LM. Effects of pulmonary rehabilitation on physiologic and psychosocial outcomes in patients with chronic obstructive pulmonary disease. *Annals of Internal Medicine*. 1995;122:823-832.

[30] Rubí, M, Renom, F, Ramis, F, Medinas, M, Centeno, MJ, Górriz, M, Crespí, E, Martín, B, & Soriano, JB. Effectiveness of pulmonary rehabilitation in reducing health resources use in chronic obstructive pulmonary disease. *Archives of Physical Medicine and Rehabilitation*. 2010;91:364-368. https://doi.org/10.1016/j.apmr.2009.09.025.

[31] Seymour JM, Moore L, Jolley CJ. Outpatient pulmonary rehabilitation following acute exacerbations of COPD. *Thorax*. 2010;65:423-428.

[32] MayoClinic. *Advancing care in chronic obstructive pulmonary disease*. MayoClinic Online 2022. https://www.mayoclinic.org/medical-professionals/pulmonary-medicine/news/advancing-care-in-chronic-obstructive-pulmonary-disease/mac-20471608.

[33] Vogiatzis, I, Terzis, G, Nanas, S, Stratakos, G, Simoes, DCM, Georgiadou, O, Zakynthinos, S, & Roussos, C. Skeletal muscle adaptations to interval training in patients with advanced COPD. *Chest*. 2005;128:3838-3845.

[34] Coppola S, Wood W. Occupational therapy to promote function and health-related quality of life. In: Hodgkin JE, Celli BR, Connors GL, editors. *Pulmonary Rehabilitation: Guidelines to Success*. 4th ed. St. Louis: Mosby; 2009.

[35] Redelmeier, DA, Bayoumi, AM, Goldstein, RS, & Guyatt, GH. Interpreting small differences in functional status: The six minute walk test in chronic lung disease patients. *American Journal of Respiratory and Critical Care Medicine*. 1997;155:1278-1282.

[36] Martín-Valero R, Cuesta-Vargas AI, Labajos-Manzanares MT. Types of physical exercise training for COPD patients. In: Ong K-C, editor. *Chronic Obstructive Pulmonary Disease-Current Concepts and Practice*. Croacia: Intechweb.org; 2012. pp. 351-374.

[37] Gimenez, M, Servera, E, Vergara, P, Bach, JR, & Polu, JM. Endurance training in patients with chronic obstructive pulmonary disease: A comparison of high versus moderate intensity. *Archives of Physical Medicine and Rehabilitation*. 2000;81:102-109.

[38] Coppoolse, R, Schols, AMWJ, Baarends, EM, Mostert, R, Akkermans, MA, Janssen, PP, & Wouters, EFM. Interval versus continuous training in patients with severe COPD: A randomized clinical trial. *The European Respiratory Journal*. 1999;14:258-263.

[39] American Thoracic Society Committee on Pulmonary Function Standards. Guidelines for methacholine and exercise challenge testing—1999. *American Journal of Respiratory and Critical Care Medicine*. 2000;161:309-329.

[40] Datta D, ZuWallack R. High versus low intensity exercise training in pulmonary rehabilitation: Is more better? *Chronic Respiratory Disease*. 2004;1:143-149.

[41] Puente-Maestu L, Sanz ML, Sanz P, Cubillo, JM, Mayol, J, Casaburi, R. Comparison of effects of supervised versus self-monitored training programs in patients with chronic obstructive pulmonary disease. *The European Respiratory Journal*. 2000;15:517-525.

[42] Hassanein SE, Narsavage GL. The dose effect of pulmonary rehabilitation on physical activity, perceived exertion, and quality of life. *Journal of Cardiopulmonary Rehabilitation and Prevention*. 2009;29:255-260.

[43] American College of Sports Medicine, Thompson WR, Gordon NF, Pescatello LS. *ACSM's Guidelines for Exercise Testing and Prescription*. 8th ed. Philadelphia: Lippincott Williams & Wilkins; 2009.

[44] Garvey C, Madeline Paternostro Bayles, Larry F Hamm, Kylie Hill, Anne Holland, Trina M Limberg, Martijn A Spruit. Pulmonary rehabilitation exercise prescription in chronic obstructive pulmonary disease: Review of selected guidelines: An official statement from The American Association of Cardiovascular and Pulmonary Rehabilitation. *Journal of Cardiopulmonary Rehabilitation and Prevention*. 2016;36:75-83.

[45] American College of Sports Medicine, Pescatello LS, Arena R, Riebe D, Thompson PD. *ACSM's Guidelines for Exercise Testing and Prescription*. 9th ed. Philadelphia: Lippincott Williams & Wilkins; 2014.

[46] Plankeel JF, McMullen B, MacIntyre NR. Exercise outcomes after pulmonary rehabilitation depend on the initial mechanism of exercise limitation among non-oxygen-dependent COPD patients. *Chest*. 2005;127:110-116.

[47] Sneed NV, Paul SC. Readiness for behavioral changes in patients with heart failure. *American Journal of Critical Care*. 2003;12:444-453.

[48] Holland, AE, Hill, CJ, Nehez, E, & Ntoumenopoulos, G. Does unsupported upper limb exercise training improve symptoms and quality of life for patients with chronic obstructive pulmonary disease? *Journal of Cardiopulmonary Rehabilitation*. 2004;24:422-427.

[49] Ortega, F., Toral, J., Cejudo, P., Villagomez, R., Sánchez, H., Castillo, J., & Montemayor, T. Comparison of effects of strength and endurance training in patients with chronic obstructive pulmonary disease. *American Journal of Respiratory and Critical Care Medicine*. 2002;166:669-674.

[50] Spruit MA, Gosselink R, Troosters T, De Paepe C, Decramer M. Resistance versus endurance training in patients with COPD and skeletal muscle weakness. *The European Respiratory Journal*. 2002; 19:1072-1078.

[51] Costi, S, Crisafulli, E, Degli Antoni, F, Beneventi, C, Fabbri, LM, & Clini, EM. Effects of unsupported upper extremity exercise training in patients with COPD: A randomized clinical trial. *Chest*. 2009; 136:387-395.

[52] Porto, EF, Castro, AAM, Velloso, M, Nascimento, O, Dal Maso, F, & Jardim, JR. Exercises using the upper limbs hyperinflate COPD patients more than exercises using the lower limbs at the same metabolic demand. *Monaldi Archives for Chest Disease*. 2009;71:21-26.

[53] Biskobing DM. COPD and osteoporosis. *Chest*. 2002;12:609-620.

[54] Dias CS, Kirkwood RN, Parreira VF, Sampaio RF. Orientation and position of the scapula, head and kyphosis thoracic in male patients with COPD. *Canadian Journal of Respiratory Therapy*. 2009;45:30-34.

[55] Greendale, GA, Huang, MH, Karlamangla, AS, Seeger, L, & Crawford, S. Yoga decreases kyphosis in senior women and men with adult-onset hyperkyphosis: Results of a randomized controlled trial. *Journal of the American Geriatrics Society*. 2009;57:1569-1579.

[56] Munro, PE, Holland, AE, Bailey, M, Button, BM, & Snell, GI. Pulmonary rehabilitation following lung transplantation. *Transplantation Proceedings*. 2009;41:292-295.

[57] Make B. Collaborative self-management strategies for patients with respiratory disease. *Respiratory Care*. 1994;39:566-579.

[58] Rice, KL, Dewan, N, Bloomfield, HE, Grill, J, Schult, TM, Nelson, DB, Kumari, S, Thomas, M, Geist, LJ, Beaner, C, Caldwell, M, & Niewoehner, DE. Disease management program for chronic obstructive pulmonary disease: A randomized controlled trial. *American Journal of Respiratory and Critical Care Medicine*. 2010;182:890-896.

[59] Puhan, MA, Gimeno-Santos, E, Cates, CJ, & Troosters, T.Pulmonary rehabilitation following exacerbations of chronic obstructive pulmonary disease. *Cochrane Database of Systematic Reviews*. 2009;21(1):CD005305. http://doi.org/10.1002/14651858.CD005305.pub2.

[60] Norweg A, Bose P, Snow G, Berkowitz ME. A pilot study of a pulmonary rehabilitation programme evaluated by four adults with chronic obstructive pulmonary disease. *Occupational Therapy International*. 2008;15:114-132.

[61] Chan SC. Chronic obstructive pulmonary disease and engagement in occupation. *The American Journal of Occupational Therapy*. 2004;58:408-415.

[62] Fraguas Cerezo MP. Terapia ocupacional en rehabilitación respiratoria [*Occupational therapy in respiratory rehabilitation*]. *Ter ocup: Rev APETO*. 2003; 31:2-4.

[63] American Occupational Therapy Association. Occupational therapy framework: Domain and process (2nd ed.). *The American Journal of Occupational Therapy*. 2008;62:625-683.

[64] Solway S, Brooks D, Lau L, Goldstein R. The short-term effect of a rollator on functional exercise capacity among individuals with severe COPD. *Chest*. 2002;122:56-65.

[65] Honeyman P, Barr P, Stubbing DG. Effect of a walking aid on disability, oxygenation, and breathlessness in patients with chronic airflow limitation. *Journal of Cardiopulmonary Rehabilitation*. 1996;16:63-67.

[66] Emery, CF, Schein, RL, Hauck, ER, & MacIntyre, NR. Psychological and cognitive outcomes of a randomized trial of exercise among patients with chronic obstructive pulmonary disease. *Health Psychology*. 1998;17:232-240.

[67] Engelen, M, Schols, A, Lamers, R, & Wouters, E.Different patterns of chronic tissue wasting among patients with chronic obstructive pulmonary disease. *Clinical Nutrition*. 1999;18:275-280.

[68] Schols AM, Slangen J, Volovics L, Wouters EF. Weight loss is a reversible factor in the prognosis of chronic obstructive pulmonary disease. *American Journal of Respiratory and Critical Care Medicine*. 1998;157:1791-1797.

[69] Shoup, R, Dalsky, G, Warner, S, Davies, M, Connors, M, Khan, M, Khan, F, Zu, R, Wallack. Body composition and health-related quality of life in patients with obstructive airways disease. *European Respiratory Journal*. 1997;10:1576-1580.

[70] Mostert, R, Goris, A, Weling-Scheepers, C, Wouters, EFM, & Schols, AMWJ. Tissue depletion and health related quality of life in patients with chronic obstructive pulmonary disease. *Respiratory Medicine*. 2000;94:859-867.

[71] Weekes CE, Emery PW, Elia M. Dietary counseling and food fortification in stable COPD: A randomised trial. *Thorax*. 2009;64:326-331.

[72] Singh, D., Agusti, A., Anzueto, A., Barnes, P. J., Bourbeau, J., Celli, B. R., Criner, G. J., Frith, P., Halpin, D., Han, M., López Varela, M. V., Martinez, F., Montes de Oca, M., Papi, A., Pavord, I. D., Roche, N., Sin, D. D., Stockley, R., Vestbo, J., Wedzicha, J. A., … Vogelmeier, C. (2019). Global Strategy for the Diagnosis, Management, and Prevention of Chronic Obstructive Lung Disease: the GOLD science committee report 2019. *The European Respiratory Journal*, 53(5), 1900164. https://doi.org/10.1183/13993003.00164-2019.

[73] Mills TL. Comorbid depressive symptomatology: Isolating the effects of chronic medical conditions on self-reported depressive symptoms among community-dwelling older adults. *Social Science & Medicine*. 2001;53:569-578.

[74] Yohannes AM, Connolly MJ. Pulmonary rehabilitation programmes in the UK: A national representative survey. *Clinical Rehabilitation*. 2004;18:444-449.

[75] Janssen, DJ, Spruit, MA, Leue, C, Gijsen, C, Hameleers, H, Schols, JM, Wouters, EF, & On behalf of the Ciro network. Symptoms of anxiety and depression in COPD patients entering pulmonary rehabilitation. *Chronic Respiratory Disease*. 2010;7:147-157.

Chapter 12

Management of Malnutrition in Stable COPD

Abdulelah M. Aldhahir[1,*], PhD, Abdullah A. Alqarni[2], PhD, Saeed M. Alghamdi[3], PhD and Ali Hakamy[1], PhD

[1]Respiratory Therapy Department,
Faculty of Applied Medical Sciences, Jazan University,
Jazan, Saudi Arabia
[2]Department of Respiratory Therapy,
Faculty of Medical Rehabilitation Sciences,
King Abdulaziz University, Jeddah, Saudi Arabia
[3]Clinical Technology Department,
Respiratory Care Program,
Faculty of Applied Medical Sciences,
Umm Al-Qura University, Makkah, Saudi Arabia

Abstract

Chronic Obstructive Pulmonary Disease is a condition of global proportions. This series of persistent respiratory illness may be common and treatable. However, the disease's progression, prevalence, and suddenness are significant points of concern as it ranks the fourth leading cause of death worldwide. Malnutrition of different forms persists and co-exists in COPD patients, further exacerbating the symptoms and leading to higher mortality. With the excessive production of Cytokines and a malnutrition-stricken body, consequences may include reduced exercise capacity, longer hospitalization, weaker body functions, and higher risk of mortality rate. Management of malnutrition included dietary advice and nutritional supplementation should be incorporated in COPD patients' management, aiming to stabilize body composition and improve functional status. Dietary advice allows for the intake of energy-dense or protein-rich foods that augments physical and weight development. Proper oral nutritional supplementation addresses malnutrition and improves the overall state of the body as it fills the gap in vitamins, amino acids, and the life necessary in maintaining the body.

Keywords: COPD, malnutrition, dietary advice, nutritional supplementation

* Corresponding Author's Email: Aldhahir.abdulelah@hotmail.com.

In: Chronic Obstructive Pulmonary Disease
Editor: Jaber S. Alqahtani
ISBN: 979-8-88697-333-4

Introduction

Chronic Obstructive Pulmonary Disease (COPD) is defined as "a common, preventable, and treatable disease that is characterized by persistent respiratory symptoms and irreversible airflow limitation that is due to airway and/or alveolar abnormalities usually caused by significant exposure to noxious particles or gases" [1]. Patients with COPD may experience a reduced quality of life due to the symptoms of the disease. Lesser exercise capacity, sudden and daily symptoms experiences, and high risk for worsening pre-existing conditions [2, 3]. Globally, COPD is a major cause of morbidity and mortality [4]. Due to its commonality and potential fatality of its aggravation, COPD is the fourth leading mortality cause globally, responsible for 3.2 million deaths in 2015 [4, 5]. Globally, 7.6% of the general population have or is diagnosed with COPD [12]. COPD may worsen its negative impact on global health without further action. By 2030, COPD will reach third place when it comes to mortality rate rankings [6, 7]. It has a severe burden on individual financial status and quality of living.

COPD is a systemic inflammatory disease; it always presents with multiple systemic manifestations and extrapulmonary effects. Malnutrition and abnormal body composition are common in individuals with COPD leading to substantial undesired outcomes such as depression, higher COPD exacerbation, deteriorated exercise tolerance, higher hospitalization, and mortality rate [8-10]. The exact causal relationship between COPD and malnutrition is complex. Still, a bidirectional link may likely exist as malnutrition is a cause and consequence of COPD simultaneously [11]. Malnourished COPD patients generally show hyperinflation, lower lung diffusion capacity, and lower exercise capacity [12]. The abnormalities may lead to several negative consequences concerning body composition and are characterized by a reduction in type I and IIa fibers, blood capillaries, oxidative enzymes, and changes in energy metabolism [12].

Due to malnutrition's consequences in individuals with COPD, several management modalities were introduced to overcome malnutrition and alert body composition in COPD patients [13, 14].

This chapter aims to provide a brief background and define malnutrition. Moreover, body composition, abnormal alteration and progression, consequences, treatment, and the like in individuals with COPD require further discussion. Additionally, screening for malnutrition and several management strategies such as dietary advice and nutritional or dietary supplementation will be detailed.

Definition and Background of Malnutrition

Malnutrition may refer to over-nutrition, overweight or obesity, under-nutrition, underweight or losing weight, or micronutrients, lacking essential vitamins and minerals. According to the European Society for Parenteral and Enteral Nutrition, malnutrition or "undernutrition" is defined as 'a state resulting from lack of intake or uptake of nutrition that leads to abnormal body composition (decreased fat free mass) and body cell mass leading to diminished physical and mental function and impaired clinical outcome from disease' [15]. Whereas the World Health Organization defines malnutrition as 'deficiencies, excesses or imbalances in a person's intake of energy and/or nutrients' [16]. In simple terms, malnutrition appertains to the imbalance of the essential vitamins, minerals, protein, and other nutrients that may adversely affect the human body's function, repair, and maintenance. In COPD patients, malnutrition accompanies more important protein requirements, energy intake, and other body nutritional needs. Reduced food intake may co-exist with malnutrition in COPD patients, potentially worsening the common symptoms of both conditions [17]. The exact relationship between malnutrition and COPD lacks proper definition and exploration, but malnutrition could possibly cause or result from an individual's case of COPD. Ezzell and Jensen reported that in a study that included 105 COPD patients, COPD patients suffering from malnutrition, especially emphysema phenotype, showed increased risks and symptoms relating to a substantial airflow blockage, diminished physical capabilities, and diffusing capacity, especially when compared to individuals of the same weight, age, and condition [18]. De Blasio et al. compared COPD symptoms in 50 COPD patients with and without malnutrition or conditions associated with inflammatory and nutritional factors. They reported that malnutrition in COPD patients worsen airflow obstruction, gas diffusion, gas exchange, vitamin D levels, and body function, as measured by the 6MWD and the COPD Assessment Test, or CAT tool [19]. Sun et al. (2019) conducted a meta-analysis to discover the potential relations between BMI and FEV_1 decline. The resulting conclusion dictates that being underweight is a significant health risk factor in the accelerated reduction of lung function in COPD patients. Higher BMI projects a slower FEV_1 decline [20]. Additionally, Marco et al. conducted a cohort study including 118 patients with COPD to predict hospitalizations and mortality in a 24 months follow-up [21]. Marco et al. proceeded with a cohort study that involved 118 COPD patients. In the determination of the projected hospitalization patterns and potential mortality within two years, after the two-year follow-up period, it was discovered that COPD patients with malnutrition were assessed to have a four times higher risk of death within the two years. Low fat free mass index (FFMI) may also be a risk identifier as it was reported that an individual is 17 times more likely to die in such conditions [21].

According to Goates et al., the projected annual cost of disease-associated malnutrition in the United States is over $15.5 billion in healthcare [22]. In the UK, comparing the treatment costs between non-malnourished and malnourished patients indicates an interesting trend. It may cost up to four times more to treat a malnourished patient [23]. Estimates show projected annual costs caused by malnutrition in the UK equate to £19.6 billion, which is 15% higher than the average healthcare spending [23].

Prevalence of Malnutrition in Stable COPD Patients

Malnutrition's progression in COPD patients may be rapid due to COPD exacerbation or gradually and consistently over a few years. Multiple healthcare and patient studies showed that malnutrition is consistently present in numerous COPD patients. Variations may be present depending on the severity of the disease, the setting of the patient, and the method of diagnosis [24]. In a prospective study conducted by Steer et al., malnutrition was prevalent in 33% of the 608 COPD patients hospitalized due to exacerbation in the UK [25]. According to Marco et al., in a prospective study conducted in Spain, which included 118 stable COPD patients free of exacerbations and hospital admissions in the previous two months, malnutrition was 24.6% [21]. Ng et al. reported that the overall persistence of malnutrition in 778 COPD patients that required pulmonary rehabilitation was denoted at 11%, 6% were at medium risk, while 5%

were at high risk in the UK [26]. Collins et al. state that in 425 outpatients with COPD screened using the Malnutrition Universal Screening Tool "MUST," 21% were at risk or had persistent malnutrition [27]. Malnutrition Pathway, a group of malnutrition experts, states that one in three hospitalized COPD patients or one in five outpatients show signs of malnutrition [23].

Causes and Consequences of Malnutrition in Stable COPD Patients

COPD refers to not only the disease of the lung but also a systemic inflammatory disorder defined by the more aggressive production of tumor necrosis factor (TNF)-α, IL-8, interleukin IL-6, chemokines, and other inflammatory cytokines [28, 29]. Inflammatory cytokines and the subsequent more outstanding production may cause or prompt hypermetabolism in COPD patients. Several studies have reported the relationship between TNF-a and weight loss in COPD population. Implications about their links and functions correlate to COPD. TNF levels were found to have been ten times higher in underweight patients compared to the average and the increase in TNF-alpha production may be the reason for weight loss in COPD patients with malnutrition [28, 30, 31]. COPD patients may experience anorexia or appetite loss due to malnutrition factors contributing to weight loss. Koehler et al. study linked the patient's lack of appetite to the IL-6 Inflammatory cytokine. IL-6 presence in higher concentrations may lead to anorexia [32] (Table 1).

Table 1. Causes and Consequences of malnutrition in COPD

Causes of malnutrition	**Consequences of malnutrition**
COPD effects, e.g., dyspnea, loss of appetite, inflammation.	Higher levels of mortality
Psychological factors, e.g., indifference, motivation, depression.	Higher healthcare costs overall
Social factors, e.g., isolation, lacking social support system, death of relatives or friends.	Lengthier hospitalization periods
Environmental factors, e.g., living space, environmental conditions, accessibility, mobility.	Consistent and frequent readmissions
Increased nutrient demand, e.g., protein, vitamins, energy.	Muscles weakness
Medication: Oxygen or inhaled therapy e.g., taste changes, mouth dryness. Frequent or prolonged utilization of corticosteroids adversely weakens bone and muscle strength	Reduced respiratory, circulatory, skeletal, and muscular function

COPD patients have high energy requirements, especially resting energy expenditure (REE). Such conditions are the cause of their malnutrition. Schols et al. measured REE in 34 healthy controls with regular weight and 68 stable COPD patients. They concluded that REE was substantially higher in malnourished COPD patients than in COPD patients with average body weight and nutritional value [33]. Wilson et al. came to the same conclusion when discovering that malnourished COPD patients had significantly higher REE levels [34]. Increased work of breathing associated with COPD may result in an increase in REE in malnourished COPD patients; however, increased breathing is not the only cause of malnutrition in COPD patients.

Corticosteroids used by COPD patients may result in malnutrition indirectly by inhibiting protein synthesis and promoting catabolism. The type of steroid, the dose, and the duration of use all significantly impact the adverse effect on muscle; thus, a higher corticosteroid dose may result in respiratory muscle weakness, resulting in abnormal muscle mass and malnutrition [35]. Researchers reported that as a result of malnutrition, hospital admissions doubled, and the six-month mortality rate tripled compared to normal-weight COPD patients [36].

According to Collins et al., the total healthcare costs for COPD patients over 12 months was two to three times high for malnourished COPD patients as it was for normal-weight and obese COPD patients c [37]. Additional consequences are listed in Table 1.

Body Composition in Stable COPD

Body composition abnormalities are common in individuals with COPD, especially those classified as moderate or severe and referred to PR. When energy expenditure exceeds available energy and food intake decreases, the body starts to lose fat, and muscle mass is impacted by a lack of balance between protein synthesis and breakdown. Typically, the BMI is calculated using the individual's weight and height. BMI is a metric determined by dividing an individual's "weight in kilograms by their height in meters squared." Individuals with a BMI less than 21 kg/m^2 are considered underweight, those with a BMI between 21 and 25 kg/m^2 are considered average weight, those with a BMI between 25 and 30 kg/m^2 are considered overweight, and those with a BMI greater than 30 kg/m^2 are considered obese. Several studies have established a link between abnormal BMI and COPD development. Marti et al. conducted a retrospective study on 128 patients with COPD to identify the relationship between body weight and respiratory related mortality. They discovered that a low BMI was associated with an increased risk of respiratory mortality [38]. Additionally, Park et al. used 437,584 Korean participants to examine the impact of BMI on the development of COPD. They discovered that having a low BMI increases the risk of developing COPD [39]. While the measurement is straightforward, it does not accurately reflect actual changes in body composition, especially in COPD patients. When measured using validated techniques, fat mass (FM) and fat-free mass (FFM), which are considered the primary components of body mass, are more specific indicators of body composition and typically reflect actual changes in body composition. Bioelectrical impedance is a well-established technique for determining the body's composition by passing an electrical current through it. It is based on FFM and FM's electrical properties. In 86 stable COPD patients, Slinde et al. investigated whether bioelectrical impedance measurements of body composition predicted one-year mortality. They discovered that bioelectrical impedance measurements of body composition were an independent predictor of mortality [40].

For many years, researchers have been concerned about accurately quantifying FFM due to its link with COPD outcomes. Hopkinson et al. conducted a study included 46 stable COPD patients to examine the relationship between body composition, exacerbation frequency over 12 months, and disease severity. They found that a decrease in FFM was associated with a decline in lung function in patients with COPD [41]. Additionally, Rutten et al. stated that persistent declines in FFM were associated with a higher rate of COPD exacerbations in patients with COPD [42]. It is well established that depleted COPD patients with a low FFM had decreased exercise capacity as measured by a 12-minute walk distance and a lower quality of life as measured by the St George's Respiratory Questionnaire (SGRQ) when compared to COPD patients with a preserved or "not depleted" FFM [43, 44].

Several studies conducted over the last decades have quantified and defined the normal range of FFM by computing FFMI, which is equal to FFM divided by height squared [45]. An FFMI of less than 16 kg/m^2 for men and less than 15 kg/m^2 for women is abnormal in COPD patients [46]. FFMI is critical in COPD patients because it is highly correlated with exercise capacity, dyspnea, respiratory muscle function, and FEV$_1$. It could be a useful predictor of COPD severity [47]. Vestbo et al. found that a low FFMI is associated with an increased risk of death, even in COPD patients with a normal BMI, in the Copenhagen City Heart Study [48]. Additionally, lower quality of life persisted in COPD patients with a low FFMI who were enrolled in a PR program [49]. As a result, it is crucial to assess COPD patients' body composition to rule out abnormalities such as muscle atrophy or malnutrition.

Screening for Malnutrition

Healthcare providers are interested in detecting and managing malnutrition throughout the population, but especially in those who have a pre-existing medical condition such as COPD that may result in malnutrition. Early detection and management of malnutrition in COPD may help reverse malnutrition, improve clinically meaningful outcomes, and reduce healthcare utilization and costs [50, 51]. The Global Leadership Initiative on Malnutrition (GLIM) introduced new malnutrition screening and diagnostic criteria in 2018, consisting of two steps [52]. The critical first step in determining nutritional status is to screen for malnutrition using a validated screening tool. The diagnosis was made using two etiologic and three phenotypic criteria. (1) Inadequate food intake or assimilation was used as an etiologic factor, as was (2) disease burden/inflammatory condition. The phenotypic criteria included a low BMI and non-voluntary weight loss, and decreased muscle mass indicative of body composition changes [52].

Several tools, including the Mini Nutritional Assessment (MNA), the Nutritional Risk Score (NRS-2002), and the Malnutrition Universal Screening Tool (MUST), have been introduced and validated in a variety of healthcare settings. The Mini Nutritional Assessment is an established tool for assessing malnutrition in older adults [53]. It includes 18 self-reported questions drawn from general, anthropometry, and self-assessment domains. The MNA-SF is a screening tool that includes six questions about food intake, weight loss, mobility, psychological stress, acute disease, dementia or depression, and BMI. The maximum score for this section is 14. A score of 12 or greater indicates that the subject is in good nutritional health, implying the absence of malnutrition or malnutrition risk; a score of 11 indicates that the complete MNA should be used [53, 54].

Two sections comprise the NRS-2002 form. The first section discusses the severity of the disease, food intake (and whether or not it has been reduced), and recent weight loss. The second section discusses malnutrition in general and the severity of the condition. Malnutrition is graded as absent (0 points), mild (1 point), moderate (2 points), or severe (3 points) (three points). Individuals who score three or higher on the total score are considered at risk of malnutrition [55].

MUST is the most frequently used, most straightforward, and most recommended screening tool for COPD adults at risk of malnutrition in various healthcare settings. It is a five-step procedure that determines an individual's BMI, recent unintentional weight loss, and the presence of disease [23]. The first step is to calculate your BMI, by determining your height and weight. The following step is to calculate and quantify the unintentional weight loss percentage that occurs. The third step is to define the symptoms and severity scores associated with acute disease. The fourth step is to add the three previous scores to determine the overall risk of malnutrition. Finally, a care plan is developed using management guidelines. Steer et al. examined whether MUST could be used to predict early readmission and mortality in 608 COPD patients hospitalized due to COPD exacerbations. They concluded that MUST is a significant predictor of in-hospital mortality and readmission and advocated for its routine assessment [25].

The National Institute for Health and Care Excellence (NICE) in the United Kingdom has advised healthcare providers to calculate BMIs for all COPD patients and monitor for unintended weight loss, especially in older adults [56]. Additionally, they recommend that healthcare providers conduct routine malnutrition risk assessments on all COPD patients using a simple screening tool. The percentage of older adults who lose weight unintentionally must be considered [56].

Management of Malnutrition in Stable COPD

Once malnutrition is identified, a risk-based management strategy should be implemented (low, medium, or high risk). The aims of managing malnutrition should increase muscle mass and body weight; a typical increase of two kilograms is recommended. Healthcare facilities offer a variety of management strategies, including dietary instruction or advice to increase nutrient intake, tailored diet plans, and oral nutritional supplements (ONS), all of which will be discussed in detail below [23].

Dietary Advice or Instruction

There is an agreement that tailored dietary advice should be provided by an experienced dietitian and be the first line of management approach when treating malnutrition, frequently over liquid ONS. However, more robust evidence introduced by the Dietetic Practice Manual's recommendation to use ONS in COPD patients [57]. Nutritional counseling to increase dietary intake is a critical dietetic skill. It is unknown whether it effectively treats malnutrition caused by disease and provides a proportional increase in energy, protein, and micronutrients.

According to Baldwin et al., dietary advice improved mortality, weight, and overall quality of life in a recent Cochrane systematic review involving 3,523 participants [58]. It may result in a more significant FFM gain than the group that did not receive advice [58]. Furthermore, Weekes et al. examined the effect of dietary counseling on 59 COPD outpatients. They were at risk of malnutrition, and they concluded that dietary advice resulted in weight gain and improvements in the St George's Respiratory Questionnaire's total score, dyspnea score, and daily living activity [59]. Additionally, Nguyen et al. discovered that when 120 malnourished

COPD patients were compared to a control group, customized dietary advice improved nutritional intake, nutritional status, functional outcomes, and quality of life [60].

As part of dietary advice, patients are encouraged to replace low energy foods with high energy foods, increasing meals frequency rather than the portion size. Additionally, dietitians should collaborate with family members and caregivers to develop a personalized nutritional care plan that incorporates dietary changes and food fortification to help an individual meet their nutritional requirements. One shortcoming of dietary advice is its frequent emphasis on the importance of increasing the macronutrient content of the diet. However, increasing protein intake significantly without increasing micronutrient intake is particularly difficult. If dietary recommendations prove ineffective, other management strategies may be necessary.

Oral Nutritional Supplementation

In clinical settings, nutritional supplements are used to treat malnutrition in patients with COPD. In malnourished COPD patients, healthy support increases exercise activity, decreases the risk of death, and strengthens muscles [61, 62].

There are both caloric and non-caloric dietary supplements available. Supplements are available in three forms: powder, liquid, and tablet. For instance, caloric supplements with a high fat and carbohydrate content increase body weight, which is especially beneficial in malnourished COPD patients with a high REE [63]. Ferreira et al. published a meta-analysis of nutritional supplementation for stable COPD in 2012. They discovered that dietary supplements increased muscle mass and body weight, improved respiratory function, and increased exercise tolerance in malnourished COPD patients [64]. Furthermore, Collins et al. demonstrated in their meta-analysis that nutritional supplements improved body weight, inspiratory and expiratory muscle strength, quality of life, handgrip strength, and exercise performance in COPD patients [65]. Several types of ONS have been successfully used in patients with COPD.

COPD patients receive supplemental protein to compensate for their low protein intake, which improves exercise performance and protein synthesis [66]. Protein synthesis is stimulated to increase body mass and muscle mass. Naz and Sahin demonstrated that protein-rich nutritional supplements improved the quality of life of COPD patients significantly [67]. Additionally, Khan et al. concluded that supplementation with a high-protein diet improved body weight and composition, exercise capacity, and overall quality of life in 60 stable COPD patients [68].

Amino acids are the protein's building blocks and are depleted in COPD patients, particularly those with low body weight [69]. Leucine has been highly effective at stimulating anabolic signaling in skeletal muscle [70].

Patients with COPD may benefit from dietary nitrate supplementation to help them overcome the exercise limitations associated with cardiopulmonary diseases [71]. In a 2021 systematic review of the effects of dietary nitrate supplementation on exercise capacity and cardiovascular parameters, Alsulayyim et al. concluded that nitrate supplementation increased exercise capacity and decreased blood pressure [71]. Additionally, Pavitt et al. concluded that dietary nitrate supplements increased exercise capacity and reduced blood pressure in COPD patients enrolled in a PR program [72].

Non-caloric supplements may also contain micronutrients. Vitamin B12 is critical, for example, because it is required for homocysteine, hematopoietic, and muscle metabolism [73].

Jonker et al. concluded from a study involving 23 COPD patients that amino acid supplementation improves whole-body protein gain compared to non-amino acid supplementation [74].

Vitamin D is essential supplementation for bone health, particularly for COPD patients predisposed to osteoporosis. Additionally, it prompts the development of antiviral and antimicrobial effector mechanisms and reduces inflammatory responses [75]. In a recent systematic review, Jolliffe et al. concluded that vitamin D supplementation might help reduce the risk and frequency of COPD exacerbations in patients with COPD [76].

Conclusion

In conclusion, malnutrition and COPD share high correlative conditions. Malnutrition and COPD have a bidirectional link that presents several implications on both sides. Malnutrition may be seen as a cause and result of COPD, while COPD patients may potentially have their conditions aggravated by malnutrition or its symptoms worsen through malnutrition. Potential biological and physical explanation exists but the focus is on the results of Malnutrition in COPD. Stable conditioning and management of COPD are necessary to improve quality of life and overall physical capabilities. Dietary advice and oral nutritional supplement intake are proper responses to managing malnutrition and preventing the potential further progression of COPD

Key Points

- COPD is a serious global health concern that must be addressed appropriately through medical research and application, owing to the fact that it is the fourth leading cause of death in the world, and it is on track to be the third leading cause.
- COPD, even though it is treatable and common, persists and has the potential to cause long-term health problems, further agitation can result in onset of severe and potentially fatal symptoms; therefore, proper management and preventive measures should be implemented in order tackle COPD progression.
- COPD has a negative impact on one's quality of life, physical abilities, and, more frequently, mental abilities. Such circumstances will result in an unfavorable situation that will have a progressive negative impact on the patient's health.
- The relationship between malnutrition and COPD is extremely strong. Malnutrition has a significant impact on the progression and overall health of COPD patients, and COPD itself can cause malnutrition. A number of additional connections were discovered. Maintaining a stable COPD patient's body in order to achieve a properly nourished body has been shown to significantly improve the condition of the COPD patient.
- The use of proper dietary advice and supplements is critical in the treatment and prevention of malnutrition and COPD. Additional routines and actions may also be implemented to improve the body's condition and biological processes.

References

[1] Vogelmeier CF, Criner GJ, Martinez FJ, Anzueto A, Barnes PJ, Bourbeau J, et al. *Global Strategy for the Diagnosis, Management and Prevention of Chronic Obstructive Lung Disease: 2020 Report.* 2020:1-141.

[2] Alqahtani JS, Njoku CM, Bereznicki B, Wimmer BC, Peterson GM, Kinsman L, et al. Risk factors for all-cause hospital readmission following exacerbation of COPD: a systematic review and meta-analysis. *European Respiratory Review.* 2020;29(156).

[3] Alqahtani JS, Aldabayan YS, Aldhahir AM, Al Rajeh AM, Mandal S, Hurst JR. Predictors of 30-and 90-day COPD exacerbation readmission: a prospective cohort study. *International Journal of Chronic Obstructive Pulmonary Disease.* 2021;16:2769.

[4] Mathers CD, Loncar D. Projections of global mortality and burden of disease from 2002 to 2030. *PLoS Med.* 2006;3(11):2011-30.

[5] Marin JM, Soriano JB, Carrizo SJ, Boldova A, Celli BR. Outcomes in patients with chronic obstructive pulmonary disease and obstructive sleep apnea: the overlap syndrome. *Am J Respir Crit Care Med.* 2010;182(3):325-31.

[6] Quaderi SA, Hurst JR. The unmet global burden of COPD. *Global Health, Epidemiology and Genomics.* 2018;3:e4-e.

[7] Alqahtani JS, Oyelade T, Aldhahir AM, Mendes RG, Alghamdi SM, Miravitlles M, et al. *Reduction in COPD Exacerbations during COVID-19: A Systematic Review and Meta-Analysis.* medRxiv. 2021.

[8] Raad S, Smith C, Allen K. Nutrition Status and Chronic Obstructive Pulmonary Disease: Can We Move Beyond the Body Mass Index? *Nutr Clin Pract.* 2019;34(3):330-9.

[9] Matkovic Z, Cvetko D, Rahelic D, Esquinas C, Zarak M, Miravitlles M, et al. Nutritional Status of Patients with Chronic Obstructive Pulmonary Disease in Relation to their Physical Performance. *Copd.* 2017;14(6):626-34.

[10] Munhoz da Rocha Lemos Costa T, Costa FM, Jonasson TH, Moreira CA, Boguszewski CL, Borba VZC. Body composition and sarcopenia in patients with chronic obstructive pulmonary disease. *Endocrine.* 2018;60(1):95-102.

[11] Collins PF, Yang IA, Chang Y-C, Vaughan A. Nutritional support in chronic obstructive pulmonary disease (COPD): an evidence update. *J Thorac Dis.* 2019;11(Suppl 17):S2230-S7.

[12] Ezzell L, Jensen GL. Malnutrition in chronic obstructive pulmonary disease. *Am J Clin Nutr.* 2000;72(6):1415-6.

[13] Alqahtani JS, Alghamdi SM, Aldhahir AM, Althobiani M, Oyelade T. Key toolkits of non-pharmacological management in COPD: during and beyond COVID-19. *Front Biosci* (Landmark Ed). 2021;26(7):246-52.

[14] Aldhahir AM, Rajeh AMA, Aldabayan YS, Drammeh S, Subbu V, Alqahtani JS, et al. Nutritional supplementation during pulmonary rehabilitation in COPD: A systematic review. *Chron Respir Dis.* 2020;17:1479973120904953-.

[15] Cederholm T, Barazzoni R, Austin P, Ballmer P, Biolo G, Bischoff SC, et al. ESPEN guidelines on definitions and terminology of clinical nutrition. *Clinical Nutrition.* 2017;36(1):49-64.

[16] Organization WH. *Malnutrition.* 2022.

[17] Stratton RJ. *Disease-related Malnutrition: An Evidence-Based Approach to Treatmen.* Rebecca J. Stratton, Ceri J. Green and Marinos Elia. Green CJ, Elia M, editors. Wallingford: Wallingford: CABI; 2003.

[18] Ezzell L, Jensen GL. Malnutrition in chronic obstructive pulmonary disease. *The American Journal of Clinical Nutrition.* 2000;72(6):1415-6.

[19] de Blasio F, Dassetto D, Ambrosanio R, Riberi L, Rella AM, Bucca C. Impact of Sarcopenia and Malnutrition on disease severity, nutritional variables and inflammatory parameters in COPD patients. *European Respiratory Journal.* 2019;54(suppl 63):PA4310.

[20] Sun Y, Milne S, Jaw JE, Yang CX, Xu F, Li X, et al. BMI is associated with FEV1 decline in chronic obstructive pulmonary disease: a meta-analysis of clinical trials. *Respiratory Research.* 2019;20(1):236.

[21] Marco E, Sánchez-Rodríguez D, Dávalos-Yerovi VN, Duran X, Pascual EM, Muniesa JM, et al. Malnutrition according to ESPEN consensus predicts hospitalizations and long-term mortality in

rehabilitation patients with stable chronic obstructive pulmonary disease. *Clinical Nutrition.* 2019;38 (5):2180-6.

[22] Goates S, Du K, Braunschweig CA, Arensberg MB. Economic Burden of Disease-Associated Malnutrition at the State Level. *PLOS ONE.* 2016;11(9):e0161833.

[23] Liz Anderson, Jo Banner, Beverley Bostock, Michaela Bowden, Peter Collins, Anne Holdoway, et al. *Managing Malnutrition in COPD. Malnutrition Pathway;* 2019. Contract No.: 2.

[24] Schols AM, Ferreira IM, Franssen FM, Gosker HR, Janssens W, Muscaritoli M, et al. Nutritional assessment and therapy in COPD: a European Respiratory Society statement. *Eur Respir J.* 2014; 44(6):1504-20.

[25] Steer J, Norman E, Gibson GJ, Bourke SC. P117 Comparison of indices of nutritional status in prediction of in-hospital mortality and early readmission of patients with acute exacerbations of COPD. *Thorax.* 2010;65(Suppl 4):A127-A.

[26] Ng MGS, Kon SSC, Canavan JL, Clark AL, Nolan CM, Jones SE, et al. Prevalence and effects of malnutrition in COPD patients referred for pulmonary rehabilitation. *European Respiratory Journal.* 2013;42(Suppl 57):P5107.

[27] Collins PF, Stratton RJ, Kurukulaaratchy R, Warwick H, Cawood AL, Elia M. Prevalence of malnutrition in outpatients with chronic obstructive pulmonary disease. *Proceedings of the Nutrition Society.* 2010;69(OCE2):E147.

[28] de Godoy I, Donahoe M, Calhoun WJ, Mancino J, Rogers RM. Elevated TNF-alpha production by peripheral blood monocytes of weight-losing COPD patients. *Am J Respir Crit Care Med.* 1996;153(2): 633-7.

[29] Gan WQ, Man SF, Senthilselvan A, Sin DD. Association between chronic obstructive pulmonary disease and systemic inflammation: a systematic review and a meta-analysis. *Thorax.* 2004;59(7):574-80.

[30] Di Francia M, Barbier D, Mege JL, Orehek J. Tumor necrosis factor-alpha levels and weight loss in chronic obstructive pulmonary disease. *Am J Respir Crit Care Med.* 1994;150(5 Pt 1):1453-5.

[31] Gorek Dilektasli A, Ulubay G, Bayraktar N, Eminsoy I, Oner Eyuboglu F. The effects of cachexia and related components on pulmonary functions in patients with COPD. *Tuberk Toraks.* 2009;57(3):298-305.

[32] Koehler F, Doehner W, Hoernig S, Witt C, Anker SD, John M. Anorexia in chronic obstructive pulmonary disease--association to cachexia and hormonal derangement. *Int J Cardiol.* 2007;119(1):83-9.

[33] Schols AM, Fredrix EW, Soeters PB, Westerterp KR, Wouters EF. Resting energy expenditure in patients with chronic obstructive pulmonary disease. *Am J Clin Nutr.* 1991;54(6):983-7.

[34] Wilson DO, Donahoe M, Rogers RM, Pennock BE. Metabolic rate and weight loss in chronic obstructive lung disease. *JPEN J Parenter Enteral Nutr.* 1990;14(1):7-11.

[35] Gosker HR, Wouters EF, van der Vusse GJ, Schols AM. Skeletal muscle dysfunction in chronic obstructive pulmonary disease and chronic heart failure: underlying mechanisms and therapy perspectives. *The American Journal of Clinical Nutrition.* 2000;71(5):1033-47.

[36] Collins PF, Elia M, Smith TR, Kurukulaaratchy R, Cawood AL, Stratton RJ. The impact of malnutrition on hospitalisation and mortality in outpatients with chronic obstructive pulmonary disease. *Proceedings of the Nutrition Society.* 2010;69(OCE2):E148.

[37] Collins PF, Stratton RJ, Elia M. An economic analysis of the costs associated with weight status in chronic obstructive pulmonary disease (COPD). *Proceedings of the Nutrition Society.* 2012;70(OCE5): E324.

[38] Marti S, Muñoz X, Rios J, Morell F, Ferrer J. Body weight and comorbidity predict mortality in COPD patients treated with oxygen therapy. *European Respiratory Journal.* 2006;27(4):689.

[39] Park HJ, Cho JH, Kim HJ, Park JY, Lee HS, Byun MK. The effect of low body mass index on the development of chronic obstructive pulmonary disease and mortality. *Journal of Internal Medicine.* 2019;286(5):573-82.

[40] Slinde F, Grönberg A, Engström C-P, Rossander-Hulthén L, Larsson S. Body composition by bioelectrical impedance predicts mortality in chronic obstructive pulmonary disease patients. *Respiratory Medicine.* 2005;99(8):1004-9.

[41] Hopkinson NS, Tennant RC, Dayer MJ, Swallow EB, Hansel TT, Moxham J, et al. A prospective study of decline in fat free mass and skeletal muscle strength in chronic obstructive pulmonary disease. *Respiratory Research.* 2007;8(1):25.

[42] Rutten EPA, Spruit MA, McDonald M-LN, Rennard S, Agusti A, Celli B, et al. Continuous fat-free mass decline in COPD: fact or fiction? *European Respiratory Journal.* 2015;46(5):1496.

[43] Schols AMWJ, Soeters PB, Dingemans AMC, Mostert R, Frantzen PJ, Wouters EFM. Prevalence and Characteristics of Nutritional Depletion in Patients with Stable COPD Eligible for Pulmonary Rehabilitation. *American Review of Respiratory Disease.* 1993;147(5):1151-6.

[44] Mostert R, Goris A, Weling-Scheepers C, Wouters EFM, Schols AMWJ. Tissue depletion and health related quality of life in patients with chronic obstructive pulmonary disease. *Respiratory Medicine.* 2000;94(9):859-67.

[45] Nici L, Donner C, Wouters E, Zuwallack R, Ambrosino N, Bourbeau J, et al. American thoracic society/European respiratory society statement on pulmonary rehabilitation. *American Journal of Respiratory and Critical Care Medicine.* 2006;173(12):1390-413.

[46] VanItallie TB, Yang MU, Heymsfield SB, Funk RC, Boileau RA. Height-normalized indices of the body's fat-free mass and fat mass: potentially useful indicators of nutritional status. *Am J Clin Nutr.* 1990;52(6):953-9.

[47] Luo Y, Zhou L, Li Y, Guo S, Li X, Zheng J, et al. Fat-Free Mass Index for Evaluating the Nutritional Status and Disease Severity in COPD. *Respiratory Care.* 2016;61(5):680.

[48] Vestbo J, Prescott E, Almdal T, Dahl M, Nordestgaard BG, Andersen T, et al. Body Mass, Fat-Free Body Mass, and Prognosis in Patients with Chronic Obstructive Pulmonary Disease from a Random Population Sample. *American Journal of Respiratory and Critical Care Medicine.* 2006;173(1):79-83.

[49] Hafner T, Sarc I, Groselj A, Zdolsek Z, Zupanc B, Kosten T. Low FFMI in COPD patients undergoing pulmonary rehabilitation. *European Respiratory Journal.* 2018;52(suppl 62):PA4125.

[50] Norman K, Pirlich M, Smoliner C, Kilbert A, Schulzke JD, Ockenga J, et al. Cost-effectiveness of a 3-month intervention with oral nutritional supplements in disease-related malnutrition: a randomised controlled pilot study. *European Journal of Clinical Nutrition.* 2011;65(6):735-42.

[51] Elia M, Normand C, Laviano A, Norman K. A systematic review of the cost and cost effectiveness of using standard oral nutritional supplements in community and care home settings. *Clinical Nutrition* (Edinburgh, Scotland). 2016;35(1):125-37.

[52] Cederholm T, Jensen GL, Correia M, Gonzalez MC, Fukushima R, Higashiguchi T, et al. GLIM criteria for the diagnosis of malnutrition - A consensus report from the global clinical nutrition community. *Clinical Nutrition* (Edinburgh, Scotland). 2019;38(1):1-9.

[53] Vellas B, Villars H, Abellan G, Soto M, Rolland Y, Guigoz Y, et al. Overview of the MNA®-Its history and challenges. *Journal of Nutrition Health and Aging.* 2006;10(6):456.

[54] Montesanto A, D'Aquila P, Rossano V, Passarino G, Bellizzi D. Mini Nutritional Assessment Scores Indicate Higher Risk for Prospective Mortality and Contrasting Correlation With Age-Related Epigenetic Biomarkers. *Frontiers in Endocrinology.* 2019;10.

[55] Kondrup J, Allison SP, Elia M, Vellas B, Plauth M. ESPEN guidelines for nutrition screening 2002. *Clinical Nutrition.* 2003;22(4):415-21.

[56] *Chronic Obstructive Pulmonary Disease in Over 16s: Diagnosis and Management NICE Guideline NG115.* The National Institute for Health and Care Excellence. 2018.

[57] Thomas B, Bishop J. *Manual of Dietetic Practice*: John Wiley & Sons; 2013.

[58] Baldwin C, de van der Schueren MAE, Kruizenga HM, Weekes CE. Dietary advice with or without oral nutritional supplements for disease-related malnutrition in adults. *Cochrane Database of Systematic Reviews.* 2021(12).

[59] Weekes CE, Emery PW, Elia M. Dietary counselling and food fortification in stable COPD: a randomised trial. *Thorax.* 2009;64(4):326-31.

[60] Nguyen HT, Pavey TG, Collins PF, Nguyen NV, Pham TD, Gallegos D. Effectiveness of Tailored Dietary Counseling in Treating Malnourished Outpatients with Chronic Obstructive Pulmonary Disease: A Randomized Controlled Trial. *Journal of the Academy of Nutrition and Dietetics.* 2020;120(5):778-91.e1.

[61] Schols A. Nutritional modulation as part of the integrated management of chronic obstructive pulmonary disease. *Proceedings of the Nutrition Society*. 2003;62(4):783-91.

[62] Efthimiou J, Fleming J, Gomes C, Spiro SG. The effect of supplementary oral nutrition in poorly nourished patients with chronic obstructive pulmonary disease. *American Review of Respiratory Disease*. 1988;137(5):1075-82.

[63] Hsieh M-J, Yang T-M, Tsai Y-H. Nutritional supplementation in patients with chronic obstructive pulmonary disease. *Journal of the Formosan Medical Association*. 2016;115(8):595-601.

[64] Ferreira IM, Brooks D, White J, Goldstein R. Nutritional supplementation for stable chronic obstructive pulmonary disease. *Cochrane Database Syst Rev*. 2012;12:1-73.

[65] Collins PF, Elia M, Stratton RJ. Nutritional support and functional capacity in chronic obstructive pulmonary disease: a systematic review and meta-analysis. *Respirology*. 2013;18(4):616-29.

[66] Ahnfeldt-Mollerup P, Hey H, Johansen C, Kristensen S, Brix Lindskov J, Jensahnfeldt-Mollerupen C. The effect of protein supplementation on quality of life, physical function, and muscle strength in patients with chronic obstructive pulmonary disease. *Eur J Phys Rehabil Med*. 2015;51(4):447-56.

[67] Naz I, Sahin H. The effect of nutritional support on pulmonary rehabilitation outcomes in COPD patients with low body mass index. *Eur Respiratory Soc;* 2018.

[68] Khan NA, Kumar N, Daga MK. Effect of Dietary Supplementation on Body Composition, Pulmonary Function and Health-Related Quality of Life in Patients with Stable COPD. *Tanaffos*. 2016; 15(4):225-35.

[69] Yoneda T, Yoshikawa M, Fu A, Tsukaguchi K, Okamoto Y, Takenaka H. Plasma levels of amino acids and hypermetabolism in patients with chronic obstructive pulmonary disease. *Nutrition*. 2001;17(2):95-9.

[70] Atherton PJ, Smith K, Etheridge T, Rankin D, Rennie MJ. Distinct anabolic signalling responses to amino acids in C2C12 skeletal muscle cells. *Amino Acids*. 2010;38(5):1533-9.

[71] Alsulayyim AS, Alasmari AM, Alghamdi SM, Polkey MI, Hopkinson NS. Impact of dietary nitrate supplementation on exercise capacity and cardiovascular parameters in chronic respiratory disease: a systematic review and meta-analysis. *BMJ Open Respiratory Research*. 2021;8(1):e000948.

[72] Pavitt MJ, Tanner RJ, Lewis A, Buttery S, Mehta B, Jefford H, et al. Oral nitrate supplementation to enhance pulmonary rehabilitation in COPD: ON-EPIC a multicentre, double-blind, placebo-controlled, randomised parallel group study. *Thorax*. 2020;75(7):547-55.

[73] Paulin FV, Zagatto AM, Chiappa GR, Muller PT. Addition of vitamin B12 to exercise training improves cycle ergometer endurance in advanced COPD patients: A randomized and controlled study. *Respiratory Medicine*. 2017;122:23-9.

[74] Jonker R, Deutz NE, Erbland ML, Anderson PJ, Engelen MP. Effectiveness of essential amino acid supplementation in stimulating whole body net protein anabolism is comparable between COPD patients and healthy older adults. *Metabolism*. 2017;69:120-9.

[75] Greiller CL, Martineau AR. Modulation of the immune response to respiratory viruses by vitamin D. *Nutrients*. 2015;7(6):4240-70.

[76] Jolliffe DA, Greenberg L, Hooper RL, Mathyssen C, Rafiq R, de Jongh RT, et al. Vitamin D to prevent exacerbations of COPD: systematic review and meta-analysis of individual participant data from randomised controlled trials. *Thorax*. 2019;74(4):337.

Chapter 13

Oxygen Therapy and Ventilatory Support Modalities in Stable COPD

Saad M. AlRabeeah*, PhD, RRT-SDS
Department of Respiratory Care,
Prince Sultan Military College of Health Sciences,
Dhahran, Kingdom of Saudi Arabia

Abstract

Chronic obstructive pulmonary disease (COPD) is a serious chronic pulmonary illness that has a considerable impact on quality of life, health care utilization, comorbidity, and mortality. Limitation of the expiratory airflow is the fundamental pathophysiological feature of COPD, which limits the respiratory system's ability to breathe appropriately. Various societies have created disease severity classifications in order to predict and manage COPD patients. Lung function, patient-reported symptoms and the frequency of exacerbations are all factors in current classification scheme. Global Initiative for Chronic Obstructive Lung Disease (GOLD) classifies airflow limitation according to predicted values of the forced expiratory volume (FEV_1 %) into four stages, ranging from mild (GOLD1) to very severe (GOLD4). Despite the severity of COPD category, COPD patients are considered stable when their symptoms are well-managed and lung deterioration is minimal. This chapter will discuss the recent approaches to oxygen therapy and ventilatory support for stable COPD patients.

Keywords: COPD, oxygen therapy, ventilatory support, oxygenation, work of breathing

Introduction

Chronic obstructive pulmonary disease (COPD) is a serious chronic disabling disease that has a substantial impact on quality of life, associated symptoms, comorbidities, health care utilization, and survival. Clinically, COPD is defined by the progressive onset of shortness of breath, cough, and phlegm production, as well as recurring incidents of severe deterioration of respiratory function known as COPD exacerbation. Tobacco usage is the leading cause of

* Corresponding Author's Email: saad.alrabeeah@psmchs.edu.sa.

In: Chronic Obstructive Pulmonary Disease
Editor: Jaber S. Alqahtani
ISBN: 979-8-88697-333-4

COPD. The primary pathophysiological characteristic of COPD is expiratory flow limitation, which decreases the respiratory system's capacity to breathe appropriately and effectively. Loss of lungs elastic recoil, inflammation and damaging of small airway walls, and mucus deposition in the small airways all contribute to the limitation of expiratory flow. Destruction of the lung parenchyma also limits the lung's capacity to engage in gas exchange. Chronic inflammation is the primary cause of COPD alterations [1].

Despite the fact that Global Initiative for Chronic Obstructive Lung Disease (GOLD) classifications of COPD severity facilitated the prediction and management of COPD patients, these classifications were based solely on objective lung function measurements. Clinicians observed that patients with comparable lung function abnormalities reported different degrees of perceived and functional limitations. The recent approaches to COPD patients' managements integrates lung function, patient-reported symptoms and the frequency of exacerbations which lead to individualize the treatment approaches in stable COPD patients [2]. In this chapter, oxygen therapy and ventilatory support modalities in stable COPD will be discussed.

Oxygen Therapy in Stable COPD

Gas exchange is impaired in COPD patients due to the progressive alveolar and airway damage. In COPD, impaired gas exchange can result in symptoms such as shortness of breath, coughing, and exhaustion. Moreover, it results in hypoxemia and hypercapnia.

COPD is commonly treated with oxygen therapy. The use of oxygen in stable COPD patients with occasional hypoxemia associated with physical activity has offered the necessary information in defining the role of oxygen in this population. Long-term oxygen treatment (LTOT) (> 15 Hrs. per day) administered at home has been shown to improve survival in patients with COPD and severe resting hypoxemia. Recent research has shown that LTOT does not improve outcomes for stable COPD patients with moderate desaturation at rest or during physical activity [3]. Oxygen treatment during physical activity and exercise has been demonstrated to reduce symptoms and maintain arterial oxygen saturation, but not to improve long-term outcomes. In COPD, oxygen therapy has numerous physiologic, functional, and biological impacts, not all of which are fully understood [3].

Oxygen Therapy in COPD Patients with Severe Hypoxemia

Early research demonstrated the benefits of LTOT for severe stable COPD PaO2 < 55 mm Hg. An earlier trail examined the use of oxygen therapy during the night (Nocturnal Oxygen Treatment Trial (NOTT) vs. continues oxygen therapy [4]. This study included 203 individuals with COPD and hypoxemia at rest. The subjects were randomly assigned to either continuous oxygen therapy or nocturnal oxygen therapy for 12 hours. At 12 months, pulmonary vascular pressures, cognitive function, and quality of life were also measured. The overall cohort had a mean survival of 19.3 months. At one year, mortality in the continuous oxygen therapy group was 11.9% and 20.6% in the nocturnal oxygen therapy group. At two years, the death rate in the continuous oxygen therapy group was 22.4 percent versus 40.8 percent in the nocturnal oxygen therapy group. At 12 months, the continuous oxygen therapy cohort experienced a higher reduction in pulmonary vascular resistance. Other outcome measures, such as FEV_1, lung volumes, gas exchange, and lung volumes, revealed no differences across groups. The finding of this study clearly supports the use of continuous oxygen therapy in stable severe COPD patients [4].

Another study involved 87 patients diagnosed with chronic emphysema or bronchitis who had significant hypoxemia at rest and carbon dioxide retention. FEV_1 and indications of high pulmonary artery pressures revealed that all individuals had irreversible air-flow blockage (cor pulmonale). Subjects were randomly assigned to either no additional oxygen (control group) or 2 L/min of nasal oxygen for at least 15 hours per day. After 5 years, the mortality rate in the control group was 67% (30 of 45) and 45 percent (19 of 42) in the oxygen therapy group. Elevated hematocrit and baseline PaCO2 were linked to mortality. Furthermore, participants in the oxygen therapy group deteriorated at a slower rate in terms of pulmonary vascular pressures and gas exchange [5]. These two landmark trails demonstrated the benefits of LTOT in patient with severe stable COPD patient. LTOT improved survival and reduced pulmonary vasculature resistance in this patient group. Therefore, early initiation of LTOT is crucial in patient with severe stable COPD patient [6].

Oxygen Therapy in COPD Patients with Moderate Hypoxemia

Moderate hypoxemia in COPD patients is defined at PaO2 57 to 68 mmHg [6]. Two landmark trials were unable to demonstrate that LTOT improves mortality in COPD patients with moderate hypoxemia. In each of these studies, participants with PaO2 > 56 mmHg were administered oxygen for a mean of 13 hours per day, whereas the control group did not receive oxygen. Subjects were tracked for three to seven years, and findings did not support LTOT in in this patient group [7, 8]. Long Term Oxygen Treatment Trial (LOTT) conducted in 2016 to assess the benefits of oxygen therapy in this patient group. The LOTT 738 participants were enrolled in the oxygen and control groups from 42 sites. There were no differences between the oxygen and control groups in terms of time to death, first hospitalization, hospitalization rates, or COPD exacerbations. In addition, there were no variations in the 6-minute walk distance, lung function, or health-related quality of life. In participants with moderate stable COPD and resting or exercise-induced oxygen desaturation, the authors concluded that LTOT did not produce a mortality benefit or significant benefits for other outcomes [6].

Although the current literature does not provide strong evidence for the use of LTOT in COPD patients with moderate hypoxemia, prescribing LTOT should be based on individual patient evaluation of lung function, patient-reported symptoms, exercise tolerance and the frequency of exacerbations.

LTOT Oxygen Delivery Systems

Oxygen Cylinders

Oxygen cylinders are the initial source of oxygen provision in residential settings. Cylinders can deliver a constant flow or be connected with demand regulators to extend the length of operation and enhance its efficacy. However, the short length of operation, weight, handling, and difficulties involved with replacing cylinders make this the least desirable alternative for home therapy. In some circumstances, small cylinders are still employed for ambulation or as backup devices [9].

Liquid Oxygen

Liquid oxygen is easier to store, carry, and fill than regular oxygen cylinders. One liter of liquid oxygen expands to produce almost 850 liters of gaseous oxygen, enabling liquid systems to operate for longer periods of time. Filling portable devices with liquids from stationary systems can facilitate patient mobility. Also capable of high flow rates, liquid systems are the ideal solution for people with increased oxygen requirements. Currently, the expense of liquid systems limits their use in home care. Portable liquid systems let patients spend more time away from home, but they cannot be utilized for air travel [9].

Oxygen Concentrators

Oxygen concentrators are the most prevalent home oxygen therapy device. These devices can offer a broad range of oxygen flows (1–10 L/min) with up to 95% oxygen concentration. Current stationary concentrators weigh up to 35 pounds and operate more effectively than their predecessors. This includes reduced energy consumption, quieter operation, and cheaper ownership expenses [7]. Typically, stationary oxygen concentrators permit a connecting tubing of up to 100 feet in length, allowing the patient mobility in the home [9].

Portable Oxygen concentrators are also another delivery system that can be used for home stationary unit and for ambulation. Major disadvantages of portable oxygen concentrator are limited battery duration and may not meet patient flow demand as the oxygen flow is only 0.5 to 3 LPM. Table 1 summarizes the advantages and disadvantages of LTOT delivery systems.

Table 1. Advantages and disadvantages of LTOT delivery systems

Oxygen delivery system	Advantages	Disadvantages
Oxygen cylinders	• Easy to use • Cost effective • Provide 5 to 10 LPM	• Limited duration • Not convenient for ambulation • Handling and storage
Portable oxygen concentrator	• Easy to use • Cost effective • Convenient for ambulation.	• Limited battery • May not patient flow demand • Require regular maintenance
Stationary oxygen concentrator	• Easy to use • Cost effective • Provide 5 to 10 LPM	• Not convenient for ambulation • Heavy • Require regular maintenance

Summary

- Clinically, COPD is defined by the progressive onset of shortness of breath, cough, and phlegm production. Tobacco usage is the leading cause of COPD.
- Oxygen treatment during physical activity and exercise has been demonstrated to reduce symptoms and maintain arterial oxygen saturation, but not to improve long-term outcomes.
- Early research demonstrated the benefits of LTOT for severe stable COPD $PaO2 < 55$ mm Hg.
- LTOT improved survival and reduced pulmonary vasculature resistance in severe stable COPD.

Ventilatory Support Modalities in Stable COPD

Ventilatory support for stable COPD is usually defined in a form of noninvasive respiratory support that include continuous positive airway pressure (CPAP), high flow nasal Cannula (HFNC) and non-invasive positive pressure ventilation (NIPPV). A recent online survey of physicians engaged in the provision of Home-NIV found that the primary benefits of NIV for COPD patients include a reduction in hospital admissions, an improvement in quality of life, and the relief of dyspnea [10]. However, there is a substantial international variation in the rate of NIV prescription for COPD patients. The indication for Home-NIV in the subgroups of COPD patients with stable chronic hypercapnic COPD has been a controversial topic over the last two decades [10].

Due to airflow limitation, the time provided for expiration in patients with (COPD) may be insufficient to allow the system to return to resting end-expiratory lung volume leading to hyperinflation. The residual inward elastic recoil causes a positive alveolar pressure at the end of expiration, described as intrinsic end expiratory pressure (intrinsic PEEP or PEEPi) [11]. The respiratory muscles must generate a negative pressure equal in magnitude to PEEPi in order to commence inspiratory airflow. Therefore, intrinsic PEEP has been described as an inspiratory threshold load on the inspiratory muscles, which increases the strain of breathing. The existence of PEEPi is also indicative of dynamic hyperinflation, with a deterioration of thoracic wall geometry and muscle tension leading to increase burden on the respiratory muscle [12]. During invasive or non-invasive ventilation, patients with COPD have been found to have intrinsic PEEPi [13].

Continuous Positive Airway Pressure (CPAP)

The benefits of CPAP in people with stable COPD may be explained by improving airflow limitation, thus a reduction in lung hyperinflation. CPAP can reduce the inspiratory load at any given volume, hence decreasing the increasing workload and enhancing lung mechanics. Some investigators suggested that a PEEP/CPAP of 5–10 cm H2O could reduce airway resistance (Raw), particularly at the end of expiration, leading to improved resting end-expiratory lung volumes [14, 15].

Lopes, Agnaldo J., et al. investigated the effect and duration of impact of CPAP on hyperinflation and Raw in patients with stable COPD and concluded that in patients with severe stable COPD, CPAP at 8 Cm H2O lowers lung volumes and Raw, and the effects extend for 15–30 minutes following CPAP [16].

Obstructive sleep apnea (OSA) is prevalent in the general population and frequently coexists with COPD (overlap OSA/ COPD) [17]. Machado, MC L., et al. in their prospective cohort study looked at how OSA treatment with CPAP affected the survival of hypoxemic COPD patients. They found that CPAP treatment was associated with increased survival in patients with moderate-to-severe OSAS with hypoxemic COPD [18].

High Flow Nasal Cannula

In a variety of clinical settings, high-flow nasal cannula (HFNC) is gaining popularity as an alternate noninvasive respiratory support method. HFNC systems provide a heated and humidified combination of air and oxygen at flow rates of up to 60 L/min, increasing patient tolerability and improving gas exchange in comparison to standard oxygenation devices [19]. The improvement in gas exchange has shown to improve of quality of life and reduce mortality.

HFNC does not offer active help for inspiration. HFNC increased tidal volume (VT) and decreased respiratory rate (RR) and minute ventilation in COPD patients compared to spontaneous breathing. HFNC also enhances the exercise capacity of COPD patients in stable condition in short term effect [20]. The long-term benefits of HFNC use in stable COPD is still not clear [21].

Non-Invasive Positive Pressure Ventilation (NIPPV)

The use of NIPPV is mostly applied on patient with chronic hypercapnic respiratory failure COPD subgroup [12, 23]. The aim is to support the inspiratory muscles leading to reduction to the overall respiratory workload. Inspiratory Positive Airway Pressures (IPAP) settings determine the benefits from the application of NIPPV. Earlier studies used IPAP from 12-14 cm H2O and results indicated no significant benefits from the use NIPPV in sever stable COPD patients [22, 23]. Recent studies showed that the use of higher IPAP setting 20- 24 cm H2O is associated with better results in terms of exercise tolerance and lung function [24, 25]. In the other hand, the use of the NIPPV is mostly indicated to liberate COPD patients from mechanical ventilation or avoid intubation, which is beyond the scope of this chapter.

Conclusion

The recent approaches to COPD patients' managements integrates lung function, patient-reported symptoms and the frequency of exacerbations which lead to individualize the treatment approaches in stable COPD patients. Long-term oxygen treatment (LTOT) (> 15 Hrs. per day) administered at home has been shown to improve survival in patients with COPD and severe resting hypoxemia. Oxygen treatment during physical activity and exercise has been demonstrated to reduce symptoms and maintain arterial oxygen saturation, but not to improve long-term outcomes. The primary benefits of home NIV for COPD patients include a reduction in hospital admissions, an improvement in quality of life, and the relief of dyspnea.

Key Points

- Ventilatory support for stable COPD is usually defined in a form of noninvasive respiratory support that include CPAP, HFNC and NIPPV.
- There is substantial international variation in the rate of NIV prescription for COPD patients.
- The indication for Home-NIV in the subgroup of COPD patients with stable chronic hypercapnic COPD has been a controversial topic over the last two decades.
- Some investigators suggested that a PEEP/CPAP of 5–10 cm H2O could reduce airway resistance (Raw), particularly at the end of expiration, leading to improved resting end-expiratory lung volumes.
- HFNC systems provide a heated and humidified combination of air and oxygen at flow rates of up to 60 L/min, increasing patient tolerability and improving gas exchange in comparison to standard oxygenation devices.
- HFNC enhances the exercise capacity of COPD patients in stable condition in short term effect.
- The use of NIPPV is mostly applied on patient with chronic hypercapnic respiratory failure.
- The aim is to support the inspiratory muscles leading to reduction on the overall respiratory workload.
- Inspiratory Positive Airway Pressures (IPAP) settings determine the benefits of the application of NIPPV.

References

[1] López-Campos, José Luis, Juan José Soler-Cataluña, and Marc Miravitlles. "Global strategy for the diagnosis, management, and prevention of chronic obstructive lung disease 2019 report: future challenges."*Archivos de bronconeumologia* 56.2 (2020): 65-67.

[2] Agrawal, R., Moghtader, S., Ayyala, U., Bandi, V., & Sharafkhaneh, A. (2019)."Update on management of stable chronic obstructive pulmonary disease." *Journal of Thoracic Disease* 11.Suppl 14 (2019): S1800.

[3] Yusen, R. D., Criner, G. J., Sternberg, A. L., Au, D. H., Fuhlbrigge, A. L., Albert, R. K., Casaburi, R., Stoller, J. K., Harrington, K. F., Cooper, J. A. D., Diaz, P., Gay, S., Kanner, R., MacIntyre, N., Martinez, F. J., Piantadosi, S., Sciurba, F., Shade, D., Stibolt, T., … Weiss, K. (2018)."The long-term oxygen treatment trial for chronic obstructive pulmonary disease: rationale, design, and lessons learned."*Annals of the American Thoracic Society* 15.1 (2018): 89-101.

[4] Nocturnal Oxygen Therapy Trial Group. "Continuous or nocturnal oxygen therapy in hypoxemic chronic obstructive lung disease: a clinical trial." *Annals of Internal Medicine* 93.3 (1980): 391-398.

[5] Report of the Medical Research Council Working Party. Long term domiciliary oxygen therapy in chronic hypoxic cor pulmonale complicating chronic bronchitis and emphysema. *Lancet* 1981; 1(8222):681-686.

[6] Long-Term Oxygen Treatment Trial Research Group. "A randomized trial of long-term oxygen for COPD with moderate desaturation." *New England Journal of Medicine* 375.17 (2016): 1617-1627.

[7] Chaouat, A., Weitzenblum, E., Kessler, R., Charpentier, C., Ehrhart, M., Schott, R., Levi-Valensi, P., Zielinski, J., delaunois, L., Cornudella, R., & Moutinho dos Santos, J. (1999). "A randomized trial of nocturnal oxygen therapy in chronic obstructive pulmonary disease patients." *European Respiratory Journal* 14.5 (1999): 1002-1008.

[8] Gorecka, D., Gorzelak, K., Sliwinski, P., Tobiasz, M., & Zielinski, J. (1997). "Effect of long-term oxygen therapy on survival in patients with chronic obstructive pulmonary disease with moderate hypoxaemia." *Thorax* 52.8 (1997): 674-679.

[9] McCoy, Robert W. "Options for home oxygen therapy equipment: storage and metering of oxygen in the home." *Respiratory Care* 58.1 (2013): 65-85.

[10] Crimi, C., Noto, A., Princi, P., Cuvelier, A., Masa, J. F., Simonds, A., Elliott, M. W., Wijkstra, P., Windisch, W., & Nava, S. (2016). "Domiciliary non-invasive ventilation in COPD: an international survey of indications and practices." *COPD: Journal of Chronic Obstructive Pulmonary Disease* 13.4 (2016): 483-490.

[11] Pepe, Paul E., and John J. Marini. "Occult positive end-expiratory pressure in mechanically ventilated patients with airflow obstruction: the auto-PEEP effect." *American Review of Respiratory Disease* 126.1 (1982): 166-170.

[12] O'Donoghue, F. J., "Effect of CPAP on intrinsic PEEP, inspiratory effort, and lung volume in severe stable COPD." *Thorax* 57.6 (2002): 533-539.

[13] Smith T C, Marini J J. Impact of PEEP on lung mechanics and work of breathing in severe airflow obstruction. *J. Appl. Physiol.* 1988;65:1488–99.

[14] Kondili E, Alexopoulou C, Prinianakis G, Xirouchaki N, Georgopoulos D. Pattern of lung emptying and expiratory resistance in mechanically ventilated patients with chronic obstructive pulmonary disease. *Intensive Care Med* 2004;30(7):1311–1318.

[15] Kaczka D W, Ingenito E P, Body SC, Duffy S E, Mentzer SJ, DeCamp M M, et al. Inspiratory lung impedance in COPD: effects of PEEP and immediate impact of lung volume reduction surgery. *J. Appl. Physiol.* 2001;90(5):1833–1841.

[16] Lopes, A. J., Nery, F. P., Sousa, F. C., Guimaraes, F. S., Dias, C. M., Oliveira, J. F., & Menezes, S. L. (2011). CPAP decreases lung hyperinflation in patients with stable COPD." *Respiratory Care* 56.8 (2011): 1164-1169.

[17] Weitzenblum E, Chaouat A. Sleep and chronic obstructive pulmonary disease. *Sleep Med. Rev.* 2004; 8: 281–294.

[18] Machado, M.-C. L., Vollmer, W. M., Togeiro, S. M., Bilderback, A. L., Oliveira, M.-V. C., Leitao, F. S., Queiroga, F., Lorenzi-Filho, G., & Krishnan, J. A. (2010). "CPAP and survival in moderate-to-severe obstructive sleep apnoea syndrome and hypoxaemic COPD." *European Respiratory Journal* 35.1 (2010): 132-137.

[19] Papazian, L., Corley, A., Hess, D., Fraser, J. F., Frat, J.-P., Guitton, C., Jaber, S., Maggiore, S. M., Nava, S., Rello, J., Ricard, J.-D., Stephan, F., Trisolini, R., & Azoulay, E. (2016). Use of high-flow nasal cannula oxygenation in ICU adults: a narrative review. *Intensive Care Med.* 2016; 42:1336–1349.

[20] Chatila W, Nugent T, Vance G, Gaughan J, Criner G J. The effects of high-flow vs low-flow oxygen on exercise in advanced obstructive airways disease. *Chest* 2004; 126:1108–1115.

[21] Pisani, Lara, and Maria Laura Vega. "Use of nasal high flow in stable COPD: rationale and physiology." *COPD: Journal of Chronic Obstructive Pulmonary Disease* 14.3 (2017): 346-350.

[22] Casanova, C., Celli, B. R., Tost, L., Soriano, E., Abreu, J., Velasco, V., & Santolaria, F. (2000). Long-term controlled trial of nocturnal nasal positive pressure ventilation in patients with severe COPD. *Chest*. 2000;118(6):1582–1590.

[23] Clini, E. c. Sturani, a. Rossi, s. Viaggi, a. Corrado, C. F. Donner, n. Ambrosino; Rehabilitation and Chronic Care Study Group, Italian Association of Hospital Pulmonologists (AIPO). The Italian multicentre study on noninvasive ventilation in chronic obstructive pulmonary disease patients. *Eur. Respir. J.* 2002;20(3): 529–538.

[24] Murphy P B, Rehal S, Arbane G, et al. Effect of home noninvasive ventilation with oxygen therapy vs oxygen therapy alone on hospital readmission or death after an acute COPD exacerbation: a randomized clinical trial. *JAMA*. 2017;317(21):2177–2186.

[25] Köhnlein T, Windisch W, Köhler D, Anna Suling. Non-invasive positive pressure ventilation for the treatment of severe stable chronic obstructive monary disease: a prospective, multicentre, randomised, controlled clinical trial. *Lancet Respir. Med*. 2014;2(9):698–705.

Chapter 14

Interventional Therapy in Stable COPD

Mihir R. Gangakhedkar[1], MD, DM
and Lokesh Kumar Saini[2,*], MD
[1]Employees State Insurance Scheme Hospital,
Vashi, Mumbai, Maharashtra, India
[2]Department of Pulmonary Medicine,
All India Institute of Medical Sciences,
Rishikesh, Uttarakhand, India

Abstract

Chronic obstructive pulmonary disease (COPD) patients face a severe challenge regarding their quality of life. Pharmacotherapy, rehabilitation, and smoking cessation form important pillars of controlling the disease. But at times, despite these efforts, the patients are not optimized to lead a comfortable, independent life. Interventions, in the form of bronchoscopic and surgical procedures to change the course of the disease, come into the picture at this point. Bronchoscopic interventions include various methods to reduce the lung volume like valves, coils, and vapor ablation. Surgical procedures range from a bullectomy to the ultimate step of lung transplantation. While surgical procedures have inherent perioperative morbidity and mortality risks, bronchoscopic procedures also carry the risks of infection, pneumothoraces, and procedural failures. The cost of these interventions is another vital dimension of the decision-making process of management. Thereby, choosing the appropriate intervention for a patient and for a budding interventionalist, choosing the appropriate patient for intervention, are key to successful management. This chapter attempts to provide evidence-based answers to basic questions like what the options for intervention are, when one should intervene and what are the challenges before and after such an intervention in a patient with stable COPD.

Keywords: bronchoscopic lung volume reduction (BLVR), bullectomy, lung transplantation, lung volume reduction surgery (LVRS), bronchoscopic valves

Introduction

The routine management of a patient with Chronic obstructive pulmonary disease (COPD) predominantly involves medical management using bronchodilators (inhaled and oral),

---

* Corresponding Author's Email address: drlssaini@gmail.com.

In: Chronic Obstructive Pulmonary Disease
Editor: Jaber S. Alqahtani
ISBN: 979-8-88697-333-4

pulmonary rehabilitation, smoking cessation, regular vaccination, adequate nutrition and as per need oxygen and non-invasive ventilation. However, the progression of the disease despite these measures or the poor existential quality of life, at times pushes patients and their physicians to explore alternative therapies.

Interventional therapy is based on understanding simple core concepts of COPD pathophysiology. COPD being a persistent disease, a patient is likely to benefit the most with either replacement, reduction or circumvention of the diseased tissue. Replacement is essentially lung transplantation, which can be accompanied by a heart transplant. Advanced COPD remains the commonest indication for transplantation. Reduction of diseased tissue can be achieved either by surgical removal or bronchoscopic lung volume reduction (BLVR) techniques, where the diseased lung volume objectively reduces post-intervention. Circumvention is essentially the use of bypass stents or valves where the airflow is directed in a manner to alter the course of the pathophysiology. The principle, however, remains the same, reducing hyperinflation and residual volume. This in turn helps reduce the metabolic cost of breathing for the patients and cascades further into improved exercise capacity, and with continued supportive management, leads to an improved quality of life. The following chapter attempts to provide a succinct summary of such interventions and reviews the evidence available for and against the same.

Screening Patients for Intervention

Screening COPD patients for further interventional therapy requires a physician to see specific signs in radiology or assess the patient's pathology accurately on pulmonary functions. As far as intervention is concerned, hyperinflated or air-trapped lungs are the predominant targets. This can be clinically estimated by surface landmarks of the lung, which will change if hyperinflated. A reduced cricosternal distance, full supraclavicular fossae, an increased subcostal angle, a prolonged forced expiratory time, a barrel chest and other characteristics may hint towards a hyperinflated lung. [1] On radiology, one may see the obvious increase in lung volume in terms of rib spaces, or one may see evident bullous disease. Additionally, one may see indirect signs in a flattened diaphragmatic contour, a tubular heart, *horizontalization* of rib spaces, pruning of peripheral vasculature or increased retrosternal space in a lateral film. [2] All of these clinical and radiological signs can further be ascertained on computed tomography (CT) imaging and pulmonary function testing. CT imaging can also provide a volumetric assessment of the lung, which may help when a patient cannot perform spirometry maneuvers. In the pulmonary function assessment, it is customary to label a lung function as hyperinflated when the total lung capacity (TLC) is more than 120% of the predicted value. [3] Similarly, one considers a lung to be air-trapped when the Residual Volume or Functional Residual Capacity is more than 120% of the predicted value. These parameters remain the cornerstones for choosing patients for interventional therapy in most trials, consensus statements and guidelines.

Interventional Therapy

Interventional therapy in stable COPD patients can broadly be classified as bronchoscopic and surgical interventions (Refer to Figure 1 for further details).

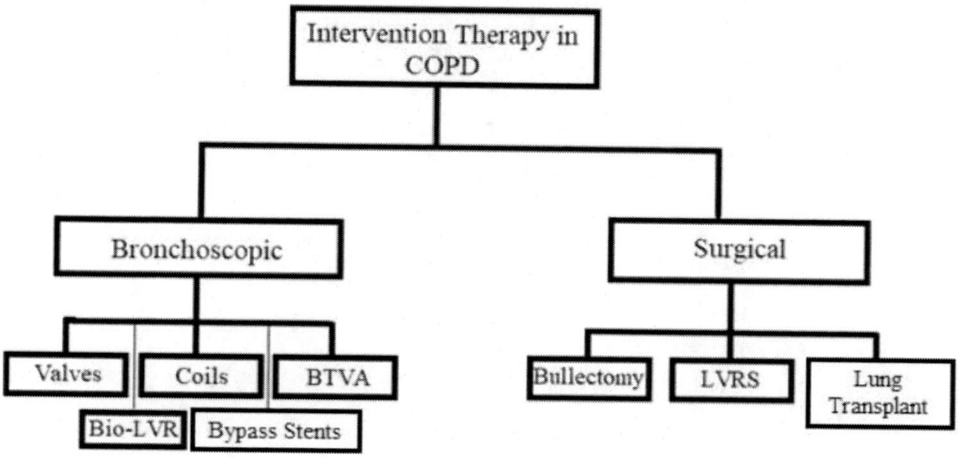

Figure 1. A simple classification of intervention therapy.
Definition of abbreviations: Bio-LVR: biologic lung volume reduction;
BTVA: bronchoscopic thermal vapor ablation; LVRS: lung volume reduction surgery.

Bronchoscopic Interventions

Historically, the strategy for BLVR was likely developed consequent to the known morbidity and mortality of surgical interventions. The bronchoscopic approach offers a lesser invasive alternative while simultaneously being a cost-effective intervention.

1. *Endobronchial Valves (EBV):*
   EBV therapy is based on the simple one-way valve system where the strategic location of these valves disallows air to enter the occluded segment but allows it to leave. [4] Thereby, there is *targeted lung volume reduction.*
   EBV is best catered to the patients having heterogenous emphysema. As the term suggests, these patients have significant areas of uninvolved lung tissue, which have separate feeding airways from the involved lung. The amount of heterogeneity has also been measured as a part of an index radiographically. Essentially, a patient with *homogenous* emphysema is more likely to benefit from another, less-targeted therapy. It is easily understood that if one puts in a one-way valve, the expectation is that the ingress of air can occur from that path alone. However, we now know that there are communications between segments beyond the regular airway. These pathways collectively form the *collateral ventilation* of the lung segments. Hence, it is best to assess the patient thoroughly for collateral ventilation before considering EBV therapy. Assessment of collateral ventilation can be done by a specialized system known as the *Chartis system,* which helps gauge the patient's eligibility. The *Chartis system* involves the introduction of a specialized assembly in which a balloon is inserted bronchoscopically in the segment of interest and inflated to occlude the segment altogether. The system then assesses the reduction in expiratory volumes of air dynamically, sensing the pressure and resistance. As can be expected, a persistent expiratory flow indicates collateral ventilation. [5]

Another indicator of collateral ventilation is the presence of discontinuous fissures on a high-resolution computed tomography (HRCT) of the thorax. The reported variation in CT fissures ranges from 17% up to 90%, with the minor fissure showing the most variation. [6, 7] However, the numbers may be affected by the lack [8-14] of uniformity in reporting.

At least four different kinds of valves have been described internationally:

- Zephyr
- Spiration
- MedLung
- Miyazawa

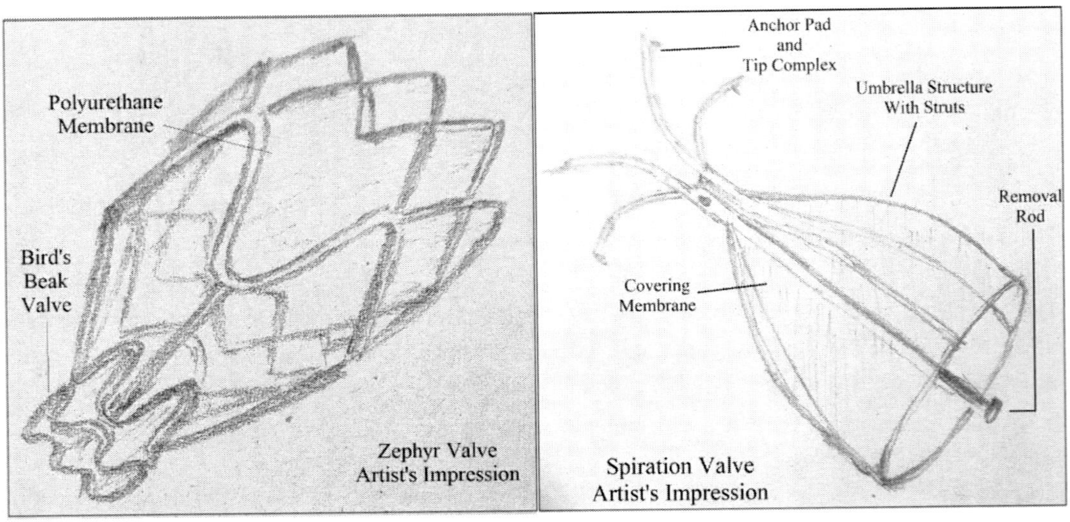

Figure 2. Endobronchial valve illustrations.

Of these, the Zephyr and Spiration valves have been studied more extensively. STELVIO, IMPACT, LIBERATE and TRANSFORM are the trials that have studied the Zephyr valve. [8-12] Of these, interestingly enough, IMPACT catered to patients with homogenous emphysema alone. In procedures where the time was recorded, the Zephyr valves were inserted in less than half an hour. On an average, a patient chosen for the procedure receives four valves. The Spiration valves were studied in detail in the REACH and EMPROVE studies, and the latter had similar results to the Zephyr studies. [13, 14] A clinically observable difference in the patients' lung functions or exercise capacity has been reported on an average at six months, while atelectasis is likely to be evident at the end of a month.

Pneumothorax, pneumonia, valve migration and exacerbations are known to occur after valve insertion. The four major studies on the Zephyr valve reported pneumothorax rates ranging from 18 to 34%. Removal, replacement or repositioning of a valve may be needed for valves which have migrated or when infective exacerbations do not respond to antibiotics or in those where atelectasis doesn't seem to have occurred at the expected time. The mortality rates reported have varied in different studies, but the LIBERATE and EMPROVE studies, which had a follow-up of 12 months each with different valves, showed 4% and 5.3% deaths, respectively. EBV therapy remains a more cost-effective modality for the patients and has lesser inherent risks than surgical interventions and thereby has a definite role in management.

2. *Coils:*

   While EBV therapy required proof of the absence of collateral ventilation, coils were developed to tackle precisely that problem. Chronologically they were developed after EBV with the necessity of solving the collateral ventilation puzzle.

   Coils are made of *Nitinol* (a nickel-titanium alloy), which retain a shape memory that allows them to return to their original double-loop form in the lung. [15] The loops of the coils end in atraumatic balls to minimize damage. The coils are placed bronchoscopically at the desired subsegmental location through a specialized loaded catheter-cartridge system which straightens the coils out. The placement is done under fluoroscopic guidance, with the middle third of the lung being the preferred location for placement. Once placed, they slowly bunch the diseased tissue together, effectively improving the elasticity of the remaining non-diseased lung. Like EBV, they are most effective in heterogenous emphysema, and each procedure has up to 14 coils placed in the targeted area. [16] Historically, patients with pulmonary hypertension, low diffusing capacity of the lungs for carbon monoxide (DLCO) values (<20%), poor six minute walk distance (6MWD) (<140 m), bullous disease, significant bronchiectasis, and ongoing anticoagulation have not been considered suitable for coils.

   In the post-procedure period, exacerbation is the commonest adverse event noted, while pneumonia, pneumothorax and lesser frequently mortalities have also been documented. It is important to note that often the consolidations seen are non-infectious as such and caused because of local coil-related inflammation. Aptly, the appearances are referred to as Coil-associated opacities (CAO). [17] Given that inflammation is intended, intuitively, the patients who have CAOs generally respond to treatment favorably in the long run.

   It is also necessary to reassure the patient that nearly 50% of them are likely to have some hemoptysis post-procedure while only 1% of the cases have a major bleed, but that too, in the subset of patients who have been taken for the procedure despite having pulmonary hypertension or who have been on anticoagulants. [15]

   The anticipation of exacerbations post-procedure has led to a practice of prescribing corticosteroids and antibiotics as a part of the protocol for at least five days post-procedure.

   Coils are an attractive alternative to EBV, especially in the presence of collateral ventilation; however, they are expensive. The associated general anesthesia may also pose additional hospitalization costs and eliminate patients with attendant anesthetic risks.

   If performed on both the lungs, the procedure is performed sequentially in two sittings, one lung at a time, at an interval of 1-2 months. Follow-up spirometry and clinical evaluation are recommended at 3,6 and 12 months at the very least.

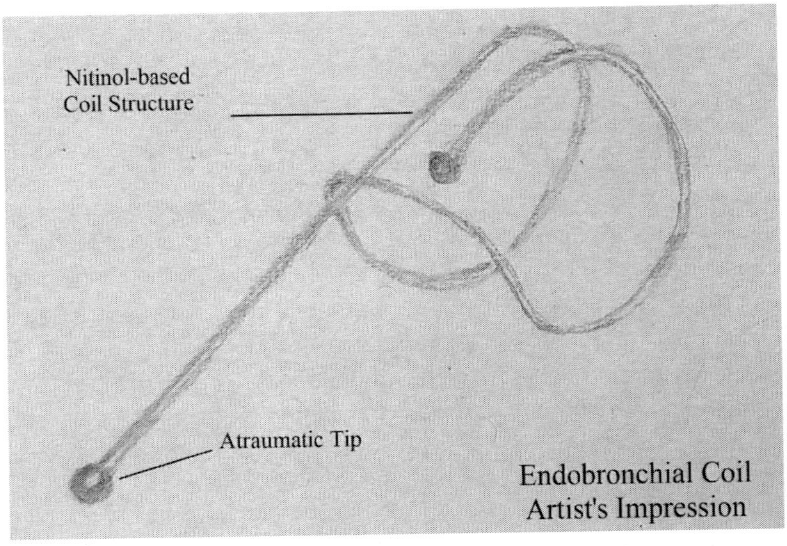

Figure 3. Endobronchial coil illustration.

3. *Bronchoscopic Thermal Vapor Ablation (BTVA)*:
While both EBV and coils leave a residual implant in the patient, BTVA is free of such remnant impact. As can be gauged, the principle of BTVA is to apply sufficient heat in the form of heated water vapor to cause local inflammation, fibrosis and closure. [18] It indeed requires a calculation for the dose of heat to be delivered, which is up to 10 calories/gram of tissue to be treated. The heat is delivered using an electronically controlled *pressure-vessel* via a specialized catheter. The analysis of the tissue to be treated is based on the CT images, Heterogeneity Index (HI) calculations and a specialized program for the same. [18, 19] The HI is essentially a ratio of ratios, that is, tissue: air ratio of the lower lobe to upper lobe. While an HI of >/= 1.2 is considered favorable for BTVA, the higher the HI, the more suitable is the patient and the more effective is the response. [18]
Like the previous two modalities, heterogenous emphysema is again the preferred sub-group of patients; however, it can be used in patients with collateral ventilation like coils. Generally performed under general anesthesia, the procedure requires an established artificial airway for the patient. Similar to coils, patients with a very poor pulmonary reserve and pulmonary hypertension are generally excluded. As are those with reduced ejection fraction, ongoing exacerbations, and Pseudomonas colonization. The catheter used for the delivery of heat has a balloon at the distal end, which occludes the segment of interest and once activated, heat is delivered via a proximal portion of the same.
Again, since the therapy principle is inciting local inflammation, patients showing a higher inflammatory response in the immediate aftermath of the procedure are generally better responders as well. Like in coils, an opacity may be seen in the areas where therapy has been instituted, and the patient may have accompanied fever, cough and sputum production.
Like in coils, these patients are often prescribed broad-spectrum antibiotics and glucocorticoids and may need extended monitoring during the inflammatory phase after the procedure.

The complications of the procedure include exacerbations and pneumonia as the commoner occurrences, while pneumothorax and death are more infrequent.
The follow-up lung functions generally start showing an improvement from one month on.

4. *Airway Bypass Stent:*
Airway bypass stents, as the name suggests, create an alternative pathway for the exhalation of air from areas with significant air trapping. [20] The procedure involves bronchoscopically inserting the stent in a trans-bronchial path which is not an existing anatomic airway. To ensure patency, drug-eluting stents using Paclitaxel have been used. [21]
Unlike the other mentioned endobronchial therapies, this option was tested in patients of predominantly homogenous emphysema.
The procedure has been associated with intra-procedural bleeding, pneumomediastinum and pneumothorax, infections, exacerbations and anesthetic complications.
However, one of the larger studies done to evaluate the efficacy of airway bypass stents (EASE) did not show an enduring effect of airway bypass stent placement. [20] A similar fitness requirement as in surgical candidates has seen the earlier endobronchial alternatives take centre-stage.
5. *Bio-LVR:*
Bio-LVR or Biologic LVR is the collective name for the instillation of biologicals-based material endobronchially to mechanically occlude the airways and promote a collapse with an inflammatory reaction. [22] The different materials used in research include fibrin-based gels, patented sealants and even autologous blood. Therapy has been attempted in homogenous and heterogenous emphysema, with or without collateral ventilation.
Understandably, the principle depends on an inflammatory reaction, and hence the patient commonly shows a *flu-like reaction*. Consequently, those who show such a reaction tend to have a more effective response to the therapy. However, the expulsion of the sealant with cough, intraprocedural spillage within the tracheobronchial tree and post-procedure exacerbations are other known adverse events with the procedure.
The results of the Bio-LVR have not always been in favor of the treatment and whether it will be a recommended treatment in the future remains to be seen.

Surgical Interventions

Surgical techniques preceded bronchoscopic therapy, as has been the case with most historical treatments, but given the critical function of the lungs, the associated perioperative morbidity and mortality have been significant limiting factors. It has taken extensive research to optimize the outcomes of these procedures, and the process has been an excellent lesson in developing a systematic approach to judging the suitability of patients for surgeries with significant risks.

The three surgical approaches that find a place in the Global initiative for chronic obstructive lung disease (GOLD) guidelines will be reviewed further. [23]

1. *LVRS*:
   This surgery had become quite popular in the previous century for tackling patients with COPD. However, the lack of ample evidence made the central agencies in the United States of America take note and plan appropriate pre-procedure patient identification. This led to the famous trial called NETT – National Emphysema Treatment Trial. [24] The trial studied the difference between opting for or against LVRS while both the categories of patients received optimal medical management and rehabilitation. Consequently, the patients were grouped into five different categories based on the trial outcome, which remain a guidance for decision making. The researchers concluded that patients with an upper-lobe predominant disease and low exercise capacities seemed to show the most benefit from the surgery. By corollary, those with non-upper-lobe predominance and higher exercise capacities were considered poor candidates for surgery. Additionally, patients with homogenous emphysema and very low lung functions (FEV_1<20% and DLCO<20%) were contraindicated from the procedure thereon, owing to the relatively high mortality in the sub-group.
   To avoid the associated morbidity, older patients (>75 years), current smokers, patients with pulmonary hypertension, and severely hypoxic and hypercapnic (>60 cm Hg) patients are generally ruled out from the procedure as well.
   Lung volumes showing hyperinflation (TLC > 100%) and a low exercise capacity on cycle ergometry (<40 W for men and <25W for women) are the objective parameters considered.
   The surgery is generally performed on both lungs, and the basis of the surgery is the improved elastic recoil because of the reduction in lung volume and improved expiratory flow. Additionally, improved cardiac function has also been reported with the surgery.
   The procedure can be performed as an open surgery or by a Video-Assisted Thoracoscopic Surgery (VATS) approach. Arrhythmias, prolonged mechanical ventilation, pneumonia, persistent air leak and death are known complications of the procedure.
   The refined criteria for inclusion of the most suitable patients are backed by robust data, and thereby the evidence level for the procedure is the highest for surgical interventions.
2. *Bullectomy*:
   As the name suggests, the procedure involves the removal of a large bulla from the lung. [25] A giant bulla is defined as one which occupies more than 30% of the hemithorax, and the surgery involves removing one or more of the same. The compressive effect on the normal lung, the diaphragmatic compromise, the increased residual volume and consequently the increased work of breathing are all countered by removing the giant bulla/e. The procedure would generally be considered in patients who perceive breathlessness despite maximal medical management or while managing a secondary spontaneous pneumothorax in a patient with a giant bulla. In one of the largest case series published, ~52% of the patients taken up for the surgery had presented with a pneumothorax. [25] Again, high-risk cases for operative management like elderly patients (>60 years), patients with poor lung functions (FEV_1<40%, DLCO<40%), concomitant pulmonary hypertension and comorbid coronary artery

disease, are considered to be poor candidates for surgery and are listed in the contraindications. A current smoker is also not considered for surgery.

The procedure in itself may involve one of several techniques. Staple excision is the commonest method used, while the other techniques include plication and experimental ablation techniques. During the surgery, small bullae in close proximity to the giant bulla are often removed. The common postoperative complications of the surgery in the descending order of frequency include air leaks, atrial fibrillation, pneumonia, prolonged mechanical ventilation and bleeding. The reported mortality is below 3.5%

A significant improvement in the patient's FEV_1 (on an average of 300 ml or 10%) is observed in the post-operative period.

3. *Lung transplant:*

Transplantation was the final frontier to conquer in many ways. Though the first transplant was for a patient with a lung malignancy, most lung transplants occur for patients with COPD in the present day and age. The enormity of the surgery demands that patient selection, pre-procedural optimization and post-procedure rehabilitation and care should be pitch-perfect to ensure the best results.

The International Society for Heart and Lung Transplantation (ISHLT) has recently (2021) revised its document published in 2014, laying down consensus statements for patient selection for transplantation. [26]

The process is streamlined in such a manner that it is recommended to start the process of *referral* at an earlier point in the chronology of the chronic respiratory disease before it reaches the end stage when the patient is *listed.* The screening process for these patients is based on the well-known BODE (Body mass index, Obstruction, Dyspnea and Exercise) index [27] (Table 1).

The latest ISHLT guidelines acknowledge that the BODE index may predict higher mortality at times than observed but continue to recommend its usage for both referral and listing. Other indications for transplantation are listed in the table, as adapted from the ISHLT consensus statement.

Lung transplantation also involves appropriate donor selection. Cadaveric donor selection is a challenge given the high rates of pneumonia in intubated patients, reducing the number of eligible donor candidates to less than half. Given the large number of patients eligible for transplant, there is a severe shortage of donor lungs. An upcoming area in this regard is Ex Vivo Lung Perfusion (EVLP) technology, which helps optimize the donor's lungs and thereby increase organ utilization. [28] Briefly, an eligible donor is a young person with less smoke exposure, good oxygenation on the ventilator, no apparent tracheal mucosal or thoracic injury, no previous thoracic surgery and otherwise normal lung radiology.

The United Network for Organ Sharing (UNOS) allots eligible patients' donor lungs based on a comprehensive Lung Allocation Score (LAS), which is a score from 0-100 that estimates the relative benefit of the candidate patient. [29] It is based on mathematical models which estimate the patient's survival without the transplant and the survival with a transplant within the subsequent year. This helps appropriate and optimal utilization of the donor organs.

Table 1. Parameters for referral and listing for lung transplant

Referral	Listing
BODE score 5-6 AND one of the following: • Frequent acute exacerbations • Increase in BODE score > 1 in 24 months • PA to Ao diameter >1 on CT scan • FEV_1 20-25%	BODE score 7-10
Clinical deterioration despite medical treatment.	• FEV_1<20% • Moderate-Severe Pulmonary Hypertension • Chronic Hypercapnia • Severe Exacerbations
Perception of poor quality of life on existent appropriate treatment.	
Any candidate for BLVR or LVRS	

Definition of abbreviations: BODE, Body mass index, Obstruction, Dyspnea and Exercise; BLVR, biologic lung volume reduction; FEV_1, Forced expiratory volume in one second; PA, Pulmonary Artery; Ao, Aorta; LVRS, lung volume reduction surgery.

While single-lung transplants can be performed in certain conditions (about 30% of the transplants presently are single-lung transplants), the current practice is to consider a double-lung transplant wherever feasible, given the longer survival. In addition, one may consider a heart transplant if the patient has left ventricular dysfunction, coronary artery disease which cannot be surgically corrected or an irreparable shunt with Eisenmenger syndrome. [26]

The anesthetic challenges to the procedure are unique, while the post-procedure immunosuppression is modelled on the lines of the regimen for other organ transplants.

Several complications are possible with this major surgery, not limited to the technique itself. The surgical complications include hemorrhage, ischemia, pneumothorax and pleural effusions due to mismatch in cage and lung sizes. Primary graft dysfunction may be seen in up to a fifth of the patients. Post-procedure atrial arrhythmias and gastrointestinal complications are also fairly common. The immunosuppression makes the patient susceptible to infective complications, with bacterial pneumonia being the commonest. Bronchiolitis Obliterans Syndrome (BOS) is a well-known immunological complication. [30] Post-transplant lymphoproliferative disease (PTLD) is a similarly known neoplastic disorder seen, causally associated with an EBV infection as a complication of immunosuppression. [31] An increase in the number of solid tumors like squamous cell carcinomas of the skin, perineum, Kaposi's sarcoma and other soft tissue tumors has also been noted.

The survival rates after lung transplant at 1 and 5 years presently are about 85% and 59%, respectively, and with the rapidly increasing awareness and expanding expertise, these are expected to increase in the future. Presently, the median survival for bilateral and unilateral transplants is around 7 and 5 years, respectively. [32]

Conclusion

There have been several advances in intervention therapy for COPD patients, and the techniques continue to be refined. It is essential to know which patient is eligible for a particular treatment modality and analyse its true benefit while counselling them. Every successful intervention relies on the continuation of optimal medical management and pulmonary rehabilitation.

Key Points

- A COPD patient has several options for interventional therapy apart from routine medical management and pulmonary rehabilitation. The decision to consider an intervention must be a shared decision-making process which involves informing the patient about the choices and the known risks and benefits of each of them.
- The interventional therapy of choice depends on the patient's baseline lung function and the radiological distribution pattern of the disease in the lungs. Very poor lung functions may negate the possibility of most interventions other than lung transplantation.
- Bronchoscopic procedures are lesser invasive and cost-effective alternatives to surgical interventions. The proven effective procedures include endobronchial valves, endobronchial coils and bronchial thermal vapor ablation. Of these, bronchial thermal vapor ablation is the only procedure with no residual implanted material in the patient's lung.
- Bronchoscopic Lung Volume Reduction is a targeted lung volume reduction technique that requires appropriate planning and patient selection. Assessment of the presence or absence of collateral ventilation is necessary for choosing the appropriate therapy.
- Surgical techniques chiefly include Lung Volume Reduction Surgery, Bullectomy and Lung Transplantation. All the procedures carry the inherent risks of anaesthesia in a patient with compromised lung functions, and perioperative management of these patients is a skill in itself.

References

[1] Sarkar M, Bhardwaz R, Madabhavi I, Modi M. Physical signs in patients with chronic obstructive pulmonary disease. *Lung India*. 2019;36(1):38-47.

[2] Washko GR. Diagnostic imaging in COPD. *Semin Respir Crit Care Med*. 2010;31(3):276-85.

[3] O'Donnell DE, Webb KA, Neder JA. Lung hyperinflation in COPD: applying physiology to clinical practice. *COPD Research and Practice*. 2015;1(1):4.

[4] Slebos DJ, Shah PL, Herth FJ, Valipour A. Endobronchial Valves for Endoscopic Lung Volume Reduction: Best Practice Recommendations from Expert Panel on Endoscopic Lung Volume Reduction. *Respiration*. 2017;93(2):138-50.

[5] Gesierich W, Samitas K, Reichenberger F, Behr J. Collapse phenomenon during Chartis collateral ventilation assessment. *Eur Respir J*. 2016;47(6):1657-67.

[6] Hayashi K, Aziz A, Ashizawa K, Hayashi H, Nagaoki K, Otsuji H. Radiographic and CT appearances of the major fissures. *Radiographics*. 2001;21(4):861-74.

[7] Manjunath M, Sharma MV, Janso K, John PK, Anupama N, Harsha DS. Study on Anatomical Variations in Fissures of Lung by CT Scan. *Indian J Radiol Imaging*. 2021;31(4):797-804.

[8] Criner GJ, Sue R, Wright S, Dransfield M, Rivas-Perez H, Wiese T, et al. A Multicenter Randomized Controlled Trial of Zephyr Endobronchial Valve Treatment in Heterogeneous Emphysema (LIBERATE). *Am J Respir Crit Care Med*. 2018;198(9):1151-64.

[9] Hartman JE, Vanfleteren L, van Rikxoort EM, Klooster K, Slebos DJ. Endobronchial valves for severe emphysema. *Eur Respir Rev.* 2019;28(152).

[10] Kemp SV, Slebos DJ, Kirk A, Kornaszewska M, Carron K, Ek L, et al. A Multicenter Randomized Controlled Trial of Zephyr Endobronchial Valve Treatment in Heterogeneous Emphysema (TRANSFORM). *Am J Respir Crit Care Med.* 2017;196(12):1535-43.

[11] Klooster K, ten Hacken NH, Hartman JE, Kerstjens HA, van Rikxoort EM, Slebos DJ. Endobronchial Valves for Emphysema without Interlobar Collateral Ventilation. *N Engl J Med.* 2015;373(24):2325-35.

[12] Valipour A, Slebos DJ, Herth F, Darwiche K, Wagner M, Ficker JH, et al. Endobronchial Valve Therapy in Patients with Homogeneous Emphysema. Results from the IMPACT Study. *Am J Respir Crit Care Med.* 2016;194(9):1073-82.

[13] Criner GJ, Delage A, Voelker K, Hogarth DK, Majid A, Zgoda M, et al. Improving Lung Function in Severe Heterogenous Emphysema with the Spiration Valve System (EMPROVE). A Multicenter, Open-Label Randomized Controlled Clinical Trial. *Am J Respir Crit Care Med.* 2019;200(11):1354-62.

[14] Li S, Wang G, Wang C, Gao X, Jin F, Yang H, et al. The REACH Trial: A Randomized Controlled Trial Assessing the Safety and Effectiveness of the Spiration(R) Valve System in the Treatment of Severe Emphysema. *Respiration.* 2019;97(5):416-27.

[15] Slebos DJ, Ten Hacken NH, Hetzel M, Herth FJF, Shah PL. Endobronchial Coils for Endoscopic Lung Volume Reduction: Best Practice Recommendations from an Expert Panel. *Respiration.* 2018;96(1):1-11.

[16] Deslee G, Klooster K, Hetzel M, Stanzel F, Kessler R, Marquette CH, et al. Lung volume reduction coil treatment for patients with severe emphysema: a European multicentre trial. *Thorax.* 2014;69(11):980-6.

[17] Sciurba FC, Criner GJ, Strange C, Shah PL, Michaud G, Connolly TA, et al. Effect of Endobronchial Coils vs Usual Care on Exercise Tolerance in Patients With Severe Emphysema: The RENEW Randomized Clinical Trial. *JAMA.* 2016;315(20):2178-89.

[18] Gompelmann D, Shah PL, Valipour A, Herth FJF. Bronchoscopic Thermal Vapor Ablation: Best Practice Recommendations from an Expert Panel on Endoscopic Lung Volume Reduction. *Respiration.* 2018;95(6):392-400.

[19] Valipour A, Shah PL, Gesierich W, Eberhardt R, Snell G, Strange C, et al. Patterns of Emphysema Heterogeneity. *Respiration.* 2015;90(5):402-11.

[20] Shah PL, Slebos DJ, Cardoso PF, Cetti E, Voelker K, Levine B, et al. Bronchoscopic lung-volume reduction with Exhale airway stents for emphysema (EASE trial): randomised, sham-controlled, multicentre trial. *Lancet.* 2011;378(9795):997-1005.

[21] Cardoso PF, Snell GI, Hopkins P, Sybrecht GW, Stamatis G, Ng AW, et al. Clinical application of airway bypass with paclitaxel-eluting stents: early results. *J Thorac Cardiovasc Surg.* 2007;134(4):974-81.

[22] Refaely Y, Dransfield M, Kramer MR, Gotfried M, Leeds W, McLennan G, et al. Biologic lung volume reduction therapy for advanced homogeneous emphysema. *Eur Respir J.* 2010;36(1):20-7.

[23] Global Initiative for Chronic Obstructive Lung Disease (GOLD). *Global Strategy for the Diagnosis, Management, and Prevention of chronic Obstructive Pulmonary Disease.* 2022 Report. http://www.goldcopd.org/.

[24] Weinmann GG, Chiang YP, Sheingold S. The National Emphysema Treatment Trial (NETT): a study in agency collaboration. *Proc Am Thorac Soc.* 2008;5(4):381-4.

[25] Krishnamohan P, Shen KR, Wigle DA, Allen MS, Nichols FC, 3rd, Cassivi SD, et al. Bullectomy for symptomatic or complicated giant lung bullae. *Ann Thorac Surg.* 2014;97(2):425-31.

[26] Crespo MM, Lease ED, Sole A, Sandorfi N, Snyder LD, Berry GJ, et al. ISHLT consensus document on lung transplantation in patients with connective tissue disease: Part I: Epidemiology, assessment of extrapulmonary conditions, candidate evaluation, selection criteria, and pathology statements. *J Heart Lung Transplant.* 2021;40(11):1251-66.

[27] Celli BR, Cote CG, Marin JM, Casanova C, Montes de Oca M, Mendez RA, et al. The body-mass index, airflow obstruction, dyspnea, and exercise capacity index in chronic obstructive pulmonary disease. *N Engl J Med.* 2004;350(10):1005-12.

[28] Machuca TN, Cypel M. Ex vivo lung perfusion. *J Thorac Dis.* 2014;6(8):1054-62.

[29] Lyu DM, Goff RR, Chan KM. The Lung Allocation Score and Its Relevance. *Semin Respir Crit Care Med.* 2021;42(3):346-56.

[30] Meyer KC, Raghu G, Verleden GM, Corris PA, Aurora P, Wilson KC, et al. An international ISHLT/ATS/ERS clinical practice guideline: diagnosis and management of bronchiolitis obliterans syndrome. *Eur Respir J.* 2014;44(6):1479-503.

[31] Al-Mansour Z, Nelson BP, Evens AM. Post-transplant lymphoproliferative disease (PTLD): risk factors, diagnosis, and current treatment strategies. *Curr Hematol Malig Rep.* 2013;8(3):173-83.

[32] Thabut G, Mal H. Outcomes after lung transplantation. *J Thorac Dis.* 2017;9(8):2684-91.

Chapter 15

Pharmacological Management of Stable COPD

Abdullah A. Alqarni[1,*], PhD, Abdulelah M. Aldhahir[2], PhD, Saeed M. Alghamdi[3,4], PhD, Rayan Siraj[5], PhD and Abdulkareem A. AlGarni[6,7], MD

[1]Department of Respiratory Therapy,
Faculty of Medical Rehabilitation Sciences,
King Abdulaziz University, Jeddah, Saudi Arabia
[2]Respiratory Therapy Department,
Faculty of Applied Medical Sciences,
Jazan University, Jazan, Saudi Arabia
[3]Clinical Technology Department,
Respiratory Care Program, Faculty of Applied Medical Sciences,
Umm Al-Qura University, Makkah, Saudi Arabia
[4]National Heart and Lung Institute, Imperial College London, UK
[5]Department of Respiratory Therapy,
College of Applied Medical Sciences,
King Faisal University, Al Ahsa, Saudi Arabia
[6]King Abdulaziz Hospital, MNGHA, Al Ahsa, Saudi Arabia
[7]King Saud bin Abdulaziz University for Health Sciences,
COAMS-A, Al Ahsa, Saudi Arabia

Abstract

Chronic obstructive pulmonary disease (COPD) is a common cause of morbidity and mortality worldwide, and its burden is expected to increase over the next decade. Proper management of COPD symptoms is vital for preventing disease progression and improving outcomes, particularly minimizing the risk of COPD exacerbation. Although non-pharmacologic management approaches are valuable and should be employed alongside pharmacologic management, this chapter focuses mainly on managing symptoms and dyspnea in patients with stable COPD using pharmacotherapy based on the best available evidence. Besides reviewing the current evidence of the value of using a pharmacologic approach (including bronchodilators and inhaled corticosteroids, either alone or in combination) to reduce the frequency and severity of COPD exacerbation and improve overall quality of life, this chapter discusses the potential of using a pharmacologic approach to improve the survival rate of patients with stable COPD.

---

* Corresponding Author's Email: aaalqarni1@kau.edu.sa.

In: Chronic Obstructive Pulmonary Disease
Editor: Jaber S. Alqahtani
ISBN: 979-8-88697-333-4

Keywords: stable COPD, pharmacological intervention, muscarinic antagonists, β2-agonists

Introduction

Chronic obstructive pulmonary disease (COPD) is a treatable group of chronic lung conditions caused by airway and/or alveolar abnormalities that lead to persistent pulmonary symptoms. Worsening of these symptoms may result in deteriorating lung function and accelerating disease progression unless the COPD symptoms are controlled and managed appropriately [1]. Evidence suggests that pharmacologic interventions can improve both quality of life and lung function, thereby reducing the frequency and severity of COPD exacerbation and unnecessary hospitalization.

This chapter discusses some of the most promising pharmacologic therapies for the management of patients with stable COPD, including bronchodilators (β2 agonists alone, antimuscarinic drugs alone, or dual combined bronchodilator therapy), anti-inflammatory agents (inhaled corticosteroids alone, dual combined therapy with inhaled corticosteroids and bronchodilators, and triple combined therapy with inhaled corticosteroids and bronchodilators), methylxanthines, and phosphodiesterase-4 (PDE4) inhibitors. This chapter also reviews the ability of these inhaled and oral therapies to preserve optimal lung function and manage COPD symptoms based on the available literature.

Muscarinic Receptor Antagonists and Stable COPD

Acetylcholine is the predominant parasympathetic neurotransmitter in the airways and has long been reported to play a key role in the pathogenesis of chronic obstructive airway diseases, including COPD, leading to bronchoconstriction, increased mucus secretion, and airway inflammation and remodeling [2]. Acetylcholine is produced from both neuronal and nonneuronal sources and regulates important physiological functions in the airways of patients with COPD (e.g., airway smooth muscle constriction and airway inflammation and remodeling) by binding to muscarinic receptors.

In human lungs, muscarinic receptors are expressed by tissue-forming cells in the airways, predominantly by smooth muscle, epithelium, and fibroblasts [3]. Once released by cholinergic nerves, acetylcholine activates these muscarinic receptors, leading to functional changes in the airways. There are five well-known subtypes of muscarinic receptors: M1, M2, M3, M4, and M5. Among these receptors, studies have shown that M1, M2, and M3 are found primarily in the peripheral airway smooth muscle [4-6] and play important roles in airway physiology [7, 8].

From a therapeutic perspective, blocking the activation of muscarinic receptors by using competitive muscarinic antagonists (also known as antimuscarinic or anticholinergic agents) has been shown to be effective in the management of stable COPD, considering that the cholinergic tone represents the major reversible component of airway narrowing in patients with COPD [9]. Currently, several long-acting muscarinic receptor antagonist (LAMA) and short-acting muscarinic receptor antagonist (SAMA) agents are available and approved for the management of stable COPD. A summary of the commonly used LAMAs and SAMAs for patients with stable COPD is shown in Table 1.

Among the approved LAMA agents, tiotropium bromide is the most commonly used therapy for the treatment of COPD because it was the first to be introduced for the treatment of patients with stable COPD [10]. A randomized, double-blind clinical trial involving 7,376 patients compared the efficacy of tiotropium bromide with that of the long-acting β2 agonist (LABA) salmeterol on the incidence of moderate or severe exacerbation. It has been demonstrated that tiotropium bromide is more effective than salmeterol in reducing exacerbation events in patients with stable COPD [11]. In addition, a systematic review of randomized controlled trials concluded that tiotropium bromide improves COPD symptoms, health status, and quality of life and reduces exacerbation in patients with moderate to severe COPD [12]. Consistent with these observations, it has been reported that the use of tiotropium bromide can reduce exacerbation compared with the LABA indacaterol [13] and can also improve the effectiveness of pulmonary rehabilitation in patients with stable COPD [14, 15].

Table 1. A summary of commonly used LAMAs and SAMAs for patients with COPD

Long-acting muscarinic receptor antagonists (LAMAs)			
Generic Name	Brand name	Type of Inhaler	Duration of action
Tiotropium bromide	Spiriva	SMI, MDI, DPI	24 hours
Aclidinium bromide	Tudorza Pressair, Eklira Genuair	DPI, MDI	24 hours
Umeclidinium bromide	Incruse Ellipta	DPI	24 hours
Glycopyrronium bromide	Magnair	Nebulization	12 hours
Revefenacin	Yupelri	Nebulization	24 hours
Short-acting muscarinic receptor antagonists (SAMAs)			
Generic Name	Brand name	Type of Inhaler	Duration of action
Ipratropium bromide	Atrovent	MDI, Nebulization	6–8 hours
Oxitropium bromide	Oxivent	MDI	7–9 hours

MDI = Metered dose inhaler.
DPI = Dry Powder Inhaler.
SMI = Soft Mist Inhaler.

These observations were further strengthened by two recent systematic reviews and meta-analyses of randomized controlled trials that compared other LAMA agents (e.g., glycopyrronium, aclidinium, and umeclidinium) with LABAs. These studies demonstrated the superiority of LAMAs over LABAs for the prevention of COPD exacerbation [16, 17]. Together, these results suggest that tiotropium bromide is beneficial for patients with stable COPD and should be recommended as an initial therapy to prevent frequent and severe exacerbation.

Besides its well-known bronchodilatory property, findings from an *in vitro* study suggest that the use of the LAMA tiotropium bromide has an anti-inflammatory effect [18] by inhibiting neutrophilic inflammation through the suppression of IL-8 production by airway epithelial cells. This may explain the beneficial effects of tiotropium bromide in reducing COPD exacerbation, considering that neutrophilic airway inflammation is generally accepted as a major factor in the pathogenesis of COPD [19]. These observations, together with the proven bronchodilatory effect of tiotropium bromide, support the current international global initiative for chronic obstructive lung disease (GOLD) recommendations of LAMA use for patients with stable COPD who are at risk of experiencing more than one COPD exacerbation per year (GOLD grade groups C and D).

Altogether, the activation of muscarinic receptors by acetylcholine-induced airway smooth muscle contraction and the release of proinflammatory mediators in COPD provide the rationale for using LAMA agents in the management of patients with stable COPD. The international guidelines strongly recommend the use of LAMA agents to prevent COPD exacerbation based on the best available evidence highlighting the positive effects on lung function and COPD symptoms reported with the use of LAMA agents. Further studies are needed to assess the effect of the currently available LAMA agents on survival rates of patients with COPD.

β2 Agonists and Stable COPD

Adrenaline—a hormone produced within the adrenal gland—acts on nearly all body tissues by binding to adrenergic receptors (α1–2 and β1–2). Adrenaline is mediated in the lungs by the β2 receptor, which is found mainly in airway smooth muscle cells. Activation of the β2 adrenergic receptor by a β2 agonist is known to have a potent airway smooth muscle relaxation effect, and it is a commonly used therapeutic pathway for managing the symptoms of pulmonary diseases, including COPD. β2 agonists are generally classified into two main categories based on the duration of action and the time of peak effect. The short-acting β2 agonist (SABA) and LABA agents commonly used to treat patients with COPD are listed in Table 2.

Table 2. Commonly used LABA and SABA agents for patients with COPD

Long-acting β2 agonists (LABAs)			
Generic Name	Brand name	Type of Inhaler	Duration of action
Indacaterol	Onbrez, Arcapta	DPI	24 hours
Olodaterol	Striverdi	SMI	24 hours
Formoterol	Foradil, Atimos, Oxis	DPI, MDI, Nebulization	12 hours
Salmeterol	Serevent	DPI, MDI	12 hours
Arformoterol	Brovana	Nebulization	12 hours
Short-acting β2 agonists (SABAs)			
Generic Name	Brand name	Type of Inhaler	Duration of action
Albuterol	Ventolin	DPI, MDI, Nebulization	4–6 hours
Fenoterol	Berotec N	MDI, Nebulization	4–6 hours
Levalbuterol	Xopenex	MDI, Nebulization	6–8 hours
Terbutaline	Bricanyl	DPI	4–6 hours

MDI = Metered dose inhaler.
DPI = Dry Powder Inhaler.
SMI = Soft Mist Inhaler.

β2 adrenergic receptor agonists exert bronchodilatory effects by stimulating the intracellular activity of adenylyl cyclase, which eventually leads to increased production of cyclic adenosine monophosphate (cAMP) and functional antagonism to bronchoconstriction. *In vitro* studies have shown that the use of β2 adrenergic receptor agonists (e.g., salmeterol) can inhibit the production of a wide range of inflammatory mediators (e.g., chemokines and cytokines) in human airway cells, particularly airway smooth muscle cells [20–22]. This suggests that β2 adrenergic receptor agonists may have anti-inflammatory properties besides their well-known bronchodilatory effects. However, the exact mechanisms remain unclear.

LABAs (e.g., salmeterol and formoterol) are used as long-term maintenance therapies to control the symptoms of patients with moderate to severe COPD. A systematic review of 26 parallel, randomized controlled clinical trials showed that the use of inhaled LABAs can improve quality of life and reduce exacerbation and hospitalization, although no significant reduction in mortality was observed [23]. A more recent systematic review and meta-analysis of 33 randomized controlled trials was conducted to compare the efficacy of LABA monotherapies and reported that indacaterol was the most effective LABA monotherapy for patients with moderate to severe COPD [24].

Collectively, β2 agonists, particularly LABAs, are commonly used for the management of patients with stable COPD, as this class of drug can produce bronchodilation by stimulating β2 receptors and anti-inflammatory effects through the inhibition of inflammatory mediators. Although the use of β2 agonists, such as salmeterol and formoterol, can improve quality of life and reduce exacerbation and unnecessary hospitalization, the current evidence suggests that β2 agonists do not influence morbidity in patients with COPD.

Dual Therapy with β2 Agonists and Muscarinic Receptor Antagonists for Stable COPD

Table 3. Commonly used combinations of acting β2 agonist and muscarinic receptor antagonist agents for patients with COPD

Combined LABA and muscarinic receptor antagonist agents			
Generic Name	Brand name	Type of Inhaler	Duration of action
Indacaterol and Glycopyrronium bromide	Ultibro Breezhaler	DPI	12-24 hours
Formoterol and Glycopyrronium bromide	Bevespi Aerosphere	MDI	12 hours
Formoterol and Aclidinium bromide	Duaklir pressair	DPI	12 hours
Olodaterol and Tiotropium bromide	Stiolto Respimat	SMI	24 hours
Vilanterol and Umeclidinium bromide	Anoro Ellipta	DPI	24 hours
Combined SABA and muscarinic receptor antagonist agents			
Generic Name	Brand name	Type of Inhaler	Duration of action
Albuterol and Ipratropium bromide	Combivent, Duoneb	MDI, SMI, Nebulization	6–8 hours
Fenoterol and Ipratropium bromide	Duovent	SMI	6–8 hours

MDI = Metered dose inhaler.
DPI = Dry Powder Inhaler.
SMI = Soft Mist Inhaler.

β2 agonists and muscarinic antagonists are considered the mainstays of pharmacologic therapy for managing patients with stable COPD. Although both agents as single therapies have been shown to be effective for managing COPD symptoms, a recent systematic review and meta-analysis of 19 randomized control trials involving 28,211 patients with stable COPD showed that the use of LAMAs can significantly reduce rates of exacerbation compared with LABAs [16]. Given their different mechanisms and durations of action, combined LABAs and LAMAs are likely to enhance the bronchodilatory effect in patients with COPD who require additional therapy to maintain bronchodilation, thereby improving lung function and reducing exacerbation. A summary of the commonly used combinations of acting β2 agonist and muscarinic receptor antagonist agents for patients with COPD is shown in Table 3.

The combination of a β2 agonist and a muscarinic antagonist is available as a dual therapy with either long-acting or short-acting bronchodilator medication, based on the duration of action and the time of peak effect. Both combination types have been shown to be effective in improving lung function in patients with stable COPD. In the early 1990s, a 12-week prospective, double-blind, parallel-group involving 534 patients showed that the use of dual-inhaler therapy with a SABA and a muscarinic antagonist (albuterol or ipratropium bromide) could improve lung function compared with either agent alone in patients with stable COPD [25]. This finding was further strengthened by a double-blind, randomized, positive-control trial involving 863 patients, which revealed a greater improvement in lung function in response to a nebulized combination of albuterol and ipratropium bromide compared to either agent alone [26]. These findings strongly indicate that dual-inhaler therapy should be recommended for patients with stable COPD as reliever/rescue first-line therapy to relieve airflow obstruction.

Recently, analysis of seven clinical trials comprising 3,821 patients evaluated the efficacy and safety of a LAMA plus LABA combination. The study reported that dual-inhaler therapy with the bronchodilators umeclidinium and vilanterol demonstrated greatly improved lung function compared with tiotropium or fluticasone propionate/salmeterol [27]. Additionally, a systematic review and meta-analysis of clinical trials involving 5,921 participants showed that combined aclidinium and formoterol improved dyspnea and lung function in people with stable COPD, compared with aclidinium and formoterol individually or a placebo [28]. A recent meta-analysis showed that the use of three different combinations of LABAs and muscarinic antagonists (tiotropium bromide and olodaterol, umeclidinium bromide and vilanterol, and glycopyrronium bromide and indacaterol) achieved clinically significant improvements in lung function and quality of life in people with COPD compared with a placebo [29]. These observations strongly suggest that dual-inhaler therapy with LABAs and LAMAs should be recommended over the use of either agent alone for patients with stable COPD as a maintenance first-line therapy to improve lung function and overall quality of life.

In summary, the combination of a β2 agonist and a muscarinic receptor antagonist appears to play a key role in maximizing bronchodilatory effects. Recent studies have shown that the addition of a β2 agonist to muscarinic antagonists reduces exacerbation rates and dyspnea and improves health status and lung function in patients with stable COPD compared with individual drugs used alone. The current studies to date indicate the positive effects of dual therapy with bronchodilators.

Inhaled Corticosteroids Alone And Stable COPD

Long-term exposure to noxious particles or gases (e.g., in cigarette smoke) can cause pulmonary inflammation, which is mediated mainly by inflammatory cells (such as neutrophils) in response to the production of inflammatory mediators. In turn, these pathophysiological changes may worsen existing COPD symptoms, ultimately leading to unnecessary hospitalizations. An increase in inflammatory mediators in the pulmonary system provides the rationale for using anti-inflammatory medications to treat patients with COPD.

Corticosteroids—a group of anti-inflammatory drugs—can inhibit the production of inflammatory mediators, thereby reducing airway inflammation and preventing the worsening of common COPD symptoms. Although oral corticosteroids, such as hydrocortisone, methylprednisolone, prednisolone, prednisone, and dexamethasone, have anti-inflammatory properties, they are not recommended for use in patients with stable COPD due to the minimal benefits and severe systemic complications associated with the use of oral corticosteroids. It should be noted that the use of oral corticosteroids for managing acute exacerbation during emergency treatment has been shown to be effective, as reported in a systematic review of 16 randomized controlled trials [30]. Alternatively, inhaled corticosteroids, such as ciclesonide, beclomethasone, fluticasone, budesonide, and mometasone, can be directly applied to the pulmonary system. This selectively targets airway inflammation while minimizing the risk of systemic side effects. A summary of the commonly used inhaled corticosteroids for patients with COPD is shown in Table 4.

Table 4. Commonly used inhaled corticosteroids for patients with COPD

Inhaled corticosteroids		
Generic Name	Brand name	Type of Inhaler
Ciclesonide	Alvesco	MDI
Beclomethasone	Qvar	MDI
Fluticasone Propionate	Flovent	MDI, DPI
Budesonide	Pulmicort	DPI, nebulization
Mometasone	Asmanex	DPI, MDI
Flunisolide	Aerospan	MDI

MDI = Metered dose inhaler.
DPI = Dry Powder Inhaler.
SMI = Soft Mist Inhaler.

Growing evidence has shown that the use of inhaled corticosteroids as monotherapy improves COPD symptoms and reduces exacerbation [31–33]. However, long-term studies of inhaled corticosteroids alone have shown that these agents fail to improve pulmonary function in patients with stable COPD [34–37]. Moreover, a systematic review of 11 double-blind, randomized controlled trials reported that inhaled corticosteroids failed to influence one-year all-cause mortality in individuals with stable COPD [38]. Interestingly, the same authors also concluded that the use of inhaled corticosteroid therapy is associated with a greater risk of pneumonia [38]. Additionally, high-quality evidence from randomized controlled trials of 55 primary studies with 16,154 participants confirmed the previous reports that long-term use of inhaled corticosteroids (for more than six months) did not consistently improve lung function in patients with COPD. More importantly, a higher prevalence of oral candidiasis, hoarse voice, skin bruising, and/or pneumonia was observed with the use of inhaled corticosteroids in patients with COPD [39]. The risk of developing these side effects of inhaled corticosteroids in COPD patients is particularly associated with older age and a lower body mass index. Therefore, careful consideration of these risk factors is needed when including inhaled corticosteroids as maintenance therapy for patients with COPD. Given the potential side effects associated with inhaled corticosteroid use and the absence of evidence of its benefits when used alone, the available findings suggest that inhaled corticosteroids alone are not recommended for use in patients with COPD.

Collectively, lung and airway inflammation play a central role in the development of COPD. Thus, pharmacologic interventions aimed at reducing or reversing inflammation could be effective for treating patients with stable COPD. Inhaled corticosteroids can reduce pulmonary inflammation by binding to glucocorticoid receptors within the airways. Although studies suggest a reduction in the rate of exacerbation and dyspnea in response to inhaled corticosteroids, their routine use as a single, stand-alone therapy is not recommended for managing patients with stable COPD due to minimal benefits and the association of their prolonged use with increased risks of severe pneumonia. Further studies are needed to explore the survival benefits of inhaled corticosteroids for people with stable COPD.

Combined Dual Therapy with LABAs and Inhaled Corticosteroids for Stable COPD

Studies have shown that an inhaled corticosteroids alone do not improve lung function or reduce exacerbation rates [34–37], probably due to corticosteroid resistance in COPD [40]. Interestingly, *in vitro* studies suggest that the addition of LABAs to inhaled corticosteroids may facilitate corticosteroid sensitivity in COPD [40]. These observations are supported by evidence from randomized control trials demonstrating that the use of inhaled corticosteroids combined with LABAs can reduce exacerbation rates [41–45]. Furthermore, it has been suggested that COPD individuals with increased levels of blood eosinophils (≥ 300 cells/μl) are most likely to benefit from the addition of inhaled corticosteroids to LABAs [46]. A summary of the commonly used combinations of acting β2 agonist agents and inhaled corticosteroids for patients with COPD can be found in Table 5.

Table 5. Commonly used combinations of LABA agents and inhaled corticosteroids for patients with COPD

Combined LABAs and inhaled corticosteroids			
Generic Name	Brand name	Type of Inhaler	Duration of action
Formoterol and Beclomethasone	Fostair	MDI, DPI	12 hours
Salmeterol and Fluticasone propionate	Advair	MDI, DPI	12 hours
Formoterol and Budesonide	Symbicort	MDI, DPI	12 hours
Formoterol and Mometasone	Dulera	MDI	12 hours
Vilanterol and Fluticasone furoate	Breo Ellipta	DPI	24 hours

MDI = Metered dose inhaler.
DPI = Dry Powder Inhaler.

A meta-analysis combining data from 19 randomized and double-blind studies with 10,400 participants demonstrated that combined inhaled corticosteroids and LABAs is more effective than the use of inhaled corticosteroids alone for improving lung function and health status and reducing exacerbation [47], although increased risk of pneumonia is also observed with the combined use of inhaled corticosteroids and LABAs. It should be noted that pneumonia symptoms resulting from the addition of inhaled corticosteroids to LABAs did not lead to hospital admission in patients with stable COPD. These observations strongly support the international GOLD recommendation that inhaled corticosteroids combined with LABAs should be initiated for COPD patients with increased levels of blood eosinophils (≥ 300 cells/μl) who have experienced 2 or more exacerbations of COPD per year and have a history of frequent hospitalizations as a result of COPD exacerbations. Limited evidence suggests the initiation of inhaled corticosteroids combined with LABAs if blood eosinophil levels are < 300 cells/μl to ≥ 100 cells/μl. It should be noted that the international GOLD guidelines do not recommend the use of inhaled corticosteroids combined with LABAs if levels of blood eosinophils are less than 100 cells/μl).

In summary, although the currently available evidence does not support the use of inhaled corticosteroid monotherapy due to unproven benefits and the association of its use with an increased risk of pneumonia, several lines of evidence suggest that certain subtypes of COPD may benefit from the addition of LABAs to inhaled corticosteroids. A summary of the available combined corticosteroids and LABAs in one inhaler can be found in Table 5. Further prospective head-to-head comparative evidence is needed to assess the risks and benefits of the different available combinations of LABAs and inhaled corticosteroids.

Triple Therapy with LABAs, LAMAs and Inhaled Corticosteroids for Stable COPD

Given the positive effects on lung function and COPD symptoms of using LAMAs as single therapies [12] and dual-inhaler therapy containing inhaled corticosteroids and LAMAs [41–45], triple therapy has been developed for administration with a single device. Single-inhaler triple therapy with an inhaled glucocorticoid, a LAMA, and a LABA has been developed. Details of these medications are provided in Table 6.

Table 6. Commonly used triple combination therapy with LABAs, LAMAs and inhaled corticosteroids for patients with COPD

Triple combination therapy with LABAs, LAMAs, and inhaled corticosteroids			
Generic Name	Brand name	Type of Inhaler	Duration of action
Formoterol, Glycopyrronium and Beclomethasone	Trimbow	MDI	24 hours
Formoterol, Glycopyrronium and Budesonide	Breztri	MDI	12 hours
Vilanterol, Umeclidinium and Fluticasone furoate	Trelegy Ellipta	DPI	24 hours

MDI = Metered dose inhaler.
DPI = Dry Powder Inhaler.

The addition of a LABA to a LAMA and an inhaled glucocorticoid is indicated for use in patients with COPD who require additional bronchodilation for relief of airflow obstruction. The international GOLD recommendation is for the use of this triple therapy for COPD patients with a history of frequent hospitalization due to COPD exacerbation, despite the use of dual LABA + LAMA or LABA + inhaled corticosteroid inhaler therapy.

Evidence from a large, randomized trial involving 10,355 patients with COPD demonstrated that single-inhaler triple therapy (using combined fluticasone furoate, umeclidinium, and vilanterol) can reduce the rate of moderate or severe COPD exacerbation and improve lung function and overall quality of life compared with dual therapy (fluticasone furoate + vilanterol) or (umeclidinium + vilanterol) [48]. This observation is further supported by a recent randomized trial that investigated the efficacy and safety of triple-inhaler therapy compared with dual-inhaler therapy. The trial showed that triple-inhaler therapy (with budesonide, glycopyrrolate, and formoterol) at two dose levels of inhaled corticosteroids (a 160 μg and a 320 μg dose) reduced the rate of moderate or severe COPD exacerbation compared with a glycopyrrolate–formoterol or budesonide–formoterol combination [49]. More importantly, a large one-year randomized controlled trial showed a significant reduction in all-cause mortality risk in COPD patients who used triple-inhaler therapy (with fluticasone furoate/umeclidinium/vilanterol) compared with dual-inhaler therapy using a LABA and a LAMA (umeclidinium/vilanterol) [50].

Together, the available evidence strongly suggests that the use of fixed-dose combinations of LABAs, LAMAs, and inhaled corticosteroids not only improves lung function and reduces COPD symptoms and exacerbation rates, but also has the potential to improve survival rates in patients with COPD. Although the international GOLD recommendation is for the use of triple therapy as a backup when other dual therapies fail to improve COPD symptoms, the promising effect of triple-inhaler therapy suggests that triple therapy should be considered as a first-line therapy for patients with COPD. Further investigations are needed to determine whether other specific patient subgroups demonstrate better survival rates.

Phosphodiesterase-4 (PDE4) Inhibitors and Stable COPD

Phosphodiesterase (PDE) enzymes (PDE1 to PDE11) are known to catalyze the hydrolytic degradation of cAMP and cyclic guanosine monophosphate (cGMP). Among these PDE enzymes, preclinical studies have shown that PDE4 is mainly expressed in airway smooth muscle in response to inflammation [51, 52]. Selective inhibition of this enzyme (PDE4) exhibits functional antagonism to bronchoconstriction and has anti-inflammatory properties by increasing levels of cAMP. It is generally accepted that increasing cAMP levels serves as a therapeutic option for managing severe COPD.

Two placebo-controlled, double-blind, multicenter trials involving 1,391 patients indicated that the use of selective PDE4 roflumilast can improve lung function and reduce exacerbation rates [53]. Additionally, the effect of roflumilast in combination with long-acting bronchodilators, such as LAMAs/LABAs, has been assessed, and the findings showed that dual-inhaler therapy with roflumilast and a LAMA or LABA can improve lung function in patients with moderate to severe COPD [54]. Moreover, the use of roflumilast led to reduced hospital admissions but frequent COPD exacerbations. A similar effect was observed with the addition of inhaled corticosteroids to roflumilast and long-acting bronchodilators [55]. However, increased risk of pneumonia was the most frequently reported serious side effect associated with the use of roflumilast combined with inhaled corticosteroids [55], probably due to inhaled corticosteroids. It should also be noted that some other side effects were observed with the use of roflumilast alone or in combination with LABAs and LAMAs, including nausea, diarrhea, weight loss, depression, and headache [53, 54]. Therefore, the international GOLD recommendation is to use roflumilast with caution in underweight patients and/or those with depression.

Collectively, the use of the selective PDE4 inhibitor roflumilast increases the intracellular second messenger cAMP, leading to bronchodilatory and anti-inflammatory effects. Given that roflumilast is administered orally, its use can reduce both systemic and pulmonary inflammation in patients with COPD. However, since there are several adverse effects of using systemic therapies, including roflumilast, their use is currently limited to patients with severe COPD who are likely to gain the greatest clinical benefit.

Methylxanthines and Stable COPD

Theophylline (the most commonly used methylxanthine) induces the relaxation of smooth muscle in the airways by increasing cAMP levels via the inhibition of PDE enzymes. Besides its bronchodilatory properties, oral administration of theophylline has been shown to reduce the number of inflammatory cells in the sputum of patients with COPD [56], suggesting that theophylline can also exert anti-inflammatory effects.

Several systematic reviews and meta-analyses of randomized controlled trials have assessed the effectiveness of oral theophylline in patients with stable COPD [57–59]. The findings suggested that the use of oral theophylline can improve lung function [57–59], arterial blood gas results [57, 59], and physical activity [57] in patients with clinically stable COPD. It has also been shown that the addition of oral theophylline to the LAMA agent tiotropium can improve both lung function and the symptoms and general health of patients with stable COPD [60]. Similarly, a randomized, double-blind, double-dummy, parallel-group trial, including 943 patients with COPD, concluded that oral theophylline as an add-on therapy to the LABA agent salmeterol can improve pulmonary function and reduce COPD exacerbation rates [61]. These findings support the addition of oral theophylline, a LABA, and a LAMA to reduce exacerbation rates and improve quality of life in patients with stable COPD. However, since the use of theophylline is generally associated with some adverse effects, including but not limited to nausea, loss of appetite, and vomiting [62], its use should always be weighed against the risk of adverse effects.

In contrast, a multicenter, pragmatic, double-blind, randomized, placebo-controlled clinical trial, including 1,578 patients, reported that the use of oral theophylline with inhaled corticosteroids failed to improve lung function, mortality, breathlessness, and quality of life [63]. Consistent with this finding, a recent systematic review and meta-analysis of seven randomized controlled trials involving 47,556 participants demonstrated that oral theophylline as an add-on therapy to inhaled corticosteroids increased hospitalization rates and mortality and failed to reduce exacerbation rates [64]. These observations suggest that combined inhaled corticosteroids and oral theophylline should not be recommended for managing patients with stable COPD.

In summary, theophylline (a nonselective inhibitor of PDE enzymes) has long been used to treat bronchospasm and airway inflammation in patients with chronic respiratory diseases, including COPD, because it is known to exert both bronchodilatory and anti-inflammatory effects. Although the current evidence does not support the use of oral theophylline in addition to inhaled corticosteroids in patients with clinically stable COPD, improved lung function and reduced exacerbation rates have been reported in patients with stable COPD in response to oral theophylline use, either alone or combined with bronchodilators such as LABAs and LAMAs.

Conclusion

COPD is associated with chronic airway and lung inflammation, which causes progressive obstruction of the airways and destruction of the lung parenchyma. These physiological changes eventually lead to frequent hospitalization as a result of worsening pulmonary symptoms. Generally, management of these pulmonary symptoms can be achieved using pharmacologic and nonpharmacologic interventions. Of the pharmacologic therapies, the best available evidence to date suggests bronchodilators (LABAs and LAMAs, either alone or in combination) for use as first-line maintenance treatments for patients with symptomatic COPD. Controversy continues regarding the effects of inhaled corticosteroids. Although the international GOLD recommendation is not to use inhaled corticosteroids as a single, stand-alone therapy, mainly due to unproven benefits and an increased risk of developing pneumonia, early evidence from *in vitro* studies suggests that combining LABAs with corticosteroids may reduce corticosteroid resistance. Given the key role of lung and airway inflammation in the development of COPD, further investigations are required to evaluate the efficacy of inhaled corticosteroids and other medications with anti-inflammatory properties in managing patients with stable COPD.

Key Points

- Both LAMA and LABA agents are effective in the management of COPD symptoms. However, studies demonstrate superiority of LAMAs over LABAs for the prevention of exacerbation in patients with stable COPD, likely due to the ability of LAMA agents to suppress neutrophilic airway inflammation.
- Studies suggest that dual combination therapy of LAMA and LABA agents can reduce COPD exacerbation rates and dyspnea and improve health status and lung function in patients with stable COPD as compared with individual drugs used alone.
- Inhaled corticosteroids alone are not recommended as long-term maintenance therapies to control the symptoms of patients with COPD due to unproven benefits and increased risk of adverse events.
- Although the use of inhaled corticosteroids alone is not recommended for patients with stable COPD, there is evidence to suggest that fixed-dose combinations of LABAs, LAMAs, and inhaled corticosteroids can reduce COPD symptoms and exacerbation rates and improve survival rates in patients with COPD.

References

[1] Alqahtani, JS, Njoku, CM, Bereznicki, B, Wimmer, BC, Peterson, GM, Kinsman, L, Aldabayan, YS, Alrajeh, AM, Aldhahir, AM, Mandal, S, & Hurst, JR. Risk factors for all-cause hospital readmission following exacerbation of COPD: a systematic review and meta-analysis. *Eur Respir Rev.* 2020;29(156).

[2] Kistemaker LE, Oenema TA, Meurs H, Gosens R. Regulation of airway inflammation and remodeling by muscarinic receptors: perspectives on anticholinergic therapy in asthma and COPD. *Life Sci.* 2012;91(21-22):1126-33.

[3] Roffel AF, Elzinga CR, Zaagsma J. Muscarinic M3 receptors mediate contraction of human central and peripheral airway smooth muscle. *Pulm Pharmacol.* 1990;3(1):47-51.

[4] Gosens R, Zaagsma J, Meurs H, Halayko AJ. Muscarinic receptor signaling in the pathophysiology of asthma and COPD. *Respir Res.* 2006;7:73.

[5] Mak JC, Baraniuk JN, Barnes PJ. Localization of muscarinic receptor subtype mRNAs in human lung. *Am J Respir Cell Mol Biol.* 1992;7(3):344-8.

[6] Ikeda, T, Anisuzzaman, A, Yoshiki, H, Sasaki, M, Koshiji, T, Uwada, J, Nishimune, A, Itoh, H, & Muramatsu, I. Regional quantification of muscarinic acetylcholine receptors and beta-adrenoceptors in human airways. *Br J Pharmacol.* 2012;166(6):1804-14.

[7] Gosens R, Gross N. The mode of action of anticholinergics in asthma. *Eur Respir J.* 2018;52(4).

[8] Buels KS, Fryer AD. Muscarinic receptor antagonists: effects on pulmonary function. *Handb Exp Pharmacol.* 2012(208):317-41.

[9] Scullion JE. The development of anticholinergics in the management of COPD. *International Journal of Chronic Obstructive Pulmonary Disease.* 2007;2(1):33-40.

[10] Barnes PJ. Tiotropium bromide. *Expert Opin Investig Drugs.* 2001;10(4):733-40.

[11] Vogelmeier, C, Hederer, B, Glaab, T, Schmidt, H, Rutten-van Mölken, MPMH, Beeh, KM, Rabe, KF, & Fabbri, LM. Tiotropium versus salmeterol for the prevention of exacerbations of COPD. *The New England Journal of Medicine.* 2011;364(12):1093-103.

[12] Karner C, Chong J, Poole P. Tiotropium versus placebo for chronic obstructive pulmonary disease. *Cochrane Database Syst Rev.* 2014(7):CD009285.

[13] Decramer, ML, Chapman, KR, Dahl, R, Frith, P, Devouassoux, G, Fritscher, C, Cameron, R, Shoaib, M, Lawrence, D, Young, D, & McBryan, D. Once-daily indacaterol versus tiotropium for patients with severe chronic obstructive pulmonary disease (INVIGORATE): a randomised, blinded, parallel-group study. *Lancet Respir Med.* 2013;1(7):524-33.

[14] Kesten S, Casaburi R, Kukafka D, Cooper CB. Improvement in self-reported exercise participation with the combination of tiotropium and rehabilitative exercise training in COPD patients. *International Journal of Chronic Obstructive Pulmonary Disease.* 2008;3(1):127-36.

[15] Casaburi R, Kukafka D, Cooper CB, Witek TJ, Jr., Kesten S. Improvement in exercise tolerance with the combination of tiotropium and pulmonary rehabilitation in patients with COPD. *Chest.* 2005; 127(3):809-17.

[16] Koarai, A, Sugiura, H, Yamada, M, Ichikawa, T, Fujino, N, Kawayama, T, & Ichinose, M. Treatment with LABA versus LAMA for stable COPD: a systematic review and meta-analysis. *BMC Pulm Med.* 2020;20(1):111.

[17] Chen, W-C, Huang, C-H, Sheu, C-C, Chong, I-W, Chu, K-A, Chen, Y-C, Tsai, J-R, Lee, C-H, & Wei, Y-F. Long-acting beta2-agonists versus long-acting muscarinic antagonists in patients with stable COPD: A systematic review and meta-analysis of randomized controlled trials. *Respirology.* 2017;22(7):1313-9.

[18] Wollin L, Pieper MP. Tiotropium bromide exerts anti-inflammatory activity in a cigarette smoke mouse model of COPD. *Pulm Pharmacol Ther.* 2010;23(4):345-54.

[19] Suzaki I, Asano K, Shikama Y, Hamasaki T, Kanei A, Suzaki H. Suppression of IL-8 production from airway cells by tiotropium bromide in vitro. *International Journal of Chronic Obstructive Pulmonary Disease.* 2011;6:439-48.

[20] Nie M, Knox AJ, Pang L. beta2-Adrenoceptor agonists, like glucocorticoids, repress eotaxin gene transcription by selective inhibition of histone H4 acetylation. *J Immunol.* 2005;175(1):478-86.

[21] Pang L, Knox AJ. Synergistic inhibition by beta(2)-agonists and corticosteroids on tumor necrosis factor-alpha-induced interleukin-8 release from cultured human airway smooth-muscle cells. *Am J Respir Cell Mol Biol.* 2000;23(1):79-85.

[22] Pang L, Knox AJ. Regulation of TNF-alpha-induced eotaxin release from cultured human airway smooth muscle cells by beta2-agonists and corticosteroids. *FASEB J.* 2001;15(1):261-9.

[23] Kew KM, Mavergames C, Walters JA. Long-acting beta2-agonists for chronic obstructive pulmonary disease. *Cochrane Database Syst Rev.* 2013(10):CD010177.

[24] Donohue JF, Betts KA, Du EX, Altman P, Goyal P, Keininger DL, Gruenberger JB, Signorovitch JE. Comparative efficacy of long-acting beta2-agonists as monotherapy for chronic obstructive pulmonary disease: a network meta-analysis. *International Journal of Chronic Obstructive Pulmonary Disease.* 2017;12:367-81.

[25] In chronic obstructive pulmonary disease, a combination of ipratropium and albuterol is more effective than either agent alone. An 85-day multicenter trial. *COMBIVENT Inhalation Aerosol Study Group. Chest.* 1994;105(5):1411-9.

[26] Gross N, Tashkin D, Miller R, Oren J, Coleman W, Linberg S. Inhalation by nebulization of albuterol-ipratropium combination (Dey combination) is superior to either agent alone in the treatment of chronic obstructive pulmonary disease. *Dey Combination Solution Study Group. Respiration.* 1998;65(5):354-62.

[27] Ray R, Tombs L, Naya I, Compton C, Lipson DA, Boucot I. Efficacy and safety of the dual bronchodilator combination umeclidinium/vilanterol in COPD by age and airflow limitation severity: A pooled post hoc analysis of seven clinical trials. *Pulm Pharmacol Ther.* 2019;57:101802.

[28] Ni H, Moe S, Soe Z, Myint KT, Viswanathan KN. Combined aclidinium bromide and long-acting beta2-agonist for chronic obstructive pulmonary disease (COPD). *Cochrane Database Syst Rev.* 2018;12: CD011594.

[29] Maqsood, U, Ho, TN, Palmer, K, Eccles, FJ, Munavvar, M, Wang, R, Crossingham, I, & Evans, DJ. Once daily long-acting beta2-agonists and long-acting muscarinic antagonists in a combined inhaler versus placebo for chronic obstructive pulmonary disease. *Cochrane Database Syst Rev.* 2019; 3:CD012930.

[30] Walters JA, Tan DJ, White CJ, Gibson PG, Wood-Baker R, Walters EH. Systemic corticosteroids for acute exacerbations of chronic obstructive pulmonary disease. *Cochrane Database Syst Rev.* 2014 (9):CD001288.

[31] Paggiaro PL, Dahle R, Bakran I, Frith L, Hollingworth K, Efthimiou J. Multicentre randomised placebo-controlled trial of inhaled fluticasone propionate in patients with chronic obstructive pulmonary disease. International COPD Study Group. *Lancet.* 1998;351(9105):773-80.

[32] Thompson, AB, Mueller, MB, Heires, AJ, Bohling, TL, Daughton, D, Yancey, SW, Sykes, RS, & Rennard, SI. Aerosolized beclomethasone in chronic bronchitis. Improved pulmonary function and diminished airway inflammation. *Am Rev Respir Dis.* 1992;146(2):389-95.

[33] Sin DD, McAlister FA, Man SF, Anthonisen NR. Contemporary management of chronic obstructive pulmonary disease: scientific review. *JAMA.* 2003;290(17):2301-12.

[34] Soriano, JB, Sin, DD, Zhang, X, Camp, PG, Anderson, JA, Anthonisen, NR, Buist, AS, Burge, PS, Calverley, PM, Connett, JE, Petersson, S, Postma, DS, Szafranski, W, & Vestbo, J. A pooled analysis of FEV1 decline in COPD patients randomized to inhaled corticosteroids or placebo. *Chest.* 2007;131(3):682-9.

[35] Highland KB, Strange C, Heffner JE. Long-term effects of inhaled corticosteroids on FEV1 in patients with chronic obstructive pulmonary disease. A meta-analysis. *Ann Intern Med.* 2003;138(12):969-73.

[36] Burge PS, Calverley PM, Jones PW, Spencer S, Anderson JA, Maslen TK. Randomised, double blind, placebo controlled study of fluticasone propionate in patients with moderate to severe chronic obstructive pulmonary disease: the ISOLDE trial. *BMJ.* 2000;320(7245):1297-303.

[37] Lung Health Study Research G, Wise R, Connett J, Weinmann G, Scanlon P, Skeans M. Effect of inhaled triamcinolone on the decline in pulmonary function in chronic obstructive pulmonary disease. *The New England journal of medicine.* 2000;343(26):1902-9.

[38] Drummond MB, Dasenbrook EC, Pitz MW, Murphy DJ, Fan E. Inhaled corticosteroids in patients with stable chronic obstructive pulmonary disease: a systematic review and meta-analysis. *JAMA.* 2008;300(20):2407-16.

[39] Yang IA, Clarke MS, Sim EH, Fong KM. Inhaled corticosteroids for stable chronic obstructive pulmonary disease. *Cochrane Database Syst Rev.* 2012(7):CD002991.

[40] Barnes PJ. New anti-inflammatory targets for chronic obstructive pulmonary disease. *Nat Rev Drug Discov.* 2013;12(7):543-59.

[41] Szafranski, W, Cukier, A, Ramirez, A, Menga, G, Sansores, R, Nahabedian, S, Peterson, S, & Olsson, H. Efficacy and safety of budesonide/formoterol in the management of chronic obstructive pulmonary disease. *Eur Respir J.* 2003;21(1):74-81.

[42] Calverley PM, Boonsawat W, Cseke Z, Zhong N, Peterson S, Olsson H. Maintenance therapy with budesonide and formoterol in chronic obstructive pulmonary disease. *Eur Respir J.* 2003;22(6):912-9.

[43] Calverley, PMA, Kuna, P, Monsó, E, Costantini, M, Petruzzelli, S, Sergio, F, Varoli, G, Papi, A, & Brusasco, V. Beclomethasone/formoterol in the management of COPD: a randomised controlled trial. *Respir Med.* 2010;104(12):1858-68.

[44] Kardos P, Wencker M, Glaab T, Vogelmeier C. Impact of salmeterol/fluticasone propionate versus salmeterol on exacerbations in severe chronic obstructive pulmonary disease. *Am J Respir Crit Care Med.* 2007;175(2):144-9.

[45] Ferguson GT, Anzueto A, Fei R, Emmett A, Knobil K, Kalberg C. Effect of fluticasone propionate/salmeterol (250/50 microg) or salmeterol (50 microg) on COPD exacerbations. *Respir Med.* 2008;102(8):1099-108.

[46] Agusti, A, Fabbri, LM, Singh, D, Vestbo, J, Celli, B, Franssen, FME, Rabe, KF, & Papi, A. Inhaled corticosteroids in COPD: friend or foe? *Eur Respir J.* 2018;52(6).

[47] Nannini LJ, Poole P, Milan SJ, Holmes R, Normansell R. Combined corticosteroid and long-acting beta(2)-agonist in one inhaler versus placebo for chronic obstructive pulmonary disease. *Cochrane Database Syst Rev.* 2013(11):CD003794.

[48] Lipson, DA, Barnhart, F, Brealey, N, Brooks, J, Criner, GJ, Day, NC, Dransfield, MT, Halpin, DMG, Han, MK, Jones, CE, Kilbride, S, Lange, P, Lomas, DA, Martinez, FJ, Singh, D, Tabberer, M, Wise, RA, & Pascoe, SJ. Once-Daily Single-Inhaler Triple versus Dual Therapy in Patients with COPD. T*he New England Journal of Medicine.* 2018;378(18):1671-80.

[49] Rabe, KF, Martinez, FJ, Ferguson, GT, Wang, C, Singh, D, Wedzicha, JA, Trivedi, R, St. Rose, E, Ballal, S, McLaren, J, Darken, P, Aurivillius, M, Reisner, C, & Dorinsky, P. Triple-inhaler Therapy at Two Glucocorticoid Doses in Moderate-to-Very-Severe COPD. *The New England Journal of Medicine.* 2020;383(1):35-48.

[50] Lipson, David A, Courtney Crim, Gerard J Criner, Nicola C Day, Mark T Dransfield, David M G Halpin, MeiLan K Han, C Elaine Jones, Sally Kilbride, Peter Lange, David A Lomas, Sally Lettis, Pamela Manchester, Neil Martin, Dawn Midwinter, Andrea Morris, Steven J Pascoe, Dave Singh, Robert A Wise, Fernando J Martinez. Reduction in All-Cause Mortality with Fluticasone Furoate/Umeclidinium/ Vilanterol in Patients with Chronic Obstructive Pulmonary Disease. *Am J Respir Crit Care Med.* 2020;201(12):1508-16.

[51] Mehats C, Jin SL, Wahlstrom J, Law E, Umetsu DT, Conti M. PDE4D plays a critical role in the control of airway smooth muscle contraction. *FASEB J.* 2003;17(13):1831-41.

[52] Barnette MS. Phosphodiesterase 4 (PDE4) inhibitors in asthma and chronic obstructive pulmonary disease (COPD). *Prog Drug Res.* 1999;53:193-229.

[53] Calverley, PM, Rabe, KF, Goehring, U-M, Kristiansen, S, Fabbri, LM, & Martinez, FJ. Roflumilast in symptomatic chronic obstructive pulmonary disease: two randomised clinical trials. *Lancet.* 2009;374 (9691):685-94.

[54] Fabbri, LM, Calverley, PM, Izquierdo-Alonso, JL, Bundschuh, DS, Brose, M, Martinez, FJ, & Rabe, KF. Roflumilast in moderate-to-severe chronic obstructive pulmonary disease treated with longacting bronchodilators: two randomised clinical trials. *Lancet.* 2009;374(9691):695-703.

[55] Martinez FJ, Calverley PM, Goehring UM, Brose M, Fabbri LM, Rabe KF. Effect of roflumilast on exacerbations in patients with severe chronic obstructive pulmonary disease uncontrolled by combination therapy (REACT): a multicenter randomised controlled trial. *Lancet.* 2015;385(9971):857-66.

[56] Hirano, T, T Yamagata, M Gohda, Y Yamagata, T Ichikawa, S Yanagisawa, K Ueshima, K Akamatsu, M Nakanishi, K Matsunaga, Y Minakata, and M Ichinose. Inhibition of reactive nitrogen species production in COPD airways: comparison of inhaled corticosteroid and oral theophylline. *Thorax.* 2006;61(9):761-6.

[57] Ram, FS, Jones, P, Jardim, J, Castro, AA, Atallah, ÁN, Lacasse, Y, Goldstein, R, & Cendon, S. Oral theophylline for chronic obstructive pulmonary disease. *Cochrane Database Syst Rev.* 2002(4): CD003902.

[58] Molfino NA, Zhang P. A meta-analysis on the efficacy of oral theophylline in patients with stable COPD. *International Journal of Chronic Obstructive Pulmonary Disease.* 2006;1(3):261-6.

[59] Ram, FSF, Jardin, JR, Atallah, A, Castro, AA, Mazzini, R, Goldstein, R, Lacasse, Y, & Cendon, S. Efficacy of theophylline in people with stable chronic obstructive pulmonary disease: a systematic review and meta-analysis. *Respir Med.* 2005;99(2):135-44.

[60] Xiong XF, Fan LL, Wu HX, Zhu M, Cheng DY. Effects of Tiotropium Combined with Theophylline on Stable COPD Patients of Group B, D and its Impact on Small Airway Function: A Randomized Controlled Trial. *Adv Ther.* 2018;35(12):2201-13.

[61] ZuWallack, RL, Mahler, DA, Reilly, D, Church, N, Emmett, A, Rickard, K, & Knobil, K. Salmeterol plus theophylline combination therapy in the treatment of COPD. *Chest.* 2001;119(6):1661-70.

[62] Ohta, K, Fukuchi, Y, Grouse, L, Mizutani, R, Rabe, KF, Rennard, SI, & Zhong, N-S. A prospective clinical study of theophylline safety in 3810 elderly with asthma or COPD. *Respir Med.* 2004; 98(10):1016-24.

[63] Devereux, G, Cotton, S, Fielding, S, McMeekin, N, Barnes, PJ, Briggs, A, Burns, G, Chaudhuri, R, Chrystyn, H, Davies, L, Soyza, AD, Gompertz, S, Haughney, J, Innes, K, Kaniewska, J, Lee, A, Morice, A, Norrie, J, Sullivan, A, Price, D. Low-dose oral theophylline combined with inhaled corticosteroids for people with chronic obstructive pulmonary disease and high risk of exacerbations: a RCT. *Health Technol Assess.* 2019;23(37):1-146.

[64] Shuai, T, Zhang, C, Zhang, M, Wang, Y, Xiong, H, Huang, Q, & Liu, J. Low-dose theophylline in addition to ICS therapy in COPD patients: A systematic review and meta-analysis. *PLoS One.* 2021;16(5):e0251348.

Chapter 16

Palliative and End-of-Life Care in COPD

Rosana Mara da Silva[1,*] and Thales Cantelle Baggio[2,†]
[1]Municipal Health Department,
Estácio de Sá University Medical School,
Jaraguá do Sul (SC), Brazil
[2]Hospital Jaraguá and Hospital São José,
Estácio de Sá University Medical School,
Jaraguá do Sul (SC), Brazil

Abstract

Palliative and end-of-life care focuses on preventing and alleviating suffering through early identification, assessment and treatment of all physical, psychosocial and spiritual issues that affect the patient and their families. Chronic obstructive pulmonary disease (COPD) is characterized as a chronic and progressive disorder that, in its advanced stages, can be associated with significant physical, psychological and social damage. Patients with advanced COPD should receive palliative care to improve their quality of life and that of their families. A problem that makes care difficult is based on establishing a prognosis, making it necessary for the team to educate patients about palliative care, in addition to understanding and respecting their preferences. The end-of-life period for COPD patients is characterized by a progressive decline in health status, increasing symptoms, and greater dependence on family and caregivers to perform daily activities, such as personal hygiene and self-care. The role of palliative and end-of-life care must have an approach that focuses on managing symptoms, maintaining quality of life, and good communication between physician and patient, and family.

Keywords: chronic obstructive pulmonary disease, communication, end-of-life care, palliative care, doctor patient relationship, quality of life

Introduction

The presence of acute or chronic respiratory failure is often seen as a terminal phase of chronic obstructive pulmonary disease (COPD). Palliative care is a practice observed with these

* Corresponding Author's Email: rosanamara.fisio@gmail.com.
† Corresponding Author's Email: thalesbaggio@gmail.com.

In: Chronic Obstructive Pulmonary Disease
Editor: Jaber S. Alqahtani
ISBN: 979-8-88697-333-4

patients [1]. Within medical practice, there is a need for a clear discussion on early decision making about the management of acute respiratory failure. Several studies point to the need to start palliative care earlier, together with curative and restorative care, when there is an increase in the intensity of symptoms [1, 2, 3]. Patients eligible for palliative care are those who complain of shortness of breath, pain, fatigue and depression, which in some studies represented a prevalence much higher than 50% [1].

Palliative care focuses on preventing and alleviating suffering through early identification and impeccable assessment and treatment of all physical, psychosocial and spiritual issues that affect the patient and their families [4, 5, 6]. All palliative care provided in the last 12 months of life is considered to be end-of-life care, that is, the last phase of palliative care [6, 7]. However, the difficult prognosis in COPD and the correct identification of patients who are likely to die within 6 months represent a major barrier to early palliative care delivery [6, 8].

Palliative and End-of-Life Care in COPD

The World Health Organization (WHO) defines palliative care as "the total active care of patients whose disease does not respond to curative treatment" [2, 4, 5, 9], a definition that certainly describes the care of patients with COPD. The WHO states that this type of care should include "an approach that improves the quality of life of patients and their families" [2, 5]. Suffering relief must also include effective communication between physician and staff, and must be patient- and family-centered, identifying patient care goals, shared decision-making, and advance care planning [9].

Chronic obstructive pulmonary disease (COPD) is characterized as a chronic [6] and progressive disorder, with persistent airflow obstruction, progressive dyspnea and chronic productive cough, which in its advanced stages can be associated with significant physical, psychological and social damage [10]. It is associated with anxiety, depression, lack of energy, anorexia and restricted mobility [2, 4]. People suffering from life-threatening illnesses such as advanced COPD should receive palliative care to improve their quality of life and that of their families [2, 4, 5].

Gore et al. report in their study that patients with end-stage COPD suffer from several severe symptoms, such as shortness of breath, anxiety and depression; only a small proportion of these patients receive palliative care and social support; with a high prevalence of mortality in Intensive Care Units due to aggressive treatments [10]. Based on this condition, and recognizing the difficulties of establishing a prognosis, it is up to the team to educate patients about palliative care and understand and respect their preferences [2, 8].

The end of life for people who die from COPD is characterized by their last month's often having a progressive decline in health status, increasing symptoms and greater dependence on family and caregivers to perform daily activities, such as personal hygiene and self-care [11]. The role of palliative and end-of-life care must have an approach that focuses on managing symptoms, maintaining quality of life, and good communication.

The Role of the Team in Palliative and End-of-Life Care

Doctor-patient communication about prognosis, preferences for life-sustaining treatments, and palliative care are essential to ensure that COPD patients receive quality care at the end of life.

The uncertain trajectory of the disease, which often involves unexpected deterioration of health status, makes advance care planning essential [12].

Palliative care should be provided with the aim of reducing the high burden of chronically debilitating symptoms such as dyspnea and anxiety. Healthcare professionals should consider patients' opinions and preferences when developing treatment escalation plans, emergency and resuscitation decisions, and palliative care interventions [2, 8].

Tavares et al. [2], Curtis [13] and Hansen-Flaschen [14] report that physicians should be encouraged to identify patients with COPD for whom discussions about treatment preferences or end-of-life care are especially important. This profile may include an assessment of forced expiratory volume in one second (FEV_1) <30% predicted; oxygen dependence; one or more hospital admissions in the previous year for an acute exacerbation of COPD; left heart failure or other comorbidities; weight loss or cachexia; decreased functional status; increasing dependence on others; and age >70 years. The presence of two or more of these prognostic indicators should be a reason for such discussions. Several criteria increase the relevance and urgency of the discussion, as they increase the risk of a life-threatening exacerbation and of receiving end-of-life care that is not consistent with informed treatment preferences.

Even when given optimal medical therapy, many COPD patients continue to experience distressing dyspnea and fatigue and often suffer from insomnia, panic, anxiety, and depression. Palliative approaches to these symptoms are effective and their use should not be restricted to end-of-life situations. It is entirely logical to introduce palliative care together with therapies aimed at correcting underlying pathophysiological abnormalities and reducing the risk of exacerbations [11].

For Halpin [11] and Andreas and Alt-Epping [15] the use of opiates and non-invasive ventilation (NIV) alleviate the sensation of shortness of breath. The use of oxygen therapy provides relief to the patient and an integrated multidisciplinary approach (physiotherapy, nursing, occupational therapy, psychology, speech therapy) to palliative and respiratory care helps to minimize dyspnea and fatigue, as well as allowing the adaptation of activities of daily living. Anxiety and depression can be reduced by appropriate pharmacotherapy and psychological therapy and mind-body interventions (mindfulness, yoga and relaxation).

Planning Palliative and End-of-Life Care for COPD Patients

Palliative care has a lot to offer for people living with advanced COPD and includes more than just terminal care. It involves attention to the emotional, spiritual and practical needs of patients and their families, including determining their opinions about future care through advance directives of will [11].

While the ability to use palliative and end-of-life approaches should be part of the skills of all clinicians dealing with people with COPD, patients also benefit from being referred to specialist palliative care teams, whose multidisciplinary approach can improve the patient's quality of life. Referral needs to be discussed sensitively with patients, with an emphasis on positive aspects of the palliative care specialist's contribution, such as help with symptom control and family support [6, 9, 11, 13].

Communication between physician, patient, family, and caregivers is extremely important to establish palliative and end-of-life care for the patient with COPD. Understanding that the care plan and the need for integration with the multidisciplinary team provides the integration of care and quality of life for the patient. An important point to understand in building this plan is that even when receiving optimal medical therapy, many COPD patients continue to experience distressing shortness of breath and fatigue and often suffer from insomnia, panic, anxiety, and depression, and that medication use will help so that these issues do not exacerbate [11, 15].

Palliative approaches to these symptoms are effective and their use should not be restricted to end-of-life situations. It is entirely logical to introduce palliative care alongside therapies aimed at correcting underlying pathophysiological abnormalities and reducing the risk of exacerbations.

Physiotherapy, working in rehabilitation and respiratory care, aims to integrate palliative care and provide support and adaptation, together with the multidisciplinary team, the active restorative care and activities of daily living, promoting quality of life for patients, families and caregivers.

Tavares et al. [11] report that conversations with patients should be initiated early in the course of the disease or opportunities to initiate discussions and treatment planning should be identified and this will help to build a therapeutic relationship with the patient.

These opportunities/triggers can be:

- The presence of cor pulmonale;
- The need for mechanical ventilation in the previous year;
- Arterial carbon dioxide partial pressure >45 mmhg or fev $_1$ <30% [13];
- Recent hospitalization or consultation [13];
- Oxygen dependence or weight loss;
- Observed deterioration in the patient's condition;
- Age over 70 years [13];
- Assessment of therapy options.

Discussions must be prepared and include the implications of the diagnosis and the possible outcomes of life-sustaining treatments [2, 6]. The patient's understanding of their condition and desired information needs should be sought. The patient's family members should be included in the discussions, if the patient so wishes, and as a result, physicians must identify and recognize the patient's preferences [2, 6, 11, 13].

The treatment plan must consider the patient's needs and desires [2, 6], and during this process the observation of the patient's emotional state is of paramount importance for the necessary adjustments, measuring their expectations, limitations and understanding.

Palliative care also involves honest discussion of prognosis and issues such as advance directives about the patient' s will regarding admission, ventilation, and resuscitation in case of cardiac arrest. Surprisingly, many patients do not understand that in most cases COPD is a progressive, life-limiting condition [2, 4, 5, 11]. Patients who are aware of the prognosis often have concerns about the manner of their death with a predominant fear of dying from shortness of breath or asphyxia, but rarely discuss these fears with doctors, and doctors often do not talk to patients about these issues.

Advance care planning improves end-of-life care, increases patient and family satisfaction, and reduces stress, anxiety, and depression in surviving relatives [2, 6, 7, 11, 13], in addition to reducing care costs. It is important that the details of advance directives are regularly reviewed with patients to ensure that their instructions reflect their current wishes [11, 16].

While often uncomfortable for clinicians, open communication about death is important in alleviating patients' fears and enabling them to make decisions about managing their end-of-life care [16]. COPD patients find it particularly difficult to make early decisions about limits of care. Even when they have had previous experience of interventions such as non-invasive ventilation, they trust their physician to make the right decision about their use in the future, rather than making their own decision [2, 6, 7, 11, 13, 16].

The progressive decline in activities of daily living and social isolation for patients with end-stage COPD are reflected by changes in the roles and responsibilities of spouses and family members. They often assume several new roles as the disease progresses, including caring for the patient and taking over all household chores, needing the psychosocial support that palliative care offers, as well as grief counseling after the patient's death [16].

The Global Strategy for the Diagnosis, Management and Prevention of Chronic Obstructive Pulmonary Disease (GOLD) report recommends "that all clinicians treating patients with COPD should be aware of the effectiveness of palliative approaches to symptom control and use them in their practice" [11, 16].

Elements of Effective Palliative Care

The management of palliative care with COPD patients often triggers disagreement among medical professionals in the identification of patients suitable for this type of care. Oliveira and Junior [17] refer that the early introduction of palliative care can improve the functionality and quality of life of patients with limitations imposed by the disease. The inability to manage symptoms such as pain and dyspnea in critically ill patients, associated with communication difficulties throughout the treatment [17], are factors that worsen the "end of life" quality of these patients.

Knowledge of the trajectory of a disease allows for effective care planning and planning with family and caregivers, and there are three recognizable patterns of function and well-being in diseases: (a) diseases with a high level of function and a short period of decline (cancer); (b) diseases with long-term functional limitation with intermittent severe episodes requiring emergency admissions (COPD); (c) diseases with low functional level and prolonged decline with associated problems (stroke, dementia) [18].

The physical, social and psychological needs of patients vary considerably according to the type of disease trajectory [19]. COPD is characterized by a decline in function with acute exacerbations, which can lead to sudden death and intermittent care needs. Therefore, Oliveira and Junior [17] refer to the need to analyze the introduction of early care with the onset of symptoms, as they state that the palliative and curative approaches are complementary throughout the course of the disease. In the initial phase, the priority is the curative treatment and, with the progression and deterioration of the condition, the control of the symptoms becomes the main focus. The advanced stage presents treatments to control the progression of the disease, which can be performed as long as they do not cause even more suffering (Figure 1).

Patients with COPD follow a chronic disease trajectory, with long periods of slow decline in health, with occasional acute exacerbations that can lead to fatal disease [19].

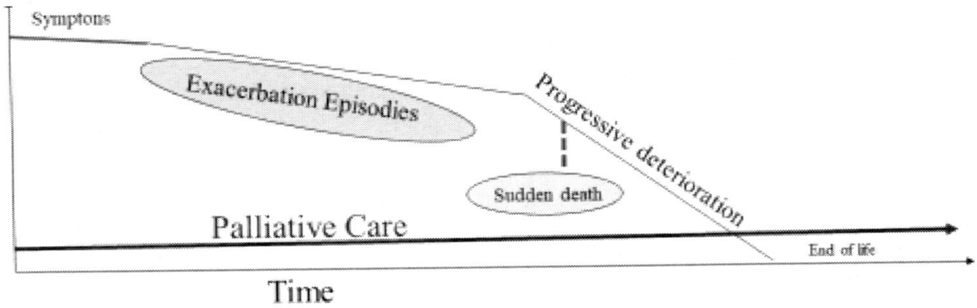

Figure 1. The disease trajectory expected in a patient with COPD and palliative care. Adapted from [17, 19].

For Choudhuri [18] and Landers et al. [19] the objective of palliative care in COPD patients is to reduce symptoms, improve quality of life and increase participation in daily activities.

Table 1. Elements of effective palliative care [18, 19]

a.	Management of dyspnea
b.	Oxygen Therapy/Non-Invasive Mechanical Ventilation (NIV)
c.	Nutritional support
d.	Emotional state: anxiety and depression
e.	Advance care planning

Management of Dyspnea

There are many possible causes of dyspnea, and proper management varies by etiology; relief of pleural obstructions or effusions may be helpful, in addition to medications, supplemental oxygen, or other indicated treatments [20]. Patients with end-stage COPD have drug-refractory dyspnea [20, 21]. However, the combination of long-acting beta-agonist, inhaled steroid and long-acting anticholinergic is one of the indicated treatments. The main bronchodilators indicated for these patients are beta-2 antagonists, methylxanthines and anticholinergics. But while methylxanthines are useful for reducing COPD exacerbations, their therapeutic index is low and they cannot be administered as an aerosol. Administration of aerosolized bronchodilators is most effective in decreasing airway resistance, easing the work of breathing, and relieving shortness of breath. Thus, a combination of beta-2 antagonist and anticholinergic or beta-2 antagonist with a glucocorticoid is the preferred choice in COPD [18].

Oxygen Therapy/Non-Invasive Mechanical Ventilation (NIV)

Non-invasive ventilation (NIV) is one of the few treatments in COPD that has been shown to improve survival [19]. The addition of NIV to usual care for the management of acute hypercapnic respiratory failure due to acute exacerbation of chronic obstructive pulmonary disease (COPD) significantly reduces the risks of mortality and endotracheal intubation [20]. NIV treatment is associated with a significant reduction in the mean length of hospital stay, but this finding is more often related to patients with prolonged hospital stays. NIV appears to improve respiratory acidosis within one hour of starting this therapy [21].

The need for endotracheal intubation was reduced by approximately two-thirds (64%) compared to usual care. The magnitude of benefit was clear and statistically significant for all subgroups, and no significant differences were observed for this outcome between subgroups related to admission pH or treatment site. These data clearly demonstrate the important clinical benefits associated with NIV [21].

Regarding the use of oxygen therapy, there is sufficient evidence to support its long-term use in hypoxemic COPD patients to improve their exercise capacity [19], allowing these patients to tolerate higher levels of physical activity with fewer symptoms on exertion and a general improvement in the quality of life [18].

Nutritional Support

Resting energy expenditure (REE) is elevated in COPD patients compared to healthy individuals due to the increased work of breathing, and frequent hospitalizations associated with episodes of acute exacerbations produce a state of negative energy balance [18]. Thus, nutritional support is an important aspect of palliative care in these patients. Weight loss and skeletal muscle mass are strong predictors of mortality risk in COPD [22, 23]. Ho et al. [23] reported that anthropometric indicators called "body mass index" (BMI), "low arm circumference" (LAC) and "low calf circumference" (LCC) can predict the risk of long-term mortality in COPD patients. The most common eating problems in patients with severe COPD are anorexia, dyspeptic symptoms, diarrhea, and fear of gaining weight [22].

Emotional State: Anxiety and Depression

In the emotional state of the patient with COPD, anxiety and depression are commonly observed. It was also observed that depressive symptoms are associated with an increased risk of 3-year mortality. Persistent smoking, increased symptom burden and worsening physical and social functioning are situations that worsen the condition. In patients with moderate to severe symptoms of depression and anxiety, psychological support provides significant support and improves quality of life, and it is important to emphasize the need to link mental health care to the overall COPD treatment regimen [18].

The success of pharmacological treatment for anxiety and depression in COPD has been very limited. Before starting any medication, it is important to distinguish true anxiety disorders in COPD from anxiety and panic states derived from the side effects of beta-2 agonists and high doses of corticosteroids [18].

Pollock et al. [24] present a systemic review of pharmacological interventions for the treatment of depression in patients with COPD, reporting that the evidence found in this review is insufficient to allow recommendations on the efficacy or safety in the use of drugs for these pathologies. The quality of the evidence was considered very low due to the small number of randomized clinical trials, in addition to presenting several methodological and clinical limitations. Therefore, great caution is advised when prescribing antidepressant medications to patients with COPD, as potential respiratory side effects have been shown to occur. As benzodiazepines can precipitate severe hypercapnia, their use should be restricted in these patients. However, no studies to date have elucidated the long-term effects of treating anxiety and quality of life in COPD patients. More studies are needed to understand effective treatments of anxiety and depression in COPD patients [18, 24].

Advance Care Planning

The integration of palliative care at the onset of illness, along with disease-specific therapy for COPD, is within the scope of advance care planning [18]. This not only provides a platform to coordinate integrated services, but also improves patient satisfaction and functional capabilities. When analyzing the barriers and facilitators of advance care planning in COPD patients, there is a better perception of end-of-life care. Reports from patients and family/caregivers demonstrated what care they would need and what kind of doctors and support staff could meet their needs. However, it is expected that more research will clarify which specific areas can be targeted most effectively, aiming at better planning of early care [18, 25, 26].

Table 2. Barriers and facilitators of palliative care with COPD patients [2, 11, 13, 14, 15, 16, 17, 19, 25, 26]

Barriers	*Facilitators*
Patients focused on staying alive [2]; Uncertainty as to which physician would be responsible for treatment [25]; Uncertainty about the type of care needed in the future [13, 25]; Limited understanding of palliative care and COPD [2, 25, 26]; Denial of health status and the possibility of dying [2, 11, 19]; Emotional distress [2, 14, 15, 25, 26]; Willingness of patients to talk about palliative care [2, 25, 26]; Lack of time in consultations to discuss all topics [2, 16, 17, 25]; Lack of feedback and documentation [2, 25]; Lack of in-depth knowledge of the patient [2, 14, 15, 25, 26]; View of palliative care as conditioned to the last days of life [2, 15, 16, 17, 19, 25, 26]; Prognostic uncertainty in COPD [2, 11, 13, 14, 15, 16, 17, 19, 25, 26]; Reluctance of palliative care services to care for COPD patients [2, 25]; Complex discharge planning for COPD patients [2, 11, 13, 14, 15, 16, 17, 19, 25, 26].	Patients who have had relatives or friends who have recently died [2, 25]; Patients' trust in their doctor [2, 11, 13, 14, 15, 15, 17, 19, 25]; Patients interpret doctors' skills as very good [2, 25]; Good doctor-patient relationship [2, 11, 13, 14, 15, 15, 17, 19, 25]; Doctors who cared for many patients with lung disease [2, 25]; Doctors who cared for patients with previous acute episodes [2, 25].

The concept of advance care planning (ACP) has been integrated into COPD patient care. ACP is a process of thinking about, discussing and planning an individual's future health desires, led by that person and their family with input from relevant health professionals. This practice allows for a positive effect on end-of-life care for patients with reductions in life-sustaining treatments and increased adherence to patient wishes [18, 26].

Barriers and Facilitators in Palliative Care

Patients often turn to physicians to initiate discussions about future care planning and prognosis, but there are considerable barriers to this happening [17, 25]. It is known that patients with COPD have little recollection of hospitalization and treatments received. They are willing to undergo life-saving treatments (despite the discomfort these treatments entail), generally expect to recover (as they have previously done) and have a high degree of delegation of decision-making to healthcare professionals, specifically physicians [19, 25, 26].

Identifying and overcoming barriers to communication will promote high-quality palliative care for COPD patients [25].

Conclusion

End-of-life palliative care for the patient with COPD should be started early and its planning discussed with the patient and family/caregivers. The frequency and quality of conversations about palliative care between patients and the health professionals who will provide them should be linear and comprehensive, allowing those involved to understand the role of each one and the prognosis of the disease.

Communication between patients and physicians has many barriers and most topics are not discussed. Often when conversations take place, they develop at an advanced stage of the disease, in stressful times and often there is no relationship and bond between them.

The early planning of actions and the interaction between patient/family/caregivers allows an adequate bond, in addition to good communication and the effectiveness of care, respecting the patient's wishes and conditions during palliative and end-of-life care.

The relationship between conversations about care and meeting patient preferences, by clinicians and the multidisciplinary team, will impact in the quality of care, patient satisfaction and quality of life, ensuring appropriate palliative care and planning advanced care through open discussions with everyone involved in the process.

Key Points

- An important point within the Support Therapy of COPD patients is the difficulty in identifying when to start palliative care.
- There are tools that can help the doctor identify those at risk of dying.

- It is essential that the patient's voice is heard, so that patients can describe specific events that can be used as a "trigger" for a palliative approach and discuss treatment with them and their family/caregivers for better adherence.
- Support services such as physiotherapy, speech therapy, psychology, nutritional therapy and occupational therapy are necessary for a better treatment in order to improve the quality of life of this patient.

References

[1] Carlucci A, Guerrieri A, Nava S. Palliative care in COPD patients: is it only an end-of-life issue?. *Eur Respir Rev*. 2012; 21(126):347-354. https://doi.org/10.1183/09059180.00001512. Available from: https://err.ersjournals.com/content/21/126/347. (Accessed on 10 March 2022).

[2] Tavares N, Jarrett N, Hunt K, Wilkinson T. Palliative and end-of-life care conversations in COPD: a systematic literature review. *ERJ Open Res*. 2017; 3(2):00068-2016. http://doi.org/10.1183/23120541.00068-2016.

[3] Seneff MG, Wagner DP, Wagner RP, Zimmerman JE, Knaus WA. Hospital and 1-year survival of patients admitted to intensive care units with acute exacerbation of chronic obstructive pulmonary disease. *JAMA*. 1995; 274 (23):1852-1857.

[4] World Health Association. *WHO Definition of Palliative Care. 2016.* Available from www.who.int/cancer/palliative/definition/en/. (Accessed on 10 March 2022).

[5] World Health Organization. Palliative care for older people: better practices. Denmark, 2011. Available from www.euro.who.int/__data/assets/pdf_file/0017/143153/e95052.pdf. (Accessed on 10 March 2022)

[6] Ahia CL, Blais CM. Primary palliative care for the general internist: integrating goals of care discussions into the outpatient setting. *Ochsner J*. 2014;14(4):704-711.

[7] NICE. End of life care for adults - *Quality Standard, 2011.* Available from www.nice.org.uk/guidance/qs13/resources/end-of-life-care-for-adults-2098483631557. (Accessed on 10 March 2022).

[8] Randall Curtis J. Palliative care for patients with chronic obstructive pulmonary disease. *Respir Med* 2006; 2: 86–90.

[9] Diaz-Lobato S, Smyth D, Curtis JR. Improving palliative care for patients with COPD. *Eur Respir J*. 2015; 46(3): 596-598. http://doi.org/10.1183/13993003.00987-2015.

[10] Gore JM, Brophy CJ, Greenstone MA. How well do we care for patients with end stage chronic obstructive pulmonary disease (COPD)? A comparison of palliative care and quality of life in COPD and lung cancer. *Thorax* 2000; 55: 1000–1006.

[11] Halpin DMG. Palliative care for people with COPD: effective but underused. *Eur Respir J*. 2018; 51(2):1702645. Published 2018 Feb 14. http://doi.org/10.1183/13993003.02645-2017.

[12] Gaspar C, Alfarroba S, Telo L, Gomes C, Bárbara C. End-of-life care in COPD: a survey carried out with Portuguese pulmonologists. *Rev Port Pneumol*. 2014;20(3):123-130. https://doi.org/10.1016/j.rppneu.2014.01.008.

[13] JR Curtis. Cuidados paliativos e de fim de vida para pacientes com DPOC grave [*Palliative and end-of-life care for patients with severe COPD*]. *Eur Respir* J. 2008; 32: 796-803.

[14] Hansen-Flaschen J. Chronic obstructive pulmonary disease: the last year of life. *Respir Care*. 2004; 49(1): 90-98.

[15] Andreas S, Alt-Epping B. Advance care planning in severe COPD: it is time to engage with the future. *ERJ Open Res*. 2018; 4(1): 00009-2018. https://doi.org/10.1183/23120541.00009-2018.

[16] Vogelmeier, CF, Criner, GJ, Martinez, FJ, Anzueto, A, Barnes, PJ, Bourbeau, J, Celli, BR, Chen, R, Decramer, M, Fabbri, LM, Frith, P, Halpin, DMG, López Varela, MV, Nishimura, M, Roche, N, Rodriguez-Roisin, R, Sin, DD, Singh, D, Stockley, R, Agustí, A. Global Strategy for the Diagnosis, Management, and Prevention of Chronic Obstructive Lung Disease 2017 Report: GOLD Executive Summary [published correction appears in *Eur Respir J*. 2017 Jun 22;49(6):]. *Eur Respir J*. 2017; 49(3):1700214. Published 2017 Mar 6. https://doi.org/10.1183/13993003.00214-2017.

[17] EPD, Medeiros Junior P. Cuidados paliativos em pneumologia [*Palliative care in pulmonology*]. *Jornal Brasileiro de Pneumologia.* 2020, 46 (3): e20190280.

[18] Choudhuri AH. Palliative care for patients with chronic obstructive pulmonary disease: current perspectives. *Indian J Palliat Care*. 2012;18(1): 6-11. https://doi.org/10.4103/0973-1075.97342.

[19] Landers, A, Wiseman, R, Pitama, S, & Beckert, L. Severe COPD and the transition to a palliative approach. *Breathe*. 2017; 13: 310–316.

[20] Narsavage GL, Chen YJ, Korn B, Elk R. The potential of palliative care for patients with respiratory diseases. *Breathe (Sheff)*. 2017;13(4):278-289. https://doi.org/10.1183/20734735.014217.

[21] Osadnik CR, Tee VS, Carson-Chahhoud KV, Picot J, Wedzicha JA, Smith BJ. Non-invasive ventilation for the management of acute hypercapnic respiratory failure due to exacerbation of chronic obstructive pulmonary disease. *Cochrane Database Syst Rev*. 2017;7(7):CD004104. Published 2017 Jul 13. https://doi.org/10.1002/14651858.CD004104.pub4.

[22] Marquis K, Debigaré R, Lacasse Y, Pierre LeBlanc, Jobin, J, Carrier, G, Maltais. F. Midthigh muscle cross-sectional area is a better predictor of mortality than body mass index in patients with chronic obstructive pulmonary disease. *Am J Respir Crit Care Med*. 2002;166(6):809-813. https://doi.org/10.1164/rccm.2107031.

[23] Ho SC, Wang JY, Kuo HP, Chien-Da Huang, Kang-Yun Lee, Hsiao-Chi Chuang, Po-Hao Feng, Tzu-Tao Chen, and Min-Fang Hsu. Mid-arm and calf circumferences are stronger mortality predictors than body mass index for patients with chronic obstructive pulmonary disease. *Int J Chron Obstruct Pulmon Dis*. 2016;11:2075-2080. Published 2016 Aug 31. doi:10.2147/COPD.S107326.

[24] Pollok J, van Agteren JE, Carson-Chahhoud KV. Pharmacological interventions for the treatment of depression in chronic obstructive pulmonary disease. *Cochrane Database Syst Rev*. 2018;12(12):CD012346. Published 2018 Dec 19. https://doi.org/10.1002/14651858.CD012346.pub2.

[25] Knauft E, Nielsen EL, Engelberg RA, Patrick DL, Curtis JR. Barriers and facilitators to end-of-life care communication for patients with COPD. *Chest*. 2005;127(6):2188-2196. https://doi.org/10.1378/chest.127.6.2188.

[26] Curtis JR, Engelberg RA, Wenrich MD, Au DH. Communication about palliative care for patients with chronic obstructive pulmonary disease. *J Palliat Care*. 2005;21(3):157-164.

Chapter 17

Self-Management and Education in Stable COPD

Victor Manuel Mendoza Romero[1,*], Amaury Hernán González Molina[2], Cinthia Susana Álvarez Maldonado[2] and José Luis Sandoval Gutiérrez[3]

[1]Lung Transplant Unit,
National Institute of Respiratory Diseases, Mexico City, Mexico
[2]National Institute of Respiratory Diseases, Mexico City, Mexico
[3] Auxiliary Diagnostic and Paramedical Services,
National Institute of Respiratory Diseases, Mexico City, Mexico

Abstract

The treatment of chronic diseases needs patient's engagement to be successful, therefore, clinicians involved in the treatment of patients with chronic obstructive pulmonary disease must reserve time in medical appointments to teach self-management interventions and give patients trustworthy information about their disease. The ultimate goal of self-management strategies in COPD is to give the patients the knowledge and skills to cooperate with their health provider to improve disease control, improve quality of life and prevent exacerbations.

The self-management interventions include education, the development of a COPD action plan, strategies for symptoms control, teaching adequate inhaler techniques, stimulating a healthy lifestyle and long-term oxygen therapy use when required. The evidence that supports self-management strategies is controversial but it seems to improve health related quality of life and lower the risk of respiratory related hospital admissions. More evidence regarding the benefit of the specific interventions is required.

Keywords: COPD, self-management, interventions, breathlessness, pulmonary rehabilitation, health related quality of life

* Corresponding Author's Email: dr.victormendoza.iner@gmail.com.

In: Chronic Obstructive Pulmonary Disease
Editor: Jaber S. Alqahtani
ISBN: 979-8-88697-333-4

Introduction

Definition of Self-Management

Self-management is considered an essential element of the treatment for chronic diseases, it consists in giving the patient knowledge and skills necessary to cooperate with the health provider to improve disease control and prevent future exacerbations, hospitalizations and ultimately, death. It refers to the interventions which have as their goals to motivate, engage, and support the patients to positively adapt their health behaviors and develop skills to better manage their disease. These interventions must be structured but personalized and are often multi-component [1].

The ultimate objectives of Chronic Obstructive Pulmonary Disease (COPD) self-management are:

- Optimizing and preserving physical health;
- Reducing symptoms and functional impairments in daily life and increasing emotional and social wellbeing and quality of life;
- Establishing effective communication with health-care professionals (clinicians, nurses, and physiotherapist), family and friends [2].

The basis of COPD maintenance treatment according to Global Initiative for Chronic Obstructive Lung Disease (GOLD) Guidelines includes:

(a) An individualized pharmacological regime based on symptom severity, risk of exacerbations and previous exacerbations events, costs and medical adverse events, also preference and availability must be considered.
(b) Pulmonary rehabilitation (exercise, control of breathing, airway clearance techniques, energy conservation techniques).
(c) Adequate Inhaler technique (when possible always add a spacer).
(d) Updated immunization schedule (influenza vaccine, pneumococcal vaccine when indicated).
(e) Smoking cessation (non-pharmacological and pharmacological management).
(f) Long term oxygen therapy (at least 15 hours per day) [2].

The effectiveness of all of these interventions will depend on patient comprehension and adherence. Patients living with COPD must make daily decisions regarding their own care, therefore patient education and self-management has been increasingly considered as an essential component for the efficacy of their treatment [3].

Evidence of Effectiveness of Self-Management in COPD

In 2017, a systematic review of 22 studies compared the use of an action plan for Acute Exacerbations of COPD (AECOPD) with usual care. The authors reported increased health-related quality of life (HRQoL) measured by St. George's Respiratory Questionnaire (SGRQ) and a lower risk of at least one respiratory-related hospital admission. It was also shown that having an action plan for acute exacerbations, can lower risk for at least one respiratory-related hospital admission and increases HRQoL. A greater improvement in HRQoL was demonstrated in studies that included a smoking cessation programme as part of the self-management intervention. However, there was no statistically significant difference in the probability of at least one all-cause hospital admission (OR 0.74, 95% CI 0.54 to 1.03), emergency department visits, general practitioner visits, and dyspnoea scores as measure by the (m)MRC questionnaire for participants in self-management interventions compared to usual care [4]

In 2018 K. Jolly et al. published a systematic review in the United Kingdom. Unlike other publications, which included basically patients from secondary care, they included patients receiving only primary care follow up. They found no difference in SGRQ scores, dyspnea or anxiety and depression between the two groups. However, results for the Chronic Respiratory Disease Questionnaire (CRQ) domains of dyspnea, emotions and fatigue were in the direction favoring the self-management interventions, but none reached statistical significance [5].

H. Bringsvor et al. published a randomized controlled trial in Norway. They examined the effects of COPD-specific health promoting self-management intervention domains known as "Better living with COPD" plus usual care vs usual care alone. The purpose of Better Living with COPD is to increase the participants' consciousness of their potential, their internal and external resources and their abilities to use them, and thus to improve their self-management capabilities in the context of everyday living. It consisted of weekly 2-hour long group conversations over 11 weeks. The analysis showed significant positive changes on constructive attitudes and approaches and skills and technique acquisitions as well as self-monitoring and insight, whereas no significant effects were found on the other domains [6].

A Delphi study by Korpershoek et al. was performed in order to rate the relevance and feasibility of predetermined self-management behaviors. They described a classification of phases of the COPD natural history and objectives of the self-management:

- Stable phase, "normal" day-to-day variations in symptoms and relatively low risk for an exacerbation, the aim is to prevent its occurrence and reduce frequency.
- Mild deterioration that can resolve spontaneously or might result in exacerbation. The aim is to reduce symptoms and prevent further deterioration.
- Exacerbation, sustained worsening of symptoms that may warrant medical treatment, such as add-on treatment, hospitalization or emergency department visit. The aim is to reduce its severity and recovery time.
- Recovery toward baseline symptom status and at risk of relapse. The aim is to reduce the recovery time and decrease short- and long-term impact.
- Stable phase, high risk period for recurrent exacerbations (8 weeks after initial exacerbation). The aim is to prevent exacerbation recurrence [7].

According to this study, there were some interventions that were more beneficial according to the phase of the symptoms.

1. *Stable phase (low risk):*
   (a) Adherence to pharmacotherapy (long-acting beta-agonist (LABA), long-acting muscarinic antagonist (LAMA) and/or inhaled corticosteroid (ICS))
   (b) Annual influenza vaccination

   (c) Daily physical activity
   (d) Avoiding viral and bacterial stimuli
   (e) Managing exposure to air quality
   (f) Smoking cessation (pharmacological and non-pharmacological combination is advised in a specialized clinic)
2. *Mild deterioration*
   (a) Early detection of symptom deterioration (dyspnea, cough, wheezing, change in sputum production and characteristics, thoracic pain or tightness)
   (b) Correct increase of the short-acting beta-agonist (SABA- SAMA)
   (c) Breathing exercises and energy conservation techniques
3. *Exacerbation/flare ups*
   (a) Early detection of symptoms (worsening of dyspnea, cough, increased sputum, chest tightness, extrapulmonary symptoms, fever, malaise)
   (b) Prompt treatment with corticosteroids and/or antibiotics, increase of SABA
   (c) Management of stress and anxiety
4. *Recovery*
   (a) Completing treatment with systemic corticosteroids and/ or antibiotics
   (b) Adjusted exercise- and resistance training.
5. *Stable (at risk)*
   (a) Increased awareness for recurring exacerbation
   (b) Early (re)start of pulmonary rehabilitation [7]

Cost Effectiveness

Khdour et al. performed a cost-utility analysis alongside a randomized control trial of a pharmacy-led self-management programme for COPD in a specialized clinic in Belfast, Northern Ireland. They used data from 127 COPD patients who received a self-management programme and education or usual care. One-year costs were estimated from the perspective of the National Health Service and Personal Social Services and quality adjusted life years (QALYs) at baseline, 6 and 12 months. The primary outcome was the cost per QALYs gained. Results showed that the mean differences in costs and effect between the self-management and usual care group were -£671.59 (95 CI %: -£1,584.73 to -£68.14) and 0.065 (95% CI; 0.000–0.128). Suggesting that the intervention was less costly and more effective, emphasizing that more research is needed to determine which aspects of the intervention have the greatest impact in cost utility [8].

Another study performed by Gallefoss et al. explored the effects and heath economic consequences of patient self-management education in 1 year follow up; 62 patients with COPD from a Pulmonary Medicine Department in a University Hospital in Bergen, Norway were randomized to a 4 hour schooling, followed by a nurse or physiotherapist consultation vs usual care. The effectiveness was measured with medical consultations, patient satisfaction and use of rescue treatments. The cost effectiveness was measured with doctor visits, days off work, dispensed pharmaceuticals, hospital admissions, travel costs, educational and time costs. The control and intervention groups induced mean total costs of USD 2 044.97 and USD 1089.28 per patient, respectively. For every 0.1 USD put into patient education, there was a saving of 0.48 USD. The number needed to educate (NNE) to make one patient independent of their general practitioner was 1.7 (95% CI: 1.3--2.8) and associated with a concomitant saving of USD 1623.64. There was also a reduced use of daily doses of rescue medications with savings of USD 575.47. Arriving to the conclusion that a self-management plan for patients with COPD is cost effective for the patient and health-care system [9].

Zwerink et al. evaluated the cost-effectiveness of a community-based exercise program as a part of a self-management program. Patients participated in an 11-month exercise program, they trained 3 times/week for 6 months and 2 times/week the following 5 months. They were followed for 2 years and compared to usual care. Incremental cost-effectiveness ratios (ICER) were calculated. The ICER for preventing deterioration at least 47.5 meters on incremental shuttle walking test (ISWT) was EUR 6257, for a relevant improvement in physical activity (≥ 500 steps/day) was EUR 1564 and for an QALY was EUR 10 950. In conclusion, beneficial effects on exercise capacity with the exercise program and also it had higher costs than usual care, thus it cannot be considered cost-effective [10].

From the previously reviewed publications, we can get to the conclusion that implementing self-management for all COPD patients besides having clinical benefits, is cost effective for the patient and health care system. Nevertheless, not all self-management recommendations are cost-effective like the community-based exercise program. All clinicians should be aware of which intervention will result in the greatest benefit; clinical and economic.

Recommended Self-Management Interventions in Stable COPD

The COPD self-management interventions include:

Education

The patient should have a deep knowledge of the risk factors for COPD and an overview of the physiopathology of the disease can be useful. Also, the expected symptoms and evolution of the disease can be included with its management.

It is advised that every patient should be aware of the following information such as the respiratory system physiology, general anatomy of the lungs and airways, the role of breathing, the protection against irritants and foreign particles given by our respiratory system, especially the upper respiratory tract; what is COPD, its causes, symptoms, treatment and prognosis.

Information about lung function tests, as a diagnostic, prognosis and follow-up tool, such as the spirometry, diffusion capacity of carbon monoxide (DLCO), plethysmography, 6-minutes walking test, must be given to the patients.

Advice for smoking cessation is also an essential component of the education program. Tobacco smoking is the leading cause of COPD, clinicians should make an effort in each consultation to convince the patients to stop smoking, highlighting that this is the most important step in slowing the progression of COPD. A deep explanation of what nicotine addiction is and what are the available options for smoking cessation should be offered.

The best quitting results are achieved when medicines (nicotine replacement therapy such as gum, patches, sprays, inhalers, varenicline, bupropion) are used in combination with counseling and support. Where available, patients could benefit from a referral to a specialized stop smoking clinic program.

Besides referring patients to a quit smoking clinic; information about e-cigarettes must be clear, highlighting that e-cigarettes are still addictive (they contain nicotine) and also represent a risk for the lungs and airways. Concluding that a tobacco cigarette replaced by an e-cigarette is not a way of smoking cessation.

COPD Action Plan

Giving the patient a written action plan may help to identify disease control and flare ups, also it may help to recognize when to seek urgent medical care. When a written action plan is handed in, the patient can easily identify the steps to follow to control the disease.

This action plan must provide information to the patient about the right moment to use reliever medications.

When preferred by the patients, clinicians can use other technological teaching tools such as applications, websites, tablets and videoconferences.

Symptoms Management

The main objective of monitoring symptoms is to avoid flare ups that can lead to hospitalizations or even death. Patients must be aware of possible triggers like respiratory infections (seasonal viruses, SARS-COV-2, rhinovirus, parainfluenza, bacterial infections), smoke (cigarette, wood, oil), pollutants (dust, wood smoke, smog) and other unknown causes. In order to elude exacerbations, it is advised to develop a written COPD action plan, avoid triggers, annual influenza vaccination, and adequate adherence to COPD controller therapy and inhaler technique, good hand hygiene, and healthy habits and keep track of daily symptoms. If the patient presents worsening of symptoms, it is recommended to follow instructions of the written action plan, reduce level of physical activity, use of reliever medications, clear secretions with an adequate cough, huff technique or accessory devices, practice controlled breathing and relaxation techniques, use of additional medicine as planned by the pulmonologist and contact doctor if symptoms become more severe.

The management of breathlessness is a key component of symptom management and the purpose of all the breathing and relaxation techniques is to reduce the impact in an individual's daily life or increase the threshold of activity at which breathlessness becomes limiting. It's important to talk about this with the patient as it is unlikely that breathlessness will be completely reversible.

Sphatis et al. developed a model to help the patients and clinicians understand the pathways responsible for the generation of breathlessness. This model is also useful to plan interventions for its management. The model is called, "Breathing, Thinking, Functioning".

1) The "Breathing" refers to the ineffective breathing patterns developed by patients with COPD (rapid shallow breaths).

2) The "Thinking" cycle refers to the recurrent thoughts about breathlessness the patients have throughout the day. This can result in anxiety and perpetuation of the symptom. Finally,
3.) The "Functioning" cycle" refers to the impediment of daily life activities due to breathlessness, this turns into a vicious cycle in which the patient avoids activities to avoid breathlessness and anxiety, leading to further deconditioning [11].

According to this model the following interventions are feasible to do in a self-management program:

Breathing

Breathing techniques may improve the respiratory patterns of COPD patients. Also, the use of a hand-held fan during activities can help to reduce breathlessness.

The most noted breathing techniques for COPD patients are:

- Pursed lips breathing: It has shown to reduce respiratory rate and improve tidal volume, suggesting it may have positive effects in airway collapse, airway resistance and air trapping.
- Diaphragmatic breathing: Similar to pursed lips breathing, diaphragmatic breathing can reduce respiratory rate. Also, alone or in combination with pursed lips breathing it can reduce sympathetic activity, which may lead to a reduction in sensation of dyspnea [12].

Thinking

Teaching relaxation techniques, mindfulness or even cognitive behavioral therapy can be used. The intervention of a psychologist or psychiatrist should be considered.

Functioning

Pulmonary rehabilitation programs are the most effective intervention for dyspnea management, also it has shown to improve symptoms related to anxiety and depression. Most patients with COPD are candidates for a pulmonary rehabilitation program according to the GOLD guidelines.

Inhaler Techniques and Drug Adherence

It is recommended that the patients know their medicine, what it is for, how the medicine works, how to take it, how long its effect lasts and its side effects. Most COPD medications are inhaled, it is important to check the inhaler technique regularly and correct possible flaws. There are three types of medications usually prescribed: reliever (short acting antimuscarinic and beta-adrenergic), maintenance (LAMA, LABA, ICS) and flare up medicines (antibiotics, oral steroids, reliever bronchodilators), it is imperative that the patient understands the role of each of them and uses them properly.

When choosing an inhalation device is of paramount importance to teach the patient about the technique, add a spacer for the pMDI devices when needed and feasible and when prescribing a dry powder inhaler make sure the patient has enough inspiratory effort to make an adequate maneuver, this can be evaluated with a closed-loop spirometry. In each medical consultation, inhaler technique must be reevaluated, looking to improve or correct it if necessary and evaluating the change of the inhalation for another better suited for the patient.

Healthy Lifestyle

In order for the patients to improve their quality of life, besides having an adequate adherence to their treatment, a healthy lifestyle is desirable and advised. It is recommended to enroll the patient in a pulmonary rehabilitation program, breathing control exercises, energy conservation activities, airway clearance techniques (manual and instrumented), healthy eating with an evaluation by a nutritionist is recommended, management of stress, anxiety and depression (referring the patient to a specialist when necessary), planning sexual activities desired by the patient and traveling (when air traveling cautions should be taken, evaluation of the duration of flight, destination characteristics such as altitude are important to evaluate, in order to make sure the patient can tolerate the conditions of the destination. In some patients a hypoxic challenge test in a laboratory may be necessary [13].

Oxygen Therapy

As a part of self-management intervention, it is of paramount importance to keep a good adherence to the oxygen therapy, in order to decrease the risk of cardiovascular complications and mortality. The American Thoracic Society recommends in its guidelines "Home Oxygen Therapy for Adults with Chronic Lung Disease", the prescription of long-term oxygen therapy (LTOT) for at least 15 hours/day in those COPD patients with severe hypoxemia ($PaO2 < 55$ mmHg or $SaO2 < 88\%$) or PaO2 56-59 mmHg plus one of the following: edema, hematocrit > 55%, or cor pulmonale. In those with severe exertional room air hypoxemia (an in-laboratory oxygen titration is advised), ambulatory oxygen is recommended. Attention should be paid to the adverse effects of LTOT such as hypoventilation, oxygen toxicity, reabsorption atelectasis and others. Patients should be taught the way of monitoring their oxygen saturation and goals (SaO2 between 88-92%) with an oxygen pulse-oximeter and titration of oxygen supply. Non-hypercapnic patients on LTOT should increase their flow rate 1 L/min at night if there are no contraindications.

Patients initiating LTOT should be followed up by their clinicians at 3 months in order to obtain blood gas analysis. Flow rate should be assessed to make sure LTOT is correctly indicated. Those patients not requiring LTOT but are hypoxemic at night should not start nocturnal oxygen therapy, instead, other causes must be investigated such as obesity hypoventilation, respiratory muscle weakness, obstructive sleep apnea and others, in which most of them the resolution to nocturnal hypoxemia is the use of noninvasive mechanical ventilation. Providing information about the importance of adherence to oxygen therapy, its benefits, oxygen sources such as portable compressed gas cylinders, portable and stationary concentrators can help patients accomplish their daily life activities and adherence. Technical aspects of the oxygen therapy such as maintenance and precautions at home with the oxygen devices should be discussed during the prescription of LTOT in the contemplation of avoiding in-home accidents and making the best of the device performance [14].

Telehealth Monitoring

An intervention review by Cochrane evaluated the effectiveness of interventions delivered by computer and by mobile technology (personal computers, applications for mobile technology such as tablets, smartphones and Skype) compared to face-to-face or hard copy/digital documents in improving, supporting and educating about self-management in patients with COPD. Three studies were included with a total of 557 participants with a confirmed diagnosis of COPD, 319 received smart technology to support self-management and 238 received face-to-face verbal/written or digital information and education about self-management. All of the studies included the primary outcome of the review, health related quality of life (HRQoL) measured by the Clinical COPD Questionnaire (CCQ) or the St George's Respiratory Questionnaire (SGRQ). The secondary outcome of this review was the physical activity measured by daily step counts, studied in two of three studies.

Outcomes at week four, month four, and month six, the effect of smart technology on self-management and HRQoL in terms of symptoms and health status was significantly better than when participants received face-to-face /digital and/ or written support for self-management of COPD (SMD -0.22, 95% confidence interval (CI) -0.40 to -0.03; P = 0.02). Hospitalizations (OR 1.6, 95% CI 0.8 to 3.2; P = 0.19) and exacerbations (OR 1.4, 95% CI 0.7 to 2.8; P = 0.33) did not differ between groups in the single study that reported these outcomes at 12 months. The activity level of people with COPD at week four, month four, and month six was significantly higher when smart technology was used than when face-to-face/digital and/or written support was provided (MD 864.06 daily steps between groups, 95% CI 369.66 to 1358.46; P = 0.0006). The only study that measured activity levels at 12 months reported no significant differences between the intervention and control groups (mean -108, 95% CI -720 to 505; P = 0.73).

It was concluded that self-management via smart technology for patients with COPD significantly improved HRQoL and levels of activity up to six months compared to the face-to-face or printed interventions, nonetheless no firm conclusions can be drawn because of the high risk of bias and the poor quality of the studies. This improvement tends to wean over time and it should be individualized for patients interested in technology [15].

Conclusion

COPD is a chronic and progressive pulmonary disease with an important impact in patients´ daily routines, thus patients should be encouraged to learn about their disease and develop strategies to control their symptoms and keep their role in society. The evidence for self-management strategies in COPD is varied and controversial, with most of the studies showing an increase in health-related quality of life and decreasing risk of respiratory-related hospitalizations. With the increasing advances in technology, in those patients who feel comfortable with it, clinicians could encourage self-management of their disease via electronic devices with the goal of improving adherence and a better control of their disease. These interventions can be considered cost effective, therefore, clinicians should guarantee that patients increase the knowledge about their disease in a progressive way and in a supervised manner.

Key Points

- Self-management of COPD is an essential component of the integral treatment of this chronic and irreversible disease which consists of educating and teaching patients the knowledge and actions necessary to have a good control of their disease and an improved quality of life.
- The main objectives of a self-management program are reducing bothersome symptoms, increasing treatment adherence, improving quality of life and tolerance to daily activities, decreasing risk of exacerbations and hospitalisations, risk of death, among others.
- Evidence about the efficacy of a self-management program is controversial with some studies showing no statistically significant benefits and others showing a decrease in respiratory-related hospitalisations, improved quality of life, programs being cost-effective, increasing awareness and adherence to treatment. In some patients benefits of self-management are greater when implemented via tele-health monitoring (apps, videoconferences, tablets, personal computers). More studies are needed to achieve a conclusion regarding a self-management program effectiveness.
- Elementary components of a self-management program are an individualized treatment (controller and reliever treatment, attention should be paid to the multiple comorbidities of COPD patients), adequate inhaler technique and adherence (add a spacer when possible), pulmonary rehabilitation, airway clearance techniques either manual nor instrumented or combined, breathing control exercises, immunization schedule (annual influenza vaccine), smoking cessation (combination of pharmacological and support-counseling treatment with an specialized team is advised), long term oxygen therapy when indicated, detection and management of worsening symptoms and so on.
- More evidence is needed in an effort to discern which self-management interventions are the most beneficial and cost-effective for the patients. Nevertheless, it has been proven that important clinical and cost benefits can be achieved with a personalized well organized self-management plan for the COPD patients. Concluding with the recommendation of implementing an individualized self-management plan for all the COPD patients.

References

[1] Effing, T., Vercoulen, J., Bourbeau, J., Trappenburg, J., Lenferink, A., Cafarella, P., et al. (2016). Definition of a COPD self-management intervention: International Expert Group consensus. *European Respiratory Journal.*, 48(1), 46-54.

[2] Global initiative for chronic obstructive pulmonary disease (2020). Pocket Guide to COPD Diagnosis, Management and Prevention. 2020 Edition. Available on: https://goldcopd.org/wp-content/uploads/2020/03/GOLD-2020-POCKET-GUIDE-ver1.0_FINAL-WMV.pdf.

[3] Nici, L., Bontly, T., ZuWallack, R., and Gross, N. (2014). Self-Management in Chronic Obstructive Pulmonary Disease. Time for a Paradigm Shift? *Annals of the American Thoracic Society.*, 11(1), 101-107.

[4] Lenferink, A., Brusse-Keizer, M., van der Valk, P., Frith, P., Zwerink, M., Monninkhof, E., et al. (2017). Self-management interventions including action plans for exacerbations versus usual care in patients with chronic obstructive pulmonary disease. *Cochrane Database of Systematic Reviews.*, 2017(8).

[5] Jolly, K., Sidhu, M., Bates, E., Majothi, S., Sitch, A., Bayliss, S., et al. (2018). Systematic review of the effectiveness of community-based self-management interventions among primary care COPD patients. *npj Primary Care Respiratory Medicine.*, 28(1).

[6] Bringsvor, H., Langeland, E., Oftedal, B., Skaug, K., Assmus, J., and Bentsen S. (2018). Effects of a COPD self-management support intervention: a randomized controlled trial. *International Journal of Chronic Obstructive Pulmonary Disease.*, Volume 13, 3677-3688.

[7] Korpershoek, Y., Bruins Slot., J., Effing, T., Schuurmans, M., and Trappenburg, J. (2017). Self-management behaviors to reduce exacerbation impact in COPD patients: a Delphi study. *International Journal of Chronic Obstructive Pulmonary Disease.*, Volume 12, 2735-2746.

[8] Khdour, M., Agus, A., Kidney, J., Smyth, B., Elnay, J., and Crealey, G. (2011). Cost-utility analysis of a pharmacy-led self-management programme for patients with COPD. *International Journal of Clinical Pharmacy.*, 33(4), 665-673.

[9] GALLEFOSS, F., and BAKKE, P. (2002). Cost–benefit and cost-effectiveness analysis of self-management in patients with COPD—a 1-year follow-up randomized, controlled trial. *Respiratory Medicine.*, 96(6), 424-431.

[10] Zwerink, M., Effing, T., Kerstjens, H., van der Valk, P., Brusse-Keizer, M., Zielhuis, G., et al. (2015). Cost-Effectiveness of a Community-Based Exercise Programme in COPD Self-Management. COPD: *Journal of Chronic Obstructive Pulmonary Disease.*, 13(2), 214-223.

[11] Booth, S., and Johnson, M. (2019). Improving the quality of life of people with advanced respiratory disease and severe breathlessness. *Breathe.*, 15(3), 198-215.

[12] Ubolnuar, N., Tantisuwat, A., Thaveeratitham, P., Lertmaharit, S., Kruapanich, C., and Mathiyakom, W. (2019). Effects of Breathing Exercises in Patients With Chronic Obstructive Pulmonary Disease: Systematic Review and Meta-Analysis. *Annals of Rehabilitation Medicine.*, 43(4), 509-523.

[13] Lung Foundation (2016). Better living with COPD. https://lungfoundation.com.au/wp-content/uploads/2018/09/Book-Better-Living-with-COPD-Dec2016.pdf.

[14] Jacobs, S., Krishnan, J., Lederer, D., Ghazipura, M., Hossain, T., Tan, A., et al. (2020). Home Oxygen Therapy for Adults with Chronic Lung Disease. An Official American Thoracic Society Clinical Practice Guideline. *American Journal of Respiratory and Critical Care Medicine.*, 202(10), e121-e141.

[15] McCabe, C., McCann, M., and Brady, A. (2017). Computer and mobile technology interventions for self-management in chronic obstructive pulmonary disease. *Cochrane Database of Systematic Reviews.*

Chapter 18

The Efficacy of Aerosol Therapy in Nasal High Flow Therapy to COPD Patients

Yasmin M. Madney, PhD, Hoda Rabea, PhD, Hasnaa Osama, PhD, Mona A. Abdelrahman, PhD, Haitham Saeed, PhD, Hadeer S. Harb, PhD, Marwa Mohsen, PhD and Mohamed E. A. Abdelrahim*, PhD

Clinical Pharmacy Department,
Faculty of Pharmacy,
Beni-Suef University, Beni-Suef, Egypt

Abstract

Aerosol delivery by pressurized metered-dose inhalers (pMDIs) and nebulizers attached by an adapter or spacer into a high flow nasal cannula (HFNC) system add great benefits in the management of obstructive lung disease patients. The inhaled medication, given during HFNC, offers better and quicker clinical effects than unassisted breathing. Unfortunately, there is no specific recommendation or guidelines to guide healthcare providers in their decisions while delivering aerosols through HFNC which puts the patients at risk of receiving either a sub-therapeutic or toxic dose of their inhaled medications. This increases the urgency for the development of recommendations or guidelines by a trusted board or society for aerosol delivery to such critically ill patients.

Keywords: aerosol therapy, noninvasive ventilation, interfaces, nebulizer, pMDI

Introduction

The backbone of pulmonary resuscitation is oxygen supplementation especially in severe hypoxemic respiratory disease patients and it is considered as one of the major remedies prescribed in health care. The diversity in pitfalls of invasive ventilation has prompted the establishment of alternative methods for respiratory support in acute respiratory distress [1].

* Corresponding Author's Email: mohamedemam9@yahoo.com.

In: Chronic Obstructive Pulmonary Disease
Editor: Jaber S. Alqahtani
ISBN: 979-8-88697-333-4

Non-invasive ventilation (NIV) was firstly presented for chronic respiratory illnesses patients for prolonged home ventilation. In the 1990s, this technique, as a superior alternative to endotracheal intubation, became widely used for better management of critically ill patients with acute respiratory circumstances. Thereafter, high flow therapy (HFT), as an alternative approach to NIV, added attention as a popular therapy for control of intensive care unit (ICU) hypoxemic patients with ARF. The application of HFT involves the application of higher flow rates of gas than the ordinary low-flow oxygen methods.

Patients with respiratory distress getting oxygen via HFT or NIV systems may benefit from drug delivery by inhalation as well. Aerosol therapy is the favored route over oral and IV routes for medicine administration in pulmonary disease treatment due to its several benefits. These benefits include greater therapeutic selectivity, higher lung doses, minor systemic effects, fast onset of action, and relatively reduced doses [2].

High-level evidence supports aerosol delivery through NIV. In acute asthma, the response to inhaled bronchodilators during NIV use might be upgraded. However, the evidence is not mature enough to apply this approach as standard therapy. Evidence favors aerosol therapy delivery by nebulizers or pressurized metered-dose inhaler (pMDI) along with NIV without disruption or discontinuation of respiratory support. The available clinical studies on HFT with concomitant aerosol delivery are limited, and the in-vitro evidence is insufficient to establish a recommendation in favor of or against aerosol therapy during HFT [2].

The efficacy of aerosol delivery within a ventilation circuit is determined by several factors and the greatest consideration should be given by the health care workers to achieve the optimal treatment plan.

Physiological Rationale and Mechanism of Actions

Hypoxemia related to ARF increases the respiratory drive resulting in difficult breathing during the inspiration phase. Hypocapnia and hyperventilation are the main characteristics of blood gas profiles. Hence, consequently, hypercapnia is a warning sign of nearby pulmonary muscle fatigue which is a serious complication. So, the optimum oxygen support should be based on a combination of minimization of the respiratory muscle load and symptomatic treatment. A common dilemma arises around the choice of whether to use NIV or HFT in the ideal management of ARF [3]. There are conflicting studies about the helpful applications of HFT in comparison with NIV.

Technical Features and Oxygenation Effect

The established physiological effects of NIV include remarkable gas exchange enhancement with a decrease in the breathing effort. It supports the spontaneous activity of the pulmonary system by positive pressure application into the airways by face mask; as the most commonly used interface [4].

The HFT devices can deliver well-conditioned oxygen in terms of heat (37ºC) and humidification provided by an oxygen/air blender, connected to an adjusted flow meter at high flow rates up to 70 L/min as shown in Figure 1. Then, the high flow gas passed through nasal cannula or prongs, providing an effective and extended development in respiratory functions in ARF patients. Adequately conditioned gas, delivered at high flow encourages diverse physiological benefits. It offers the capability of independent adjustment of the fraction of inspired oxygen (FiO_2) ranging from 0.21 to 1.0. It also provides flexibility to match the inspiratory requirements of critically ill patients, thereby, it reduces room entrainment of air, which is common with conventional face masks. Another valuable effect of HFT is the generation of lower and variable positive end-expiratory pressure (PEEP) proportional to the flow rate of the delivered gas, thereby actually it improves oxygenation. In contrast, NIV is characterized by its preset steady pressure support and PEEP [4]. Unlike HFT, NIV use should be careful in patients with ARF due to high PEEP and tidal volumes (VT) which may deteriorate lung injury [5].

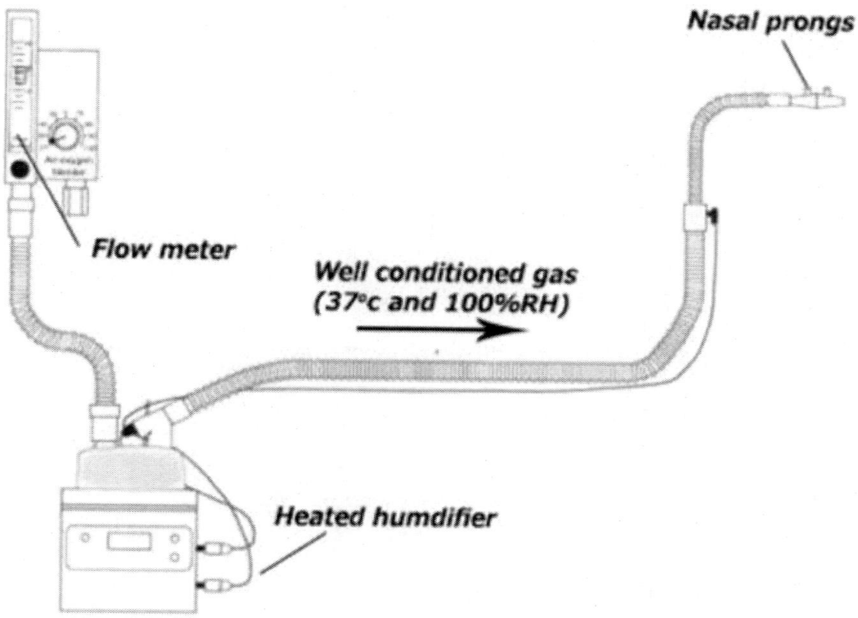

Figure 1. Setup of the high flow system.

Airways Ventilation Support

Spontaneous breathing resulting from the augmented respiratory drive-in hypoxemia may worsen lung injury through regional pressure alteration. Therefore, the term patient self-inflicted lung injury (P-SILI) was developed. NIV delivers inspiratory pressure support which is considered as a determinant of the patient's tidal volume, depending on work of breathing (WOB). Therefore, the resulting ventilation is determined by the breath efforts of patients and pressure support preset above PEEP. Although the PEEP effect is helpful in oxygenation, it has a partial effect on airway muscles unload [6].

The continuous high gas flow rate delivered by HFT systems creates dead space washout and flushes carbon dioxide out through the upper airways. Otherwise, HFT displayed a decline in the respiratory effort and mechanically improve thoracic compliance.

Humidification and Comfort

The major determinants of successful NIV strategies are tolerability and compliance. About 25% of patients with ARF display intolerance to NIV and about 10% need intubation. The delivered humidity through NIV ranges between 5 and 30 mg/L reliant on the present system. Less comfort and feeling of mucosal dryness are associated with the delivered little levels or even absence of humidification through long NIV phrases such as 12 or 24 hours.

Despite the high gas flow rate using HFT systems, it seems to display improved tolerance compared to NIV and standard oxygen therapy, enhancement of dyspnea feeling, and, consequently, well compliance. The conditioned gas delivered by HFT provides optimum physiological conditions which are relatively like those found in the alveolar system with humidity levels over 40 mg/L. [7].

Mucociliary Clearance

The inspiration of optimally conditioned gas/air in HFOT systems in standings of humidity and temperature is commonly expected to preserve mucociliary system clearance and avert mucosal dryness or desiccation to a higher degree when compared to other oxygen delivery systems with fewer conditioning features. However, evidence that supports these expectations is limited [8].

Factors Affecting Aerosol Delivery During Non-Invasive Ventilation and High Flow Therapy

Aerosol therapy delivery is commonly used with mechanical ventilation either invasive or non-invasive due to the diversity of factors affecting the delivery pattern. Optimization of settings during nebulization varies in tolerability among patients with certain respiratory illnesses such as acute respiratory distress syndrome (ARDS) or severe hypoxemic patients with Pneumonia.

Also, merging aerosol nebulization with nasal high flow cannula (NHFC) therapy was established while ordering prescribed medications mainly in patients who cannot live with temporary termination of oxygen flow [9].

However, the humidified heated gas utilization had resulted in the loss of a large amount of aerosol in the process. Hence, a newer way of aerosol delivery was recognized, enhanced condensational growth, which transports sub-micrometer-sized droplets instead of conventional micrometer-sized droplets in a high flow system by 30% to reduce aerosol loss.

Numerous factors were involved in aerosol delivery during NHFC oxygen therapy:

Airway Anatomy and Lung Disease Injury

The effect of airflow and V_T determine airway anatomy and hence, aerosol deposition. Normal clearance through the mucociliary system can be maintained by the optimal depth and composition of the mucus layer, rheology of mucus with the intact epithelial cells with ciliary structure. In patients with airway obstruction due to asthma or COPD, diminishing of mucociliary clearance with following mucous retention is common and consequently, peripheral deposition of drugs in the lungs by inertial impaction. Some drugs with insufficient trans-mucosal permeability such as inhaled aminoglycosides showed a decreased drug delivery and hence lesser efficacy; however, clinical trials approving this effect are not enough. Remodeling of the airways due to chronic inflammation can harmfully affect airflow dynamics and mucociliary clearance resulting in fewer drug deposition in the pulmonary airways [10].

Aerosol Generator Type in the Circuit

Nebulizers and pMDIs are the most commonly used aerosol generators in mechanically ventilated patients, either with spacers or without [11].

Nebulizers

The standard dose generated by nebulizers differs significantly depending on the type of nebulizer used with a considerably longer time for dose delivery compared to further devices. This effect is emphasized with the mechanics of the lung and the ventilator mode. Adequate cleaning of the nebulizer is essential to prevent the risk of nosocomial infection. Vibrating mesh nebulizers (VMNs) tend to improve delivery with an over 3-fold increase compared to jet nebulizers (JN), however, the formulation and desired site of delivery are elements of the proper nebulization choice [11].

Mode of Nebulizers

Synchronization of intermittent nebulization technique with inspiration confirmed better delivery of aerosol compared to constant nebulization mode due to the minimization of the fraction of drug missing in the exhalation phase. For better application of the intermittent nebulization with synchronization, a ventilator is recommended for better gas flow than that generated using an air compressor or gas cylinder [11].

Nebulizer Dead Volume

The residual volume in the nebulizer chamber after nebulization is called dead volume. It plays a dynamic role in determining the aerosol amount delivered to the patient. It is inversely proportional to the inhaled drug fraction. It varies from 0.1 to 2.4 ml by nebulizer type. VMNs and ultra-sonic nebulizers (UNs) left a smaller residual volume than traditional JNs. It was established by diluting the aerosolized medication with either water or saline will increase the drug delivery from JNs opposing VMNs due to their minimal residual volumes [8].

pMDIs

Pressurized metered-dose inhalers are a more practicable, cost-effective option with reliable dose delivery compared to nebulizers. Moreover, the collapsible spacer can be used easily in the circuit without the need for disconnection. The offered drugs for this device are anti-inflammatory drugs and bronchodilators. The performance of pMDIs during NIV can be enhanced by dose actuation primarily in the inspiration phase with the spacer connection to the inhaler. In HFOT, spacer-connected use displayed lesser efficacy when compared with nebulizers in this arrangement [12].

Aerosol Generators' Location within the Circuit

Nebulizer position varies according to the ventilation circuit type; in a single-limb circuit, the nebulizer is generally situated between the patient interface and expiration port close to the patient while in the dual-limb circuit, the nebulizer is typically situated on the inspiratory limb close to the ventilator, where they offered enhanced aerosol delivery and least loss [13].

Like NIV, nebulizers and pMDIs with adaptors had been used to deliver aerosols through a high-flow system. There are three probable sites to place aerosol generators within the high flow circuit. The first place is just before the humidification chamber (upstream), the second location is immediately after the humidification chamber (downstream) and the last position is immediately before the nasal cannula. The upstream position (before the inlet of the humidifier) is considered the favored one compared to the further two positions as it permits filtering out large particles inside the humidifier allowing only smaller particles to reach the cannula outlet decreasing nasal and oropharyngeal deposition and improving alveolar deposition [14].

Using pMDIs with spacer showed lesser efficiency than nebulizers within this system. The delivered dose through pMDIs was lower than itemized for the therapeutic response because aerosol delivery at this time is largely dependent on the delivered gas density.

Humidification and Heat of the Circuit

The relative humidity of the lung is assessed at up to 99.5% and it is detrimental in aerosolized particle deposition. Hygroscopic aerosols tend to increase moisture resulting in larger particle size and initial deposition in the airways. There are two major humidifier systems including active system (heated humidifier or HH) and passive system (heat and moisture exchanger or HME). It was institute that the delivery of drugs during humidified conditions can lessen to half compared to non-humidification. HME use with nebulization can result in obstruction of airflow due to particulate filters. Therefore, air filters should be routinely changed. Fisher-Paykel and Vapotherm are the two commonly high flow systems used. Studies using the Fisher-Paykel system presented higher delivery of aerosol compared to those performed using Vapotherm. Because the Vapotherm system is a closed structure with only one choice to locate the nebulizer (just before the nasal cannula), contrasting the Fisher-Paykel structure which has three configurations for aerosol generator placement [8]. The upstream position within the vapotherm system improves gas flow passing within the humidifier followed by the heating tube. So, the aerosolized medication will be enforced in the small diameter cannula that leads to a resistance change, flow turbulence, support drug buildup in the nebulizer adapter instead of leaving the cannula, and lastly low aerosol dose output to the patient.

Gas Flow Rate

The most important decision established by a high flow system over other respiratory support techniques is the ability to produce gas flows equal to 60 L/min with amplified tolerability, which is inversely proportional to the amount of drug delivered using this system [15]. The decreased portion of the drug is brought to the patient whenever the increased oxygen flow is used as greater oxygen flow creates additional turbulence and thus aerosol loss within the circuit, especially in the nasal interface due to inertial effects.

Gas Density

The medication percentage given to patients was increased by gases with a lower density than air. Heliox is a mixture of helium/oxygen with a 70/30 mixture that offers greater aerosol distribution than air as it improves lung aerosol retention for ambulatory patients. Nonetheless, the use of a mixture of helium-oxygen (low-density gases) for JNs resulted in decreased drug production from nebulizers. Oxygen accompanied by heliox (70/30 mixture) is recommended to operate JNs for the greatest drug delivery during NIV. At low flow, Heliox better drug delivery than that observed with 100% oxygen. This development may be linked to the low heliox density which, at only higher gas flows, produces less turbulence and less aerosol impaction within the system than that of oxygen. Correspondingly lower pMDI efficiency is closely correlated with rising gas density [15].

Also at low gas flow, the use of 100% oxygen (the densest possible gas mixture) with a high flow system greatly reduces the pMDI aerosol delivery. By increasing the effect of gas density by reducing the shear force applied to gas layers and particularly influencing the evaporation rate of MDI propellant, a low flow rate of 5 L/min contributes to decreasing the drug production of pMDI.

Interfaces

The direct link between the ventilation circuit and the patient is the patient interface. Nasal masks and oro-nasal masks are the best interfaces commonly found in NIV as shown in Figure 2. Nasal pillows, helmets, complete facemasks, and mouthpieces with or without the oral mask provide additional interfaces. Focusing on the proper fitting of the patient interface is important since a bad fitting decreases therapeutic efficacy by aerosol leakage or causes high facial pressure facial skin breakdown where accidental leaks are very prevalent in NIV [6].

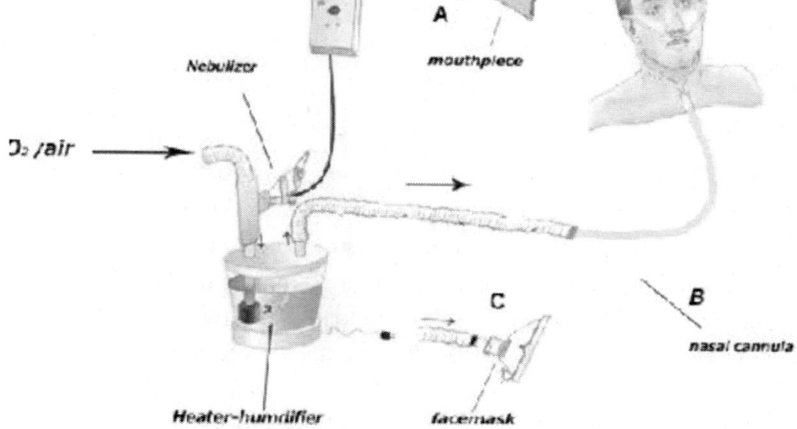

Figure 2. Different possible interfaces used in HFNC.

Via a high flow procedure, the nasal cannula is the ideal interface where the cannula size can impact the amount of aerosol administered to the patient. The dose given has been reported to be directly proportional to the cannula size. As the cannula size increases, relative to pediatric or infant size cannulas, the increased delivered dose is the most experienced delivery inside the adult cannula.

Aerosol Aerodynamic Effect

The diameter of aerosol particles and the velocity of airflow decide the distribution and deposition inside the airways. Conversely, the diameter of the particles is associated with the penetration depth of the pulmonary airways. The particle velocity through the tracheobronchial tree shows a large variety with the highest lung air velocity rates in the first 10 generations, with the highest impact compared to the terminal bronchioles and the alveolar area [2]. The effect of particles in the oropharynx reduces the amount of deposition of drugs in the lung and thus becomes less successful. With the strongest deposition features deep within the small bronchioles and alveoli, the optimal particle size array is 0.5 to 5 μm. The least preferable deposition characteristics are demonstrated by particles larger than 5 μm and smaller than 0.5 μm. Since large particles are more likely to be deposited and swallowed while the small particles are more lost during exhalation, this breath-hold cannot be tolerated by mechanically ventilating patients using NIV or HFT, unless breath-holding is done for about 5 to 10 seconds to allow deposition in the alveolar sacs.

Patient Position

The two invasively ventilator-dependent patient roles in mechanical ventilation are most usually supine or semi-recumbent. A semi-recumbent position is a more relaxed one for reducing gastric material aspiration related to the supine position in extremely exacerbated patients. A significant bronchodilator reaction might be given by the semi-recumbent set. Otherwise, standing or sitting posture is typically introduced by spontaneously breathing patients by aerosol inhalation by NIV [6].

Ventilator-Associated Factors Affecting Aerosol Delivery

In improving bronchodilator delivery by mechanical ventilation, spontaneous modes are more relaxed and efficient than controlled modes (pressure-controlled "PC" and volume-controlled "VC") as the patient can change both the size and timing of each breath, which develops synchrony with a ventilator to. For example, aerosol delivery was amplified by up to 30% by continuous positive air pressure (CPAP) compared with regulated ventilation modes at equivalent tidal volume. Therefore, when the patient is bearable, if non-bearable, regulated modes are considered, spontaneous modes of breathing are recommended [6].

Current Clinical and Pharmacological Aerosol Therapy Applications during Ventilation Using NIV and HFT

Aerosolized pharmacological agents such as corticosteroids (CS), bronchodilators, surfactants, mucolytics, and expectorants are routinely used during mechanical ventilation (NIV and HFT), with a recent interest in antibiotic aerosolization for the treatment of patients with respiratory failure.

For the control of acute COPD exacerbations and asthma, oxygenation in conjunction with inhaled bronchodilators is known to be the first-line therapy. Aerosol delivery by NHFC and NIV through pMDIs and nebulizers linked through a spacer or adapter through a ventilation circuit adds significant advantages to the treatment of patients with obstructive lung disease. The inhaled medication provided via NHFC and NIV provides medicinal properties that are faster and better than with unassisted respiration [6].

For COPD and cystic fibrosis patients, aerosolization of saline solutions is also used. In general, 0.9% of the regular saline solution is used in patients prone to bronchoconstriction in particular. Alternative acceptance of an alternative.

Acute Respiratory Distress

To prevent tissue hypoxia, HFOT may be rated as a first-line oxygenation strategy in ARF patients. It was found that as opposed to NIV, it may reduce the mortality of these patients. The beneficial effects of HFOT can be explained by its respectable tolerance and by physiological features such as the influence of PEEP, high FiO_2 delivery, and the continuous washout of dead space promoted to minimize WOB. Conversely, in patients with ARF, NIV should be used cautiously because of high VT caused by pressure support that may exacerbate existing lung injury [6].

Acute COPD Exacerbations

NIV use substantially reduced the need for intubation and mortality risk reduction in patients with acute COPD exacerbations. Compared to the conventional oxygen delivery systems and with pharmacological agents, the revised evidence strongly recommends NIV. The severity of COPD is the determinant of the anticipated benefits, especially for patients with hypercapnia and $pH<7.35$, while patients with higher pH (>7.35) have fewer NIV clinical outcomes. The data available on the use of HFT in COPD is restricted to discrepant performance. Limited numbers of studies and case reports indicated that HFT reduces $PaCO_2$ and respiratory rate, but the selection criteria of the included patients were without acute exacerbations [15].

ARF Immunocompromised Patients

In immunocompromised patients with hypoxemia, the mortality rate is relatively high. The main purpose of respiratory management is to prevent invasive ventilation. With the absolute reduction of mechanical ventilation of 29.8%, HFOT was reported to increase recovery from respiratory failure without intubation. HFOT has also reduced respiratory rate and mortality. In immunocompromised patients, both NIV and HFOT greatly improved dyspnea. HFOT has demonstrated safety and feasibility comparable to those obtained by NIV in immunocompromised patients, considering the difference in the results of the preliminary trials [6].

Cardiogenic Pulmonary Edema

For the treatment of cardiogenic pulmonary edema patients, NIV is strongly recommended, with a substantial reduction in mortality and intubation rates compared with traditional oxygen therapy. BiPAP and CPAP are similarly successful, but it is better to use BiPAP to resolve the possible WOB or in the case of comorbidities, like COPD. There is currently insufficient evidence promoting the use of HFT in patients with cardiogenic pulmonary edema and it should not be used until a clear supportive recommendation has been made.

Post-Extubation

Several studies have discussed the beneficial effects of NIV in the post-extubation period. Indeed, relative to normal oxygen systems, the risk of intubation with the use of NIV after surgery has been reduced. In such conditions, the European/American Guidelines recently recommended NIV as first-line therapy. A comparable beneficial impact and greater tolerance were seen in the emergence of HFT. Despite the hopeful outcomes of this technique in preventing or treating respiratory failure in post-operative patients, there is minimal evidence available on this issue.

Palliative Care

In patients with end-stage respiratory disorders or cancer with advanced pulmonary function loss, physicians must identify, evaluate and consider the appropriate treatment plan for dyspnea in such patients. Oxygen supplementation with the potential for symptomatic and functional enhancement is one of the common modalities in such cases. HFT has been found to outweigh the intolerance and protection of conventional oxygenation strategies. The suitability of this technique for eating and talking with ease during oxygen delivery is another benefit. It was also observed that in patients with end-stage interstitial lung disease, HFT substantially decreased cough and improved oxygenation, thereby improving living conditions and family contact. However, for end-stage respiratory failure patients who do not want intubation or resuscitation, the whole practice is still debated and NIV is recommended as superior to HFT.

Complications

As a result of the associated complications, the magnitude of NIV and HFOT usage is limited; however, it is still less than those associated with intrusive ventilation. The most common complication of NIV is facial injury and pressure necrosis, thereby adversely affecting ventilatory support. In addition to dressing use, the proper choice of the right size and form of the mask is made to outweigh the mask strain on facial skin. In addition to the danger of infections, other complications include barotrauma and hemodynamic compromise. HFT-related risks include aspiration and sometimes barotrauma and are much lower than NIV or mechanical ventilation [2].

Discontinuation

In addition to respiratory rate (RR) ≤ 25 breath/min, heart rate ≤ 120 beats/min, and systolic blood pressure ≥ 90 mmHg, the weaning plan from NIV is properly initiated upon achieving normal pH and pCO_2 estimates or patient overall improvement as calculated by the estimated parameters including pH levels that should be ≥ 7.35 and SpO_2 greater than 90 percent on FiO_2 less than 50 percent. Signs of pulmonary pressure and hypoxia can be minimized for a long time within the first 24 hours, such as agitation or anxiety [2].

Prediction of NIV and HFT Failure

Strategies for oxygen administration should not prolong tracheobronchial intubation or mask the life-threatening symptoms of ARF to prevent lung damage from worsening. Mechanical intubation decisions remain a frequent clinical concern in patients with advanced respiratory failure while on NIV or HFT. The delay of intubation in patients receiving NIV or HFT beyond approximately 48 hours is associated with higher mortality rates and prolongs the period of mechanical ventilation required. The presence of the following symptoms, including high RR, shock, progressive hypoxemia, or metabolic acidosis, will support the need for intubation. However, these are not established by the evidence as a valid indication of the decision to intubate. The SpO_2/FiO_2 index ratio, abbreviated as the ROX index relating to oxygenation of the respiratory rate, was developed as a predictor of the need for intubation. The ROX index > 4.88 after 12 hours indicates the suitability and protection of HFT usage and no need for mechanical intrusive ventilation [2].

Conclusion

Several factors are affecting aerosol delivery to patients through HFNC which necessitates certain adjustments in some situations to ensure optimum aerosol delivery to critically ill patients. Type of aerosol generator and its position, use of humidifiers, gas density, the type of interface used, and the gas flow rate in HFNC therapy are the most important influencing factors.

There are a huge number of published works related to aerosol delivery to such a critically ill patient. Physician decisions about the aerosol delivery method to such a critically ill patient based upon reading any of this released literature without a trusted recommendation and guidelines are very critical. This increases the need for the development of recommendations and guidelines, by a trusted board or society.

To summarize, inhaled drugs administered to critically ill patients is of benefit compared to stopping the HFNC therapy and delivering during spontaneous unassisted breathing. However, dependable guidelines are needed to optimize aerosol delivery.

Key Points

- Patients with obstructive pulmonary illness can benefit greatly from the aerosol delivery provided by pressurized metered-dose inhalers (pMDIs) and nebulizers attached by an adapter or spacer into a high flow nasal cannula (HFNC) system.
- In comparison to unaided breathing, the drug administered during HFNC has better and quicker clinical results.
- Several factors are affecting aerosol delivery to patients through HFNC which necessitates certain adjustments in some situations to ensure optimum aerosol delivery to critically ill patients.
- Inhaled drugs administered to critically ill patients are of benefit compared to stopping the HFNC therapy and delivering during spontaneous unassisted breathing. However, dependable guidelines are needed to optimize aerosol delivery.
- Unfortunately, while administering aerosols using HFNC, there are no clear recommendations or guidelines, which put patients at risk of receiving either a sub-therapeutic or hazardous amount of their inhaled drugs.
- This makes it much more urgent for a reputable body or society to create recommendations or guidelines for administering aerosols to such seriously ill patients.

References

[1] Seif SM, Ma E, Rabea H, Saeed H, Abdelrahim MEA. Aerosol delivery of inhalation devices with different add-on connections to invasively ventilated COPD subjects: An in-vivo study. *European Journal of Pharmaceutical Sciences.* 2021 2021/12/01/;167:105988.

[2] Madney YM, Laz NI, Elberry AA, Rabea H, Abdelrahim MEA. Aerosol delivery aspects within a high-flow therapy system in COPD patients. *ERJ Open Research.* 2021;7(1):00422-2020.

[3] Madney YM, Fathy M, Elberry AA, Rabea H, Abdelrahim ME. Aerosol delivery through an adult high-flow nasal cannula circuit using low-flow oxygen. *Respiratory Care.* 2019;64(4):453-61.

[4] Madney YM, Fathy M, Elberry AA, Rabea H, Abdelrahim ME. Nebulizers and spacers for aerosol delivery through adult nasal cannula at low oxygen flow rate: An in-vitro study. *Journal of Drug Delivery Science and Technology.* 2017;39:260-5.

[5] Seif SM, Elnady MA, Rabea H, Saeed H, Abdelrahim MEA. Effect of different connection adapters on aerosol delivery in invasive ventilation setting; an in-vitro study. *Journal of Drug Delivery Science and Technology.* 2020 2020/10/26/:102177.

[6] Madney YM, Laz NI, Elberry AA, Rabea H, Abdelrahim ME. The influence of changing interfaces on aerosol delivery within high flow oxygen setting in adults: An in-vitro study. *Journal of Drug Delivery Science and Technology.* 2020;55:101365.

[7] Saeed H, Salem HF, Rabea H, Abdelrahim ME. Effect of human error, inhalation flow, and inhalation volume on dose delivery from Ellipta® dry-powder inhaler. *Journal of Pharmaceutical Innovation.* 2019;14(3):239-44.

[8] Saeed H, Mohsen M, Eldin AS, Elberry AA, Hussein RR, Rabea H, et al. Effects of fill volume and humidification on aerosol delivery during single-limb noninvasive ventilation. *Respiratory Care.* 2018;63(11):1370-8.

[9] Saeed H, Ali AM, Elberry AA, Eldin AS, Rabea H, Abdelrahim ME. Modeling and optimization of nebulizers' performance in non-invasive ventilation using different fill volumes: comparative study between vibrating mesh and jet nebulizers. *Pulmonary Pharmacology & Therapeutics*. 2018;50:62-71.

[10] Nicola M, Elberry A, Sayed O, Hussein R, Saeed H, Abdelrahim M. The impact of adding a training device to familiar counselling on inhalation technique and pulmonary function of asthmatics. *Advances in Therapy.* 2018;35(7):1049-58.

[11] Harb HS, Elberry AA, Rabea H, Fathy M, Abdelrahim ME. Performance of large spacer versus nebulizer T-piece in single-limb noninvasive ventilation. *Respiratory Care.* 2018;63(11):1360-9.

[12] Saeed H, Abdelrahim ME, Rabea H, Salem HF. Impact of Advanced Patient Counseling Using a Training Device and Smartphone Application on Asthma Control. *Respiratory Care.* 2020;65(3):326-32.

[13] Hassan A, Rabea H, Hussein RR, Eldin RS, Abdelrahman MM, Said AS, et al. In-Vitro Characterization of the Aerosolized Dose During Non-Invasive Automatic Continuous Positive Airway Pressure Ventilation. *Pulmonary Therapy.* 2016;2:115-26.

[14] Rabea H, Ali AM, Eldin RS, Abdelrahman MM, Said AS, Abdelrahim ME. Modelling of in-vitro and in-vivo performance of aerosol emitted from different vibrating mesh nebulisers in non-invasive ventilation circuit. *European Journal of Pharmaceutical Sciences.* 2017;97:182-91.

[15] Madney YM, Ibrahim Laz N, Elberry AA, Rabea H, Abdelrahim MEA. The impact of changing patient interfaces on delivering aerosol with titrated oxygen in the high flow system. *International Journal of Clinical Practice.* 2021;74(4):e13898.

Chapter 19

Definition, Severity and Prevalence of COPD Exacerbation

Pinar Atagun Guney*
Koşuyolu High Specialızation Education and Research Hospital,
Istanbul, Turkey

Abstract

No single definition of acute (Chronic obstructive pulmonary disease) COPD exacerbation has been universally accepted. However, it can reasonably be defined as an acute change in a patient s initial shortness of breath, or sputum, that exceeds normal daily variability and needs a change in medication. The impact of exacerbations is significant and it may take several weeks for the patient s symptoms and lung function to return to baseline values. The most common causes of exacerbation are tracheobronchial tree infection and air pollution, but the cause of about a third of severe exacerbations cannot be determined. While managing the exacerbation of COPD with history, physical examination, laboratory, and imaging, alternative diagnoses that may be confused with the acute situation should also be kept in mind. Exacerbations significantly reduce the quality of life, deplete financial resources and accelerate a progressive decline in pulmonary function, causing frequent hospitalizations, relapses, and readmissions, contributing to death during or shortly after hospitalization. For this reason, patients should be made aware of exposure and should care about symptoms different from their current symptoms. It can also be controlled in the progression of the disease with the need for medical treatment support.

Keywords: chronic obstructive pulmonary disease exacerbation, exacerbation

Introduction

Exacerbations of chronic obstructive pulmonary disease place a significant burden on health systems all over the world in terms of disease-related morbidity, mortality, and health care costs [1].

A clear definition of an acute COPD exacerbation has not yet been clarified worldwide. However, the patient s initial shortness of breath, and the presence of cough or sputum, which

---

* Corresponding Author s Email: atagunpnar@yahoo.com.

In: Chronic Obstructive Pulmonary Disease
Editor: Jaber S. Alqahtani
ISBN: 979-8-88697-333-4

may be beyond the normal daily variability, can cause changes in the routine treatment of this condition. For an attack, the deterioration in general condition must have been lasting for at least a duration of 24 hours. The deterioration in the general condition of the patient is not a clear situation. The most prominent symptoms in a COPD attack can be described as increased sputum volume and/or purulence, increased dyspnea and/or wheezing, chest tightness, and fluid retention (Table 1) [2, 3]. Severity classification: Mild exacerbation is an attack in which the patient can meet the increasing need for treatment with short-acting bronchodilators. A moderate attack is an attack in which the patient applies to outpatient units for increased treatment needs such as systemic steroids or anti-biotherapies. Severe exacerbation is defined as an attack in which the patient or his/her relative notices the significant and/or rapid deterioration of the disease and requires hospital treatment [2]. COPD exacerbations may result in conditions such as impairing the quality of life of patients, worsening the course of the disease, increasing hospitalization, and increasing the risk of mortality [4].

Table 1. Classification of COPD attack according to clinical findings (Anthonisen Criteria) (3)

Basic Symptoms
• Dyspnea increase
• Increased amount of sputum
• Increase in sputum purulence
Type 1 (Severe) Attack
• The combination of all 3 symptoms
Type 2 (Moderate) Attack
• Presence of 2 symptoms
Type 3 (Mild) Attack
• Presence of 1 symptom and addition of one of the following:
- Fever not attributed to any other cause
- Increase in cough
- 20% increase in heart rate
- 20% increase in respiratory rate
- Wheezing increase
- Signs of upper respiratory tract infection in the last 5 days

Epidemiology

The observational studies of COPD patients have shown a heterogeneous distribution in exacerbations. In studies involving a large number of patients, 0 to 2 exacerbations were detected per year; while in studies conducted on fewer patients, 10 and/or more exacerbations per year were revealed. The average number of COPD exacerbations per year correlates with COPD severity, but the numbers are highly variable. On the other hand, 40% of COPD patients may not have any exacerbation. If unreported COPD exacerbations are included, the mean for severe patients (GOLD stage III) is 3.43 exacerbations/year, and the annual mean for GOLD stage II is 2.68. The COPD patients who have had frequent exacerbations in the past are more likely to experience more frequent COPD exacerbations in the future [5]. Anthonisen et al., found that 50% of the attacks were not reported to the healthcare team in their study, in which the study determined the attacks according to the symptoms. Due to the frequent changes in symptoms during the course of COPD, it is thought that patients who are accustomed to this condition care about all attacks [3].

Etiology

COPD attacks can be caused by a wide variety of etiologic factors:

a) *Infections:* Most exacerbations are caused by infections. In the initial studies, bacteria were shown as the main cause of exacerbations. During an attack, S. pneumonia, Moraxella Catarrhalis, and Haemophilus influenzae are the most frequently isolated pathogens in patients with positive bacterial cultures. However, with the development of molecular diagnostic techniques, the importance of viral agents in exacerbations has been emphasized. Rhinoviruses were the most common in most studies, accounting for 60% of all exacerbations. Influenza viruses (36%) and (Respiratory syncytial virus) RSVs (28%) are among other common viral agents. A Viral and/or bacterial infection was detected in 78% of the COPD exacerbations. In the hospital, 29.7% of such infections were bacterial, while 23.3% of them were viral, and 25% were viral/bacterial coinfections. Infectious exacerbations have been shown to cause longer hospital stays and greater deterioration in lung function tests than non-infectious exacerbations [6, 7].
b) *Environmental Factors:* The triggering role of air pollution has been known for a long time. Short-term exposure to air pollutants (trioxygen, carbon monoxide, nitrogen dioxide, sulfur dioxide, particulate matter [PM] 10, and PM 2.5) is associated with an increased risk of attacks [8]. These particles can trigger airway inflammation and increase susceptibility to infections. Therefore, exposure to air pollutants can precipitate exacerbations, which can be both infectious and non-infectious in origin [9].

Other contributing mechanisms must be excluded before exacerbations from respiratory infections and/or contaminants can be identified. These acute events can be summarized as pneumonia, pneumothorax, foreign body, atelectasis, acute ischemic heart disease and arrhythmia, pulmonary embolism, anemia, and depression (Table 2) [10].

Table 2. Most common causes of acute exacerbation of COPD

Primary: Tracheobronchial infections: Viral (Rhinovirus spp., influenza); bacteria (Haemophilus influenza, Streptococcus pneumonia, Moraxella catarhalis, Enterobacteriacease spp., Pseudomonas spp.)
• Environmental factors
• Air pollution
• Non-compliance with long-term oxygen therapy
• Pulmonary rehabilitation mismatch
Secondary (situations mimicking acute attack)
• Pneumonia
• Pneumothorax, Foreign body
• Pulmonary Embolism, Atelectasis
• Right and/or left heart failure
• Arrhythmias, Anemia, Depression

Pathology

The pathology of exacerbations is complex. The changes that may contribute to exacerbation symptoms can be stated as; increased airway inflammation, mucus production, and marked gas entrapment. A COPD attack is an acute exacerbation development with a background of chronic inflammation. This inflammation is a complex response involving multiple mediators including cytokines regulated by chemoattractant and adhesion molecules, as well as the migration, activation, and degeneration of inflammatory cells. [11]

In the sputum samples of COPD patients with frequent attacks:

- It has been shown that IL-6 and IL-8 levels are high even if the disease is stable, and there is an even greater increase in IL-6 levels during the attack.
- IL-6 level is correlated with eosinophil and lymphocyte count.
- In chronic bronchitis attacks, there are an approximately 30-fold increase activated eosinophil granule 2 (EG2+) in eosinophils, which approaches the levels observed in asthma.
- COPD and asthma attack mechanisms differ. IL-4 and IL-5, which are the 2 main determinants in asthma attacks, are not seen in COPD attacks.
- In bronchial biopsies of patients with chronic bronchitis;
  - There is an increase in eotaxin gene expression in response to cigarette smoke.
  - Monocyte chemotactic peptide (MCP)-4, another eosinophil chemoattractant, is unchanged.
  - Baseline ((Regulated on activation, normal T-cell expressed and secreted) RANTES levels are increased in smokers with COPD. However, especially during acute attack, the increase in RANTES level is higher and RANTES gene expression correlates with increased tissue eosinophil level.
  - RANTES induces CD8+ T-lymphocytes to apoptosis.
  - Viruses invade the lower respiratory tract in COPD patients. Persistent viral infections may be important in the pathogenesis of COPD.
  - Viruses provide upregulation of RANTES as well as proinflammatory cell adhesion molecules (ICAM-1, LFA-3).
  - Epithelial expression of ICAM-1 explains why neutrophils attach to the epithelium in bronchial biopsies.
- Increasing severity of COPD is associated with a decrease in the CD4/CD8 T-lymphocyte ratio (due to CD8 T-cell increase) [12].

Clinical and Laboratory Evaluation

In order to determine the severity of an acute attack, the evaluation is made in three parts: questioning the condition of the patient in previous attacks with anamnesis, symptoms, and the physical examination findings at the time of the attack, as well as laboratory tests. Cough, sputum amount and color, dyspnea, and the level of restriction in daily activities help in determining the severity of the attack. Dyspnea is the most common and important symptom of a COPD exacerbation [13]. Use of accessory respiratory muscles, paradoxical chest wall motion, worsening of central cyanosis, hemodynamic disorder, cor pulmonale signs (peripheral edema, jugular venous engorgement, and hepatomegaly) indicate the severity of the disease. Generally, there is a positive correlation between the reduction in breathing sounds and airflow limitation. Rales or rhonchi may also be heard. On cardiac auscultation, it is noticed that the heart sounds seem to originate from a depth. Arrhythmia or tachycardia may be detected. In cases where cor pulmonale develops, S3 gallop and S2 hardening, as well as murmurs due to pulmonary or tricuspid regurgitation may be heard. Coma and cardiorespiratory arrest are life-limiting attacks, and the patient must be admitted to the intensive care unit. Fever > 38.5°C, respiratory rate > 25/minute, and heart rate > 100/minute are the parameters determining the severity of the attack. In order to determine the severity of the attack, the use of the accessory respiratory muscles, paradoxical chest wall motion, new or worsening central cyanosis, the presence of peripheral edema, as well as any change in the hemodynamic and/or mental status should be checked quickly. In recent years, studies have been carried out on biomarkers that will help predict the length of hospital stay, treatment failure or mortality risk in exacerbations. In acute exacerbations, the role of procalcitonin in addition to (C-reactive protein) CRP, white blood cell (WBC), sputum cultures in the decision of antimicrobial therapy is well established [3].

In the studies of Stolz et al., conducted in hospitalized COPD attack patients, it was found that serum levels of copeptin, CRP, and procalcitonin increased at hospitalization, decreased with treatment, and procalcitonin predicted prognosis during hospitalization and requiring intensive care. It is stated that serum copeptin levels are superior to other markers in predicting long-term (6 months) prognosis as well as in the short term [14]. Blood gas analysis is important in detecting respiratory failure developing in the acute attacks of COPD. The acute exacerbation of COPD typically presents with marked hypoxia with or without hypercapnia. Severe COPD exacerbations frequently require admission to the hospital and/or intensive care unit and are associated with acute respiratory failure: arterial oxygen tension (PaO2) < 60 mm Hg with or without arterial carbon dioxide tension, (PaCO2) > 45 mm Hg, and hydrogen ion concentration (pH) < 7.35) on room air [2, 13].

Pulmonary function testing is not routinely recommended in acute exacerbations due to the difficulty of its application [2].

Radiography

(Posterioranterior) PA chest radiography is an important examination in the management of acute exacerbation of COPD. PA chest radiography can be used both in terms of differential diagnosis (chronic heart failure, pleural fluid) and to exclude causes that may mimic an exacerbation, such as pneumonia or pneumothorax due to COPD. The differential diagnosis of pulmonary embolism is difficult in severe attacks. Spiral computed tomography, angiography, and D-dimer are tests that can be used in suspected pulmonary embolism in COPD [14, 15].

Sputum

In stable chronic bronchitis, sputum is mucoid and the dominant cell is macrophage. In periods of acute attack, sputum becomes purulent. During this period, neutrophils increase.

Microorganisms can be demonstrated by Gram staining. Streptococcus pneumoniae, Haemophilus influenzae and Moraxella catarrhalis are usually responsible for acute attacks of COPD. Routine sputum culture is not required. This examination can be performed when an unknown bacteria is seen on gram stain, gram-negative bacillus or staphylococcus-like bacteria are widely observed, there is a history of antibiotic use, severe COPD or pneumonia is present [12, 16].

The symptoms during an exacerbation last for approximately seven days. It has been observed that the acute attack may last longer, and that some cases cannot return to their pre-exacerbation state at the end of eight weeks and the disease progresses as a result [2].

Clinical Course and Mortality

In the study, it was found that the factors that increase the risk of exacerbation are advanced age, (Forced expiratory volume in 1 second) FEV_1 percent value, COPD diagnosis time, productive cough, antibiotic or corticosteroid use for COPD in the previous year, theophylline use, and hospitalization for COPD in the previous year by Niewoehner et al. It has been shown that after a COPD attack, patients either do not reach their initial (Peak expiratory flow rate) PEFR or FEV_1 values at all, or this process takes months, and there are significant decreases in quality of life questionnaires. 109 patients with COPD were followed for 4 years, during which 757 attacks were observed. It was determined that the annual loss in FEV_1 and PEFR was significantly higher in cases with frequent attacks. It was found in a study that it took an average of 91 days for PEFR values to return to the starting point, and 404 attacks in 101 COPD patients were followed. In the long-term follow-up of patients hospitalized for COPD attack, 3-month, 1-year, 2-years mortality rates were found to be 13%, 22%, and 35%, respectively. The long-term prognosis after hospitalization for COPD exacerbation is poor. Factors associated with poor outcomes include low BMI, advanced age, comorbidities, previous hospitalizations for COPD exacerbations, clinical severity of exacerbation, and the need for prolonged oxygen therapy at discharge [17]. Exacerbations were measured in patients followed up, and many factors associated with exacerbations were reported in prospective cohort studies. These identified risk factors are summarized in Table 3.

Mortality rates were much higher, found in another study of 1016 patients with severe COPD with a PaCO2 above 50 mmHg: 60-day, 180-day, 1-year, and 2-year mortalities were 20%, 33%, 43%, and 49%, respectively. Risk factors for higher hospital mortality, advanced age, severity of disease, previous functional status, malnutrition, concomitant heart disease, cor pulmonale, PaO2/FiO2, hypoalbuminemia, previous mechanical disease among patients requiring hospitalization and intensive care for COPD exacerbation ventilation therapy, long-term corticosteroid therapy, and the APACHE II score at admission to the intensive care unit. In recent years, studies have been carried out on biomarkers that will help predict the length of hospital stay, treatment failure or mortality risk in exacerbations [18, 19].

COPD patients admitted to the emergency department due to an exacerbation and taken under observation should be evaluated promptly in terms of the severity of the exacerbation, hospitalization, and need for intensive care. Indications for hospitalization in exacerbation; the presence of severe symptoms can be listed such as sudden worsening in resting dyspnea, increased respiratory rate, decreased oxygen saturation, confusion, somnolence, acute respiratory failure, newly developed physical findings (cyanosis, peripheral edema), failure to respond to the initial medical treatment, presence of serious comorbidities (cardiac failure, newly developed arrhythmia, etc.) and inadequate home care [2].

Table 3. Factors associated with an increase in COPD exacerbations [20]

Risk Factor
• Ischaemic heart disease (2 studies with 2,495 participants, low quality evidence) • History of reflux or heartburn (1 study with 2,138 participants, moderate to high quality evidence) • History of pneumonia (2 studies with 1,490 participants, moderate quality evidence) • Diabetes (2 studies with 637 participants, low to moderate quality evidence) • Emphysema (1 study with 2,138 participants, moderate quality evidence) • History of asthma (2 studies with 5,942 participants, moderate quality evidence) • Overweight/obesity (1 study with 512 participants, low to moderate quality evidence)

We recommend the use of antibiotics in the treatment of patients with outpatient COPD exacerbations in patients with increased sputum purulence and an increase in dyspnea or sputum volume in at least one of the following: The choice of antibiotics for possible treatment based on local resistance patterns should be carefully chosen. Sputum cultures are generally not recommended unless the patient has been on antibiotics recently. For patients who meet the antibiotic criteria above, the choice of a specific antibiotic depends on risk factors for poor outcomes with narrower-spectrum antibiotics (eg age ≥ 65, FEV1 < 50% predicted, ≥ 2 exacerbations/year, presence of comorbid diseases) and unusual circumstances.

Pulmonary rehabilitation recommendations contribute to pulmonary rehabilitation to reduce the risk of hospitalization in patients with COPD who have recently had a COPD exacerbation. (i.e., 4 weeks after hospitalization).

Pulmonary rehabilitation is not recommended to prevent acute COPD exacerbations in patients with moderate, severe, or very severe COPD who have had exacerbations for more than 4 weeks. In patients with COPD with a previous or recent history of exacerbations, education and case management that includes direct access to a healthcare professional at least monthly to prevent severe acute exacerbations of COPD, as assessed by reductions in hospitalizations, is recommended [21].

COPD Exacerbations and COVİD-19

The reductions in face-to-face consultations due to the COVID-19 pandemic have made the routine management and diagnosis of COPD more difficult due to difficulties in spirometry applications and disruptions in traditional pulmonary rehabilitation and home care programs.

Many studies reporting comorbidities of patients admitted to hospital with COVID-19 have suggested a lower-than-expected prevalence of COPD from the population prevalence; these findings are limited by small sample sizes and missing data on comorbidities. A large study with extensive data on comorbidities showed a high prevalence of COPD (19%) among those admitted, although many patients had more than one comorbidity.

There is evidence of a decrease in hospitalization rates for COPD during the pandemic. The reasons for this are not fully clear. However, patients experiencing exacerbation symptoms should be evaluated as usual during the pandemic and hospitalized if necessary. COPD patients presenting with respiratory symptoms, fever, or other symptoms suggestive of SARS-CoV-2 infection should be tested for possible infection, even if mild. False-negative RT-PCR tests have been reported in patients with computerized tomographic (CT) scan findings of COVID-19 who eventually tested positive by serial sampling. Patients with COPD should contact their healthcare provider to determine the need for specific testing if they have been exposed to someone with a known COVID-19 infection. Antibody testing can be used to support the clinical assessment of late presenting patients.

A high index of suspicion for COVID-19 should be maintained, particularly in COPD patients presenting with exacerbation symptoms accompanied by fever, taste or smell disturbance, or gastrointestinal complaints.

Prevention and treatment of exacerbations are important goals in COPD management. COVID-19 infection has presented unique barriers to the prevention and management of exacerbations. These are limited access to treatments due to their use for patients with COVID-19 without COPD, disruptions in global supply chains, and the inability of patients to afford medicines due to economic difficulties associated with the pandemic. On the other hand, pollutant emissions have been significantly reduced and air quality has improved as countries have come under quarantine and industrial activities ceased. These factors may have contributed to the reported reductions in hospitalizations for COPD during the COVID-19 pandemic. Coronaviruses are among the respiratory viruses that trigger COPD exacerbations. To date, MERS-CoV, SARS-CoV, and SARS-CoV-2 infection have not been reported in COPD exacerbations. However, patients with COPD and SARS-CoV-2 infection presenting with respiratory symptoms requiring a change in maintenance medication would be included in the definition of exacerbation. It can be extremely difficult to distinguish the symptoms of a typical flare-up from a COVID-19 infection, as many of the symptoms overlap. If a COVID-19 infection is suspected, RT-PCR testing should be performed. If COVID-19 infection is confirmed, treatment for COVID-19 infection should be undertaken regardless of the presence of COPD. COVID-19 infection has a significant risk, including vascular injury, hypoxemia-associated pneumonia, coagulopathy, high-level systemic inflammation ("cytokine storm"), and multi-organ involvement, which lead to a different pattern of pathophysiological changes. These features are very different from typical COPD exacerbations. However, COVID-19 infection can resemble a COPD exacerbation. Fever, anorexia, myalgia, and gastrointestinal symptoms are reported more frequently in COVID-19 than COPD exacerbations, while sputum production occurs in both [22].

Preventing exacerbations in COPD is of great importance in terms of reducing morbidity, mortality and health burden. Therefore, it is among the primary goals of treatment in patients with stable COPD. Despite both pharmacological and non-pharmacological treatment methods, unfortunately, some of the patients still continue to have frequent exacerbations. In the prevention of exacerbations, studies are continuing to select the patients who will gain the most from the current treatments and to develop new treatment methods. Pharmacological treatments; inhalers, antibiotics, mucolytics, and non-pharmacological approaches; patients can be protected from acute attacks by tailoring treatments such as patient education, smoking cessation, influenza vaccination, pulmonary rehabilitation, and lung volume reduction interventions (surgical or bronchoscopic), long-term oxygen therapy and non-invasive ventilation [2].

Conclusion

COPD is an increasing cause of morbidity and mortality worldwide. Acute exacerbations negatively affect health status, hospitalization rates, disease progression, and mortality in COPD. In a COPD patient hospitalized for an acute exacerbation, the five-year mortality rate reaches 50%. In addition, hospitalizations account for more than 70% of COPD-related health care expenditures. However, since about half of acute exacerbations are not reported by patients, it becomes difficult to give the true incidence of acute exacerbations in COPD. For this reason, it is of great importance to provide adequate education to patients about the importance of exacerbation symptoms and when to admit to the hospital.

Key Points

- COPD is an increasing cause of morbidity and mortality worldwide.
- COPD exacerbation is under recognized and under reported.
- Treatment compliance of the patients should be checked as to reach positive outcomes.
- The assessment and treatment of outpatients and hospitalizations must be done in the context of accurate and evidence-based data.
- In order to assist patients in recognizing and rapidly obtaining treatment for exacerbations, self-management programs should be devised.

References

[1] Anzueto A. Impact of exacerbations on COPD. *Eur. Respir. Rev*. 2010;19(116):113-118.

[2] Singh D, Agusti A, Anzueto A, Barnes P J, Bourbeau J, Celli B R, Criner G J, Frith P, Halpin D M G, Han M, López Varela M V, Martinez F, Montes de Oca M, Papi A, Pavord I D, Roche N, Sin D D, Stockley R, Vestbo J, Wedzicha J A, Vogelmeier C. Global Strategy for the Diagnosis, Management, and Prevention of Chronic Obstructive Lung Disease: the GOLD science committee report 2019. *Eur. Respir. J*. 2019;53(5):1900164.

[3] Anthonisen N R, Manfreda J, Warren C P, Hershfield E S, Harding G K, Nelson N A. Antibiotic therapy in exacerbations of chronic obstructive pulmonary disease. *Ann. Intern. Med*. 1987;106(2):196-204.

[4] Wedzicha J A Ers Co-Chair, Miravitlles M, Hurst J R, Calverley P M A, Albert R K, Anzueto A, Criner G J, Papi A, Rabe K F, Rigau D, Sliwinski P, Tonia T, Vestbo J, Wilson K C, Krishnan Ats Co-Chair J A. Management of COPD exacerbations: a European Respiratory Society/American Thoracic Society guideline. *Eur. Respir. J*. 2017;49(3):1600 791.

[5] Caramori G, Adcock I M, Papi A. Clinical definition of COPD exacerbations and classification of their severity. *South Med. J*. 2009;102(3):277-282.

[6] Ritchie A I, Wedzicha J A. Definition, Causes, Pathogenesis, and Consequences of Chronic Obstructive Pulmonary Disease Exacerbations. *Clin. Chest Med*. 2020;41(3):421-438.

[7] MacLeod M, Papi A, Contoli M, Beghé B, Celli B R, Wedzicha J A, Fabbri L M. Chronic obstructive pulmonary disease exacerbation fundamentals: Diagnosis, treatment, prevention and disease impact. *Respirology*. 2021;26(6):532-551.

[8] Li J, Sun S, Tang R, Qiu H, Huang Q, Mason T G, Tian L. Major air pollutants and risk of COPD exacerbations: a systematic review and meta-analysis. *Int. J. Chron. Obstruct. Pulmon. Dis*. 2016;1 1:3079-3091.

[9] Pfeffer P E, Donaldson G C, Mackay A J, Wedzicha J A. Increased Chronic Obstructive Pulmonary Disease Exacerbations of Likely Viral Etiology Follow Elevated Ambient Nitrogen Oxides. *Am. J. Respir. Crit. Care Med.* 2019;199(5):581-591.

[10] Beghé B, Verduri A, Roca M, Fabbri LM. Exacerbation of respiratory symptoms in COPD patients may not be exacerbations of COPD. *Eur. Respir. J.* 2013;41(4):993-995.

[11] MacLeod M, Papi A, Contoli M, Beghé B, Celli B R, Wedzicha J A, Fabbri L M. Chronic obstructive pulmonary disease exacerbation fundamentals: Diagnosis, treatment, prevention and disease impact. *Respirology*. 2021;26(6):532-551.

[12] Papi A, Luppi F, Franco F, Fabbri L M. Pathophysiology of exacerbations of chronic obstructive pulmonary disease. *Proc. Am. Thorac. Soc.* 2006;3(3):245-251.

[13] Stolz D, Christ-Crain M, Morgenthaler N G, Leuppi J, Miedinger D, Bingisser R, Müler C, Struck S, Müler B, Tamm M. Copeptin, C-Reactive Protein, and Procalcitonin as prognostic biomarkers inith chroxacerbation of COPD. *Chest* 2007; 131:1058-67.

[14] O Brien C, Guest P J, Hill S L, Stockley R A. Physiological and radiological characterisation of patients diagnosed with chronic obstructive pulmonary disease in primary care. *Thorax*. 2000;55(8):635-642.

[15] Stockley R A, O Brien C, Pye A, Hill S L. Relationship of sputum color to nature and outpatient management of acute exacerbations of COPD. *Chest*. 2000;117(6):1638-1645.

[16] Vogelmeier C F, Criner G J, Martinez F J, Anzueto A, Barnes P J, Bourbeau J,·Celli B R, Chen R,·Decramer M,·Fabbri L M, Frith P, Halpin D M G, López Varela M V, Nishimura M,·Roche N,·Rodriguez-Roisin R, Sin D D, Singh D, Stockley R, Vestbo J, Wedzicha J A, Agustí A. Global Strategy for the Diagnosis, Management, and Prevention of Chronic Obstructive Lung Disease 2017 Report. GOLD Executive Summary. *Am. J. Respir. Crit. Care Med.* 2017;195(5):557-582.

[17] Connors A F Jr, Dawson N V, Thomas C, Harrell F E, Desbiens N, Fulkerson W J, Kussin P, Bellamy P, Goldman L, Knaus W A. Outcomes following acute exacerbation of severe chronic obstructive lung disease. *AJRCCM* 1996;154: 959-67.

[18] Niewoehne D E, Lokhnygina Y, Rice K, Kuschner W G, Sharafkhaneh A, Sarosi GA, Krumpe P, Pieper K, Ketsen S. Risk Indexes for exacerbations and hospitalizations due to COPD. *Chest* 2007; 131:20-8.

[19] Seemungal T A, Donaldson G C, Bhowmik A, Jeffries D J, Wedzicha J A. Time course and recovery of exacerbations in patients with chronic obstructive pulmonary disease. *AJRCCM* 2000; 161:1608-13.

[20] *Predicting and preventing exacerbations: Chronic obstructive pulmonary disease in over 16s: diagnosis and management*. London: National Institute for Health and Care Excellence (NICE); December 2018.

[21] Criner G J, Bourbeau J, Diekemper R L, Ouellette D R, Goodridge D, Hernandez P, Curren K, Balter M S, Bhutani M, Camp P G, Celli B R, Dechman G, Dransfield M T, Fiel S B, Foreman M G, Hanania N A, Ireland B K, Marchetti N, Stickland M K. Prevention of acute exacerbations of COPD: American College of Chest Physicians and Canadian Thoracic Society Guideline. *Chest*. 2015;147(4):894-942.

[22] Halpin D M G, Criner G J, Papi A, Singh D, Anzueto A, Martinez F J, Agusti A A, Vogelmeier C F. Global Initiative for the Diagnosis, Management, and Prevention of Chronic Obstructive Lung Disease. The 2020 GOLD Science Committee Report on COVID-19 and Chronic Obstructive Pulmonary Disease. *Am. J. Respir. Crit. Care Med.* 2021;203(1):24-36.

Chapter 20

Acute Exacerbation of COPD: Differential Diagnosis

Habib Md Reazaul Karim[1,*]
and Mahesh S Kurwe[2]

[1]Department of Anaesthesiology,
Critical Care and Pain Medicine,
All India Institute of Medical Sciences, Raipur, India
[2]Department of Anaesthesia and Intensive Care,
Peoples College of Medical Sciences,
Bhopal, India

Abstract

Chronic obstructive pulmonary disease (COPD) is widely prevalent in patients aged beyond the fourth decade across the globe. It has significant morbidity and impact on quality of life. Acute exacerbation of COPD (AECOPD) has even significant mortality if not detected and treated on time. It is characterized by the acute deterioration of the cough and shortness of breath, often requiring increasing medication and even emergency department visits and hospitalization. Multiple factors can predispose a COPD patient to AECOPD. Many cardiorespiratory conditions also co-exist and even mimic AECOPD when present as an isolated condition. These conditions need to be considered as differentials of AECOPD and managed accordingly. The present chapter briefly enumerates the differentials of AECOPD and puts forward a bedside algorithmic approach to reaching a differential diagnosis.

Keywords: COPD, Asthma, Differential Diagnosis, Lung Ultrasound, Emergency

Introduction

An acute exacerbation of chronic obstructive pulmonary disease (AECOPD) is a clinical diagnosis made when COPD patients experience an acute and sustained increase in cough, sputum production, and/or dyspnea. Although there is an absence of homogeneity in the

[*] Corresponding Author's Email: drhabibkarim@gmail.com.

In: Chronic Obstructive Pulmonary Disease
Editor: Jaber S. Alqahtani
ISBN: 979-8-88697-333-4

definition, the Global Initiative for Chronic Obstructive Lung Disease has defined it as an acute worsening of the signs and symptoms of COPD requiring additional medication to control it [1].

However, most internationally accepted definitions have common components, i.e., acute onset and worsening symptoms; the requirement of additional therapy is not emphasized in the European Respiratory Society/American Thoracic Society guideline [2, 3]. The clinical picture of AECOPD varies from a self-limiting illness to progressive respiratory failure. On average, a COPD patient experiences two episodes of AECOPD in a year, and about 10 – 15% of these patients require hospitalization [4]. However, a COPD patient might get signs and symptoms mimicking AECOPD from either superimposed or other diseases that need to be considered differential diagnoses. The present write-up briefly describes the approach to differentiate AECOPD from other differential diagnoses.

Differential Diagnosis

Most of the common differential diagnoses are related to the cardio-respiratory systems (Table 1).

Table 1. The common differential diagnoses for COPD exacerbation

Respiratory System	Cardiovascular System	Other
Pneumonia Acute exacerbation of Bronchial Asthma Bronchiectasis Upper Airway Obstruction Pulmonary edema Pleural effusion Pneumothorax Acute pulmonary embolism	Heart failure Acute Coronary Syndrome Arrhythmia Cardio-genic pulmonary edema	Severe anemia Inappropriate oxygen therapy Coronavirus disease of 2019

Pneumonia (Community-acquired/Hospital-acquired/COVID-19)

Lung parenchymal infections, primarily by bacteria and viruses, are the primary causative factor in the majority of the cases of AECOPD; Haemophilus influenza and Streptococcus pneumonia Pseudomonas, Staphylococcus, Rhinovirus, and Respiratory syncytial virus, are common organisms. Usually, Pseudomonas and gram-negative enteric bacilli cause severe diseases [5].

Even COVID-19 causes acute pneumonia and respiratory failure and has even been implicated as a cause of AECOPD [6]. Accompanying symptoms like fever, impaired taste or smell, or gastrointestinal complaints might hint at COVID-19 pneumonia [1]. Community-acquired pneumonia (CAP) contributes to AECOPD leading to hospitalization. Many aspects of acute exacerbations, including dyspnea, cough, and sputum production, may be found in patients with pneumonia or other pulmonary pathologies, and it is often impossible to differentiate without chest imaging [7]. Inflammatory markers indicating infection, i.e., C-reactive protein and procalcitonin on admission, might be helpful in the discrimination of AECOPD cases with or without CAP [8]. Bedside lung ultrasound can help in the differentiation of the cases. Notable that such pneumonia itself can mimic AECOPD and even cause AECOPD. New-onset fever and exacerbation of COPD type feature usually hint toward pneumonia.

Bronchial Asthma (Acute exacerbation) is characterized by largely reversible airflow limitation. The patient might already be a known case of bronchial asthma, or a history of allergy, allergic rhinitis, and eczema may be present. The onset is often in childhood, and symptoms are usually predominant at night or early morning. Sputum production is usually minimal to nil and restricted to early morning in asthma. A family history of bronchial asthma is also frequently noted [8]. Wheeze is predominant, especially in the end-expiratory phase, but it might be pan-expiratory in acute exacerbation. Bedside spirometry and blood gas analysis can help deafferent it from AECOPD [9].

Asthma-COPD Overlap is another entity that bears both COPD and bronchial asthma features and can present even as a syndrome. Usually, these patients present with disproportionately high wheeze, mucus production, and dispones and are diagnosed based on spirometry findings and other diagnostic criteria [10].

Bronchiectasis: Bronchiectasis is characterized by a large volume of purulent sputum. It is commonly associated with recurrent or persistent bacterial infections. Clinical findings include coarse crackles on auscultation and clubbing of digits. HRCT finding of honeycomb appearance is also classical [11].

Upper airway obstruction: Upper airway obstruction caused by bronchogenic or metastatic cancer, lymphadenopathy, and scarring from endotracheal tube may also present like AECOPD. On clinical examination, monophonic wheeze or stridor can be evident. Flow volume loop of spirometry show variable inspiratory or fixed slowing loop. Chest radiographs might not represent the finding, but a three-dimensional reconstruction of the HRCT scan is diagnostic [12].

Pulmonary edema: Both cardiogenic and non-cardiogenic pulmonary edema can mimic AECOPD.

Cardiogenic cases usually have a feature of heart failure. Chest auscultation of patients with pulmonary reveals coarse crepitation in the lung field, more in the dependent areas. Sputum might have characteristic color, and lung ultrasound shows significant B-lines, which can help in differentiating from AECOPD [13].

Pleural effusions and Pneumothorax: Both pleural effusion and pneumothorax may mimic AECOPD because it presents with dyspnea. Such patients often have other lung pathology, and cough is frequently noted. Physical examination may demonstrate absent or decreased breath sounds; percussion helps differentiate the conditions. While dullness to percussion is found in cases with pleural effusion, hyper resonance to percussion is the feature of pneumothorax.

Tracheal deviation might also be present. Although chest x-ray can be diagnostic in both cases, bedside lung ultrasound takes less time, has good accuracy in diagnosing both conditions, and is increasingly used nowadays.

Congestive heart failure: Acute onset of left or right-sided heart failure may present like acute COPD exacerbation. Ventricular dysfunction is frequently noted in all classes of COPD patients and is difficult to diagnose [14]. Right-sided heart failure (cor pulmonale) can be precipitated by pulmonary hypertension induced by hypoxia, pulmonary embolism, or pneumonia.

Reduced cardiac output will hamper oxygen delivery, causing respiratory decom-pensation in patients with COPD [15]. Heart failure is even a risk factor for AECOPD; adjusted hazard ratio of 1.5 [16]. While left-sided heart failure is challenging to differentiate clinically, heart failure patients usually have pitting pedal edema, basal crepitations, and raised jugular pressure. Bedside lung ultrasound, B-type natriuretic peptide, and screening echocardiography can help reach the diagnosis.

Acute Coronary Syndrome: Chest pain and shortness of breath are mimicking features. Even many patients with COPD have coronary artery disease and hypertensive heart disease, which may lead to acute coronary syndrome (ACS). Therefore, ACS in a patient with or without COPD can be a differential diagnosis of AECOPD. Chest pain in such patients is usually typical, and radiation is frequent. Bedside electrocardiogram and cardiac enzymes card-tests can help in reaching a diagnosis.

Cardiac arrhythmias: These patients can also present with chest tightness, shortness of breath, and even cough. Differentiating features from AECOPD may include palpitations, light-headedness, loss of consciousness, and/or collapse. The electrocardiogram is often diagnostic.

Pulmonary embolism: Pulmonary embolism may present with signs and symptoms like AECOPD. It should be considered a cause of the acute symptoms if no other identifiable trigger for the exacerbation is evident. People with prior thrombo-embolic disease or underlying malignancy may be at particular risk. A low systolic blood pressure and/or the inability to increase the $PaO_2 > 60$mmHg with oxygen may indicate the presence of a pulmonary embolism [17]. Electrocardiogram, arterial blood gas analysis, and bedside screening echocardiography might help reach a diagnosis and differentiate it from AECOPD.

Oxygen toxicity and inappropriate oxygen use: Oxygen therapy is frequently indicated for many COPD patients. Excessive oxygen therapy interferes with the patient's respiratory physiology. Exposure to oxygen leads to a decrease in hypoxic pulmonary vasoconstriction, leading to the decreased blood supply to poorly ventilated spaces, increasing the degree of ventilation-perfusion mismatch and/or intrapulmonary shunt [18]. An excess of oxygen may also decrease the capacity of erythrocytes to carry CO_2 (Haldane effect). These changes may then worsen the patient's hypercarbia and respiratory acidosis.

Anemia: Unrecognized severe anemia can present with shortness of breath and decreased exercise tolerance [19]. However, isolated anemia is unlikely to cause cough or fever. Mild anemia in stable COPD or AECOPD patients has not been reported to impact the six-minute walk test [20] significantly; severe anemia in stable COPD or even mild pneumonia can mimic AECOPD. A bedside clinical examination and point-of-care hematocrit testing can easily detect anemia.

Bedside Approach for Differentiation

While the above-mentioned brief descriptions can help differentiate the differential diagnosis of a COPD patient presenting to the hospital with acute exacerbation, there is a significant overlap of signs and symptoms. Recently lung ultrasound is gaining popularity as a point-of-care device, and its diagnostic utility for reaching a diagnosis for different causes of acute respiratory failure is well evaluated [21]. The details of the lung ultrasound findings for different cardiopulmonary conditions are beyond the present chapter's scope. However, a simple and easy to perform lung ultrasound might detect the presence or absence of B-lies or lung slides, lung point, stratosphere sign, quad sign, sinusoid sign, etc., which can help in reaching a diagnosis of different lung pathologies with good sensitivity and specificity [21]. We are presenting an algorithm (Figure 1) for different differential diagnoses of AECOPD based on salient clinical features and mention the need for different bedside tests, which might be helpful for the bedside approach.

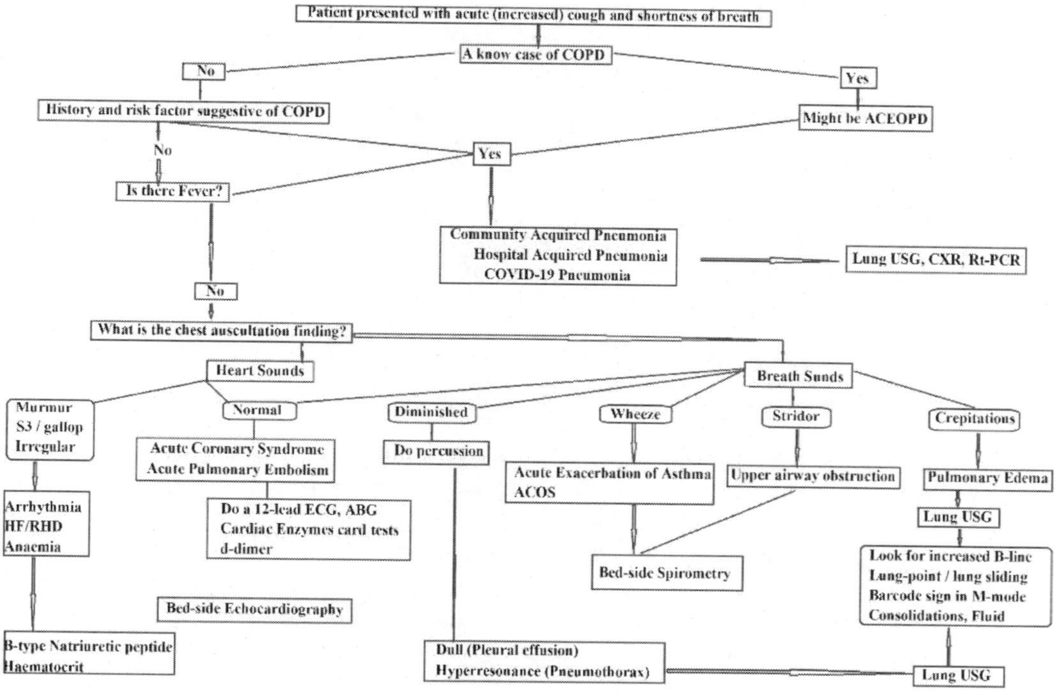

Figure 1. An algorithm for different differential diagnoses of AECOPD based on salient clinical features.

Conclusion

Many diseases can co-exist when present as isolated and can mimic AECOPD. Symptom complex, clinical characteristics, and bedside evaluation tools can help differentiation.

Key Points

- Acute exacerbation of COPD is a common clinical condition in the emergency department or intensive care unit.
- The clinical features mimic many cardio-respiratory conditions, including COVID-19-related pneumonia.
- Timely and appropriate differentiation from the other differential diagnosis can help better management planning.

- Signs, symptoms, and point of care testing-based algorithms might help narrow down the differentials.
- Bedside lung ultrasound and screening echocardiography might aid in early diagnosis.

References

[1] Global Initiative for Chronic Obstructive Lung Disease. *Global Strategy for the Diagnosis, Management, and Prevention of Chronic Obstructive Pulmonary Disease: 2022 Report*. 2022 [internet publication] (last accessed Apr 29, 2022). Available from https://goldcopd.org/2022-gold-reports-2/.

[2] Crisafulli E, Barbeta E, Ielpo A, Torres A. Management of severe acute exacerbations of COPD: An updated narrative review. *Multidiscip Respir Med*, 2018 Oct 2;13:36. https://doi.org/10.1186/s40248-018-0149-0.

[3] Wedzicha JA, Miravitlles M, Hurst JR, Calverley PMA, Albert RK, Anzueto A, Criner GJ, Papi A, Rabe KF, Rigau D, Sliwinski P, Tonia T, Vestbo J, Wilson KC, Krishnan JA. Management of COPD exacerbations: A European Respiratory Society/American Thoracic Society guideline. *Eur Respir J,* 2017 Mar 15; 49(3):1600791. https://doi.org/10.1183/13993003.00791-2016.

[4] Sullivan SD, Ramsey SD, Lee TA. The economic burden of COPD. *Chest*, 2000;117:5S-9S. doi: 10.1378/chest.117.2_suppl.5s.

[5] Fein A, Fein AM. Management of acute exacerbations in chronic obstructive pulmonary disease. *Curr Opin Pulm Med,* 2000 Mar; 6(2):122-6. https://doi.org/10.1097/00063198-200003000-00007.

[6] Poonuraparampil JA, Karim HMR, Kesavankutty MP, Nayak PP. Successful noninvasive ventilation in a severely acidotic and hypercapnic comatose COVID-19 patient with multiple comorbidities: a case report. *Acute Crit Care,* 2022 Feb; 37(1):120-123. https://doi.org/10.4266/acc.2020.00983.

[7] Rangelov BA, Young AL, Jacob J, Cahn AP, Lee S, Wilson FJ, Hawkes DJ, Hurst JR. Thoracic Imaging at Exacerbation of Chronic Obstructive Pulmonary Disease: A Systematic Review. *Int J Chron Obstruct Pulmon Dis,* 2020 Jul 22; 15:1751-1787. https://doi.org/10.2147/COPD.S250746.

[8] Niu Y, Xing Y, Li J, Shui W, Gu Y, Zhang C, Du H. Effect of Community-Acquired Pneumonia on Acute Exacerbation of Chronic Obstructive Pulmonary Disease. *COPD,* 2021 Aug; 18(4):417-424. https://doi.org/10.1080/15412555.2021.1950664.

[9] Cukic V, Lovre V, Dragisic D, Ustamujic A. Asthma and Chronic Obstructive Pulmonary Disease (COPD) - Differences and Similarities. *Mater Sociomed,* 2012; 24(2):100-5. https://doi.org/10.5455/msm.2012.24.100-105.

[10] Mekov E, Nuñez A, Sin DD, Ichinose M, Rhee CK, Maselli DJ, Coté A, Suppli Ulrik C, Maltais F, Anzueto A, Miravitlles M. Update on Asthma-COPD Overlap (ACO): A Narrative Review. *Int J Chron Obstruct Pulmon Dis,* 2021 Jun 17; 16:1783-1799. https://doi.org/10.2147/COPD.S312560.

[11] MacIntyre N, Huang YC. Acute exacerbations and respiratory failure in chronic obstructive pulmonary disease. *Proc Am Thorac Soc*, 2008; 5(4):530-535. doi: 10.1513/pats.200707-088ET.

[12] Hill AT, Haworth CS, Aliberti S, Barker A, Blasi F, Boersma W, Chalmers JD, De Soyza A, Dimakou K, Elborn JS, Feldman C, Flume P, Goeminne PC, Loebinger MR, Menendez R, Morgan L, Murris M, Polverino E, Quittner A, Ringshausen FC, Tino G, Torres A, Vendrell M, Welte T, Wilson R, Wong C, O'Donnell A, Aksamit T. Pulmonary exacerbation in adults with bronchiectasis: A consensus definition for clinical research. *Eur Respir J,* 2017; 49: 1700051. https://doi.org/10.1183/13993003.00051-2017.

[13] Volpicelli G, Cardinale L, Garofalo G, Veltri A. Usefulness of lung ultrasound in the bedside distinction between pulmonary edema and exacerbation of COPD. *Emerg Radiol*, 2008 May; 15(3):145-51. https://doi.org/10.1007/s10140-008-0701-x.

[14] Tinè M, Bazzan E, Semenzato U, Biondini D, Cocconcelli E, Balestro E, Casara A, Baraldo S, Turato G, Cosio MG, Saetta M. Heart Failure is Highly Prevalent and Difficult to Diagnose in Severe Exacerbations of COPD Presenting to the Emergency Department. *J Clin Med,* 2020 Aug 14; 9(8):2644. https://doi.org/10.3390/jcm9082644.

[15] Ernst A, Feller-Kopman D, Becker HD, Mehta AC. Central airway obstruction. *Am J Respir Crit Care Med,* 2004; 169:1278-1297. https://doi.org/10.1164/rccm.200210-1181SO.

[16] Axson EL, Bottle A, Cowie MR, Quint JK. Relationship between heart failure and the risk of acute exacerbation of COPD. *Thorax,* 2021 Apr 29; 76(8):807-14. https://doi.org/10.1136/thoraxjnl-2020-216390.

[17] Tillie-Leblond I, Marquette CH, Perez T, Scherpereel A, Zanetti C, Tonnel A-B, Remy-Jardin M. Pulmonary embolism in patients with unexplained exacerbation of chronic obstructive pulmonary disease: Prevalence and risk factors. *Ann Intern Med,* 2006 Mar 21; 144(6):390-6. https://doi.org/10.7326/0003-4819-144-6-200603210-00005.

[18] Robinson TD, Freiberg DB, Regnis JA, Young IH. The role of hypoventilation and ventilation-perfusion redistribution in oxygen-induced hypercapnia during acute exacerbations of chronic obstructive pulmonary disease. *Am J Respir Crit Care Med,* 2000 May; 161(5):1524-9. https://doi.org/10.1164/ajrccm.161.5.9904119.

[19] Hetzel TM, Losek JD. Unrecognized severe anemia in children presenting with respiratory distress. *Am J Emerg Med,* 1998 Jul; 16(4):386-9. https://doi.org/10.1016/s0735-6757(98)90135-8.

[20] Nowiński A, Kamiński D, Kram M, Korzybski D, Stokłosa A, Górecka D. impact of mild anaemia on dyspnoea during exertion and exercise tolerance in patients with acute exacerbation of chronic obstructive pulmonary disease. *Pneumonol Alergol Pol,* 2013; 81(3):200-6.

[21] Wallbridge P, Steinfort D, Tay TR, Irving L, Hew M. Diagnostic chest ultrasound for acute respiratory failure. *Respir Med,* 2018 Aug; 141:26-36. https://doi.org/10.1016/j.rmed.2018.06.018.

Chapter 21

Acute Exacerbations of COPD: A Pathophysiology Overview

Maria Bragança[1,*], MD, Miguel Guia[1,2,3], MD, Paula Pinto[1,2,3], MD, PhD and Raffaele Scala[4], MD

[1]Thorax Department;
Centro Hospitalar Universitário Lisboa Norte,Lisbon, Portugal
[2]Sleep and Non-Invasive Ventilation Unit,
Centro Hospitalar Universitário Lisboa Norte, Lisbon, Portugal
[3]Instituto de Saúde Ambiental (ISAMB),
Faculty of Medicine, Lisbon University, Lisbon, Portugal
[4]Pulmonology and Respiratory Intensive Care Unit,
S. Donato Hospital, Arezzo, Italy

Abstract

Although Chronic Obstructive Pulmonary Disease (COPD) is mainly a chronic disease, during its natural disease course, a significant number of patients suffer from COPD exacerbations, with consequences in terms of lower quality of life and higher morbidity and mortality rates in frequent exacerbators and particularly in severe exacerbations.

The most prevalent triggers for COPD exacerbations are airway infections (viruses and bacteria) and air pollution. Some risk factors like bronchiectasis, eosinophilia and frequent prior exacerbations are important predictors for exacerbations.

The pathophysiological hallmark of COPD exacerbation is increased airway inflammation, consequent expiratory flow limitation, reduced lung recoil pressure, and small airway obstruction. Thus, the ventilation (especially the expiratory time) is compromised, preventing end-expiratory lung volume from achieving natural relaxation volume at the end of a tidal expiration, leading to lung overinflation.

This chapter intends to give insight into relevant aspects of COPD exacerbations in terms of its pathophysiology to expand our understanding of the disease further and hopefully improve our clinical and therapeutic approach.

Keywords: emphysema, expiratory flow limitation, dynamic hyperinflation, PEEPi, muscle fatigue

---

* Corresponding Author's Email: maria.luis.braganca@gmail.com.

In: Chronic Obstructive Pulmonary Disease
Editor: Jaber S. Alqahtani
ISBN: 979-8-88697-333-4

Introduction

Pathology of COPD

In terms of pathological alterations in COPD, the lung parenchyma is characterized by abnormal, permanent enlargement of the airspaces distal to the terminal bronchiole, the alveoli, accompanied by destruction of their walls, which is termed emphysema. The classification of emphysema is determined based on the involvement of the acini. The emphysema can be panacinar/panlobular (in which the acinus is uniformly involved), centriacinar/centrilobular (in which the proximal portion of the acinus is involved), paraseptal (the proximal portion of the acinus is normal, and the distal part with the alveolar sacs and ducts is altered), and paracicatricial (acinus may be irregularly involved) [1-3].

Concerning the large airways in chronic bronchitis, the gross findings are the presence of mucus in the airway lumen and prominent circular ridges in the bronchial ducts due to bands of hypertrophic smooth muscle. On a microscopical level, the airway wall thickens, mainly due to the inner wall, internal to the muscular layer [2, 3].

On the other hand, the small airways are filled with intraluminal mucus, and there is an increase in wall thickness due to increases in the epithelium, muscle, and fibrotic tissue. However, there is also a loss of alveolar attachments to the airway wall with consequent modification of the elastic recoil of the lungs, resulting in airway collapse on expiration beyond the airway obstruction [2, 3].

Pathophysiology of Stable COPD

Considering the pathology and pathogenesis of COPD, the small airways are extensively affected not only by chronic inflammation, fibrosis, and exudates but also by an altered elastic recoil of the lungs. These alterations reduce the expiratory flow and increase the resistance of the airways, resulting in airway limitation and reduction of FEV_1 (forced expiratory volume in 1 second) and FEV_1/FVC (forced vital capacity) ratio [1, 2].

Beyond the repercussions of the airflow limitation itself, this process also causes air trapping during expiration, resulting in hyperinflation. The patient's breathing is shifted towards the upper part of the pressure/volume curve at higher end-inspiratory lung volumes. This hyperinflated state translates into an increase in total lung capacity and residual volume, which reduces the inspiratory capacity of the lung and contributes to the impairment of the respiratory muscle, further perpetuating fatigue and dyspnoea. During exercise or exacerbation, there is dynamic hyperinflation in which there is a further reduction of airflow associated with rapid breathing and reduced expiratory volume, causing increased dyspnoea and limitation of the respiratory muscle capacity [1, 2].

Gas exchange abnormalities are another hallmark of COPD, which may lead to hypoxemia and hypercapnia. In fact, there can be multiple mechanisms to justify these irregularities, namely different ventilation-perfusion patterns, varying from V/Q mismatch to alveolar shunt. Airway obstruction associated with hyperinflation and respiratory muscle dysfunction further aggravates the ventilation. In the presence of hypoxemia and hypercapnia, the physiological response is to increase the respiratory frequency to maintain minute ventilation. However, in the presence of the restrictive limitation to ventilation, with muscle fatigue, the organism adapts a "central wisdom" posture in which they choose to be eupnoeic and maintain hypercapnia but prevent exhaustion. Therefore, there is hypercapnia with increased serum bicarbonate concentration, preserving a normal pH [1, 2].

In chronic bronchitis, clinically relevant because of chronic productive cough, there is an inflammatory response to the noxious stimulus by increasing the number of goblet cells and the submucosal glands, amplifying mucus secretion [1].

From a cardiovascular point of view, there could be pulmonary arterial hypertension, primarily due to the hypoxic vasoconstriction of the pulmonary arteries. In emphysema, the destruction of the alveoli walls with the loss of the pulmonary capillary bed further contributes to the increased pressure in pulmonary circulation. Pulmonary hypertension may lead to right ventricular dilation, hypertrophy, and right-side cardiac failure [1].

Most patients with COPD have concomitant chronic diseases that can significantly impact health status and survival, such as cardiovascular, anemia, osteoporosis, cachexia, and muscle wasting. There could be many reasons for these comorbidities, like the already present risk factors for COPD (i.e., smoking, aging, and inactivity), the chronic inflammatory state, and the consequent effects on cardiac function and gas exchange [1, 2].

Pathophysiology of Acute Exacerbations of COPD

While COPD is predominantly a chronic disease, many patients experience exacerbations.

Indeed, an acute exacerbation of COPD is an episode in the natural history of the disease that is characterized by a variation in the patient's baseline dyspnoea, cough, sputum production (volume or purulence), wheezing, or chest tightness, sufficient to cause a change in management. The clinical manifestations of COPD exacerbations are highly variable in presentation and severity, reflecting the broad pathophysiology of COPD and diversity in the nature and effect of the provoking agent itself [1, 5, 6].

The most prevalent triggers for COPD exacerbations are airway infections (viral infections and bacterial infections) which are responsible for up to 50-70% of exacerbations, followed by air pollution, which is responsible for 10%, and up to 30% of unknown etiology [5, 7].

Etiology

Exacerbations are mainly triggered by respiratory infections, particularly viral infections, although bacterial infections may also initiate and amplify these events. The most common virus isolated is human rhinovirus (the cause of the common cold) and can be detected for up to a week after an exacerbation onset. Other viruses often detected are picornaviruses, respiratory syncytial virus, influenza A and B, and coronaviruses. These infections are more frequent during winter. In the presence of a virus, the organism releases proinflammatory mediators and recruits leukocytes (particularly eosinophils) and T lymphocytes, increasing airway and systemic inflammation [5, 7, 8].

Commonly isolated bacteria include *Streptococcus pneumoniae*, *Haemophilus influenzae*, *Moraxella catarrhalis, Haemophilus parainfluenza,* and *Pseudomonas aeruginosa* in more severe patients. Bacteria increase pulmonary inflammation and decrease airway function in COPD patients, and the bacterial burden determines the degree of inflammation [5, 7].

In 25 to 50% of patients with COPD, these microorganisms are found despite no evidence of infection, considered therefore colonization. The presence of these bacteria in non-exacerbated patients indicates a breach of the defense mechanisms, like impaired mucociliary clearance and immunity, and is related to increased airway inflammation, worsened airflow obstruction, and increased exacerbation frequency. Many studies showed the efficacy of long-term antibiotic treatment with macrolides in reducing exacerbation [4, 5, 7, 8].

For the development of COPD exacerbation, there could be new bacterial species, an increase in the number of colonizing bacteria, or the acquisition of a different strain from the same bacterial species. In exacerbation, the bacteria stimulate airway inflammation by activating the complement system activation and attracting leukocytes (particularly of neutrophilic type) [4].

Even if present on rare occasions, atypical bacteria have a role in acute exacerbations, including *M. Pneumoniae, C. Pneumoniae,* and *Legionella spp* [4].

COPD exacerbations can also be triggered by increases in air pollution, in particular diesel particulates, sulfur dioxide (SO2), nitrogen dioxide (NO2), and black smoke particulate matter. Though well acknowledged, it is difficult to establish a causal effect between air pollution and COPD exacerbations as the studies focus primarily on the temporal correlation. Even so, studies show that air pollution may account for 6 to 10% of COPD exacerbation. These pollutants stimulate the production of proinflammatory cytokines, neutrophilic inflammation, and reactive oxygen species resulting in airway inflammation and increased mortality in patients with COPD [2, 4, 5, 7].

As for non-infectious causes of COPD exacerbation, recent studies included pulmonary embolism (5%), congestive heart failure (2%), and discontinuation of COPD medications (1%) as some of the possible causes [2].

In terms of risk factors for an acute COPD exacerbation, there seems to be a correlation between coexistent bronchiectasis, high eosinophil count in blood (with a reduction of exacerbation on patients treated with inhaled corticosteroids), and frequent prior exacerbations (each exacerbation increases the risk for a subsequent exacerbation, with a decrease in time between exacerbations, and higher mortality) [8].

Pathogenesis of COPD Exacerbation

During COPD exacerbation, the chronic inflammatory response present in COPD patients, characterized mainly by macrophages, CD8+ T lymphocytes, and neutrophils, suffers a pattern change, with an increase in eosinophils (different from an asthmatic as the eosinophils are non-degranulated and not associated with increased IL-5), neutrophils, CD4+ T lymphocytes, and inflammatory mediators. The accumulation of the inflammatory cells in the mucosa, along with the inflammatory mediators, causes several changes in the airway. Namely, it causes airway wall thickening with smooth muscle proliferation, inflammatory damage, increased oxidative stress, and increased permeability of the bronchial mucosa, with consequent edema, protein exudation, mucus secretion (by goblet cells), and bronchial hyperresponsiveness. These changes, especially in the small airways, lead to a reduction in airway flow, with consequent breathlessness. Corresponding clinical manifestations include dyspnoea, cough, sputum production, and sputum purulence, which are the cardinal manifestations of an exacerbation [4, 5].

Pathophysiology of COPD Exacerbation

The pathophysiological hallmark of acute COPD exacerbation is expiratory flow limitation, resulting from increased airway inflammation, emphysema with reduced lung recoil pressure, and small airway obstruction. In fact, in the presence of an airflow difficulty, the ventilation, mainly the expiratory time, is compromised, being insufficient to allow end-expiratory lung volume to achieve natural relaxation volume at the end of a tidal expiration, leading to lung overinflation [5].

In stable COPD patients, lung hyperinflation is steady. However, during exacerbations, because of the inflammatory process, there are variations in the end-expiratory lung volume above baseline, called dynamic hyperinflation (Figure 1) [6, 9].

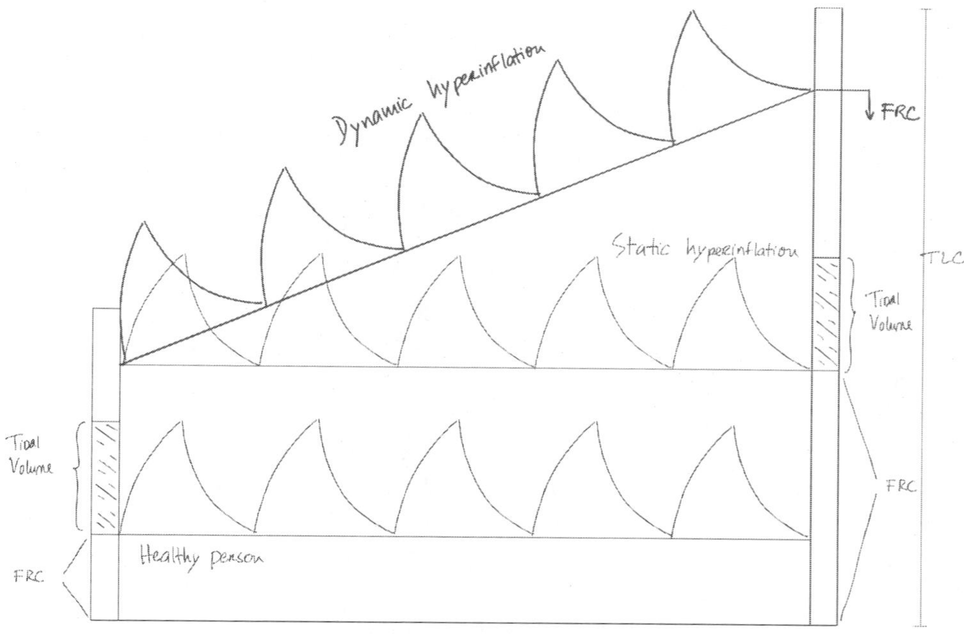

Figure 1. Dynamic and static hyperinflation (graphical representation).

In fact, in healthy individuals, the end-expiratory alveolar pressure and airway pressure are zero relative to the atmospheric pressure, and pleural pressure is negative, allowing a passive inhalation of air. On the other hand, in the presence of dynamic hyperinflation, with an increase in end-expiratory lung volume, the alveolar pressure remains positive throughout expiration, leading to an auto-positive end-expiratory pressure (auto-PEEP), also designated intrinsic PEEP or PEEPi (Figure 2). The PEEPi is a load the patient must overcome to initiate inspiration that further contributes to muscle fatigue [6, 9].

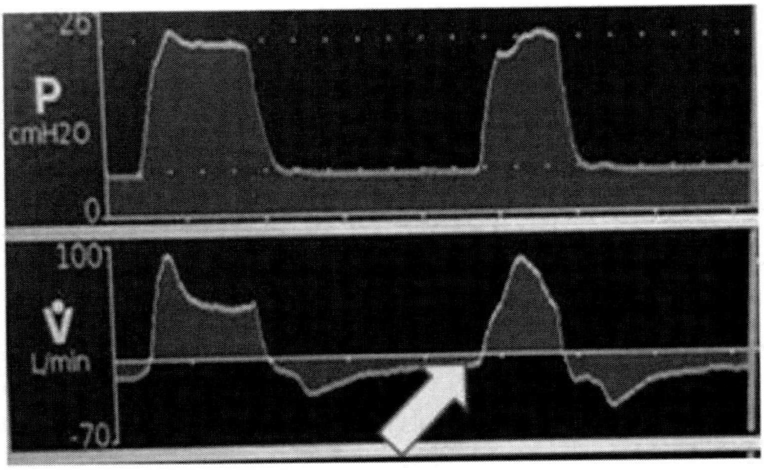

Figure 2. Auto-positive end-expiratory pressure (auto-PEEP) is evident in the flow curve on the ventilator (yellow arrow). Photographic representation of a patient with exacerbated COPD in our ward.

As an adaptive mechanism, during COPD exacerbation, the patient increases the respiratory frequency, with rapid shallow breaths, as a means to increase minute ventilation. However, it further diminishes expiratory time, reducing the expiratory volume and perpetuating hyperinflation. In this situation, the tidal volume is shifted upwards closer to the total lung capacity of the respiratory system compliance curve. Although this change optimizes expiratory flow, it forces the respiratory system to function on the flatter part of the compliance curve, where each increase in pressure generates smaller incremental volume changes. Thus, dynamic hyperinflation limits the inspiratory effort, forcing a restrictive mechanical constraint on the respiratory system. Hyperinflation, beyond requiring additional effort from the respiratory muscles, also damages the muscle's configuration diminishing their efficacy, resulting in muscle weakness and fatigue [6, 9].

Because of severe airflow limitation, dynamic hyperinflation, and PEEPi, COPD exacerbations frequently cause acute respiratory failure. Even if stable COPD patients can maintain an acceptable gas exchange, in the presence of acute decompensation, that fragile balance can easily be altered since these patients have a limited physiological reserve accordingly to the severity of the disease.

Ventilation-perfusion (V/Q) mismatch with low V/Q units and low mixed venous oxygen tension, subsequent to increased work of breathing, results in hypoxemia. In some cases, it can even be a consequence of an alveolar shunt phenomenon, but in a small percentage [4, 6, 9].

Beyond hypoxemia, COPD exacerbation can accompany carbon dioxide retention and acidaemia. In severe COPD, in the presence of increased dead space at the expense of emphysema, there are high V/Q units dispersed, resulting in a rapid shallow breathing pattern and hypercapnia. The expected response would be to increase the respiratory rate substantially to overcome the "wasted" ventilation. However, complementary to the V/Q mismatch, COPD patients usually have a hyperinflated state, which significantly alters the respiratory muscle pump, increasing the work and reducing the efficacy of breathing. Therefore, the continuous hypercapnia cannot be overcome by hyperventilation, thus needing compensating mechanisms such as increased serum bicarbonate to maintain normal pH [4, 6, 9].

In COPD exacerbations, at the cost of further airway obstruction, hypermetabolic state, dynamic hyperinflation, and muscle fatigue, there could be acid-base decompensation resulting in some cases of hypoxemia, hypercapnia, and respiratory acidaemia.

On a clinical level, it is therefore essential for an arterial blood gases analysis to evaluate if hypoxemia, hypercapnia, and acidaemia are present. One should also pay attention to serum bicarbonate. A rigorous analysis of the results can infer the presence of an acute respiratory failure or an acute on chronic respiratory failure and further help the clinician with the best treatment approach.

The neural drive to breathe increases during exacerbations. It happens at the expense of hypoxemia, hypercapnia, acidosis, fever, or increased sympathetic nervous system activation. The incentive to increase the respiratory rate is a means to increase minute ventilation. However, due to constraints related to dynamic hyperinflation, PEEPi, and weakened respiratory muscles, the ventilatory response may not be sufficient in proportion to the neural drive, resulting in neuromechanical dissociation or uncoupling of the respiratory system with significant thoracoabdominal asynchrony. This restriction limits tidal volume, resulting in dyspnoea. Rapid shallow breaths further reduce the expiratory time, aggravating hyperinflation, and the hypermetabolic state produces supplemental carbon dioxide. The additional effort required on the respiratory muscles, coupled with the decrease in supply, leads to fatigue and inefficient work. Therefore, it is easily understood why COPD exacerbation is a complex disease and a vicious cycle [6].

In terms of cardiovascular repercussions, COPD patients with emphysema, in which there is the destruction of vascular beds within the lungs and V/Q mismatch with consequent hypoxemia, have a high probability of pulmonary arterial hypertension with increased right ventricular afterload. This can lead to right ventricle dilation and right ventricle hypertrophy [6, 9].

During COPD exacerbations with expiratory flow limitation, dynamic hyperinflation, and PEEPi, there is a decrease in venous return, reducing right ventricle preload. On the other hand, dynamic hyperinflation can lead to significant negative intrathoracic pressure swings, which increase, in turn, the venous return to the right ventricle, increasing the preload [6, 9].

The right ventricle is mainly affected. However, in the presence of significant increases in right ventricular end-diastolic pressures, there could be a movement of the interventricular septum towards the left ventricle during diastole to accommodate the volume, causing left ventricular diastolic dysfunction with consequences in ejection fraction [6, 9].

Consequences of COPD Exacerbation

Studies show that the frequency of COPD exacerbations is one of the most critical determinants of quality of life, with considerably lower quality of life and increased morbidity and mortality rates in frequent exacerbators and even more in severe exacerbations. Exacerbations have been shown to accelerate the long-term decline in lung function, specifically in smokers, resulting in prolonged activity limitation, and can reverse won benefits of respiratory rehabilitation. From the standpoint of recovery, studies show that the functional respiratory losses developed during COPD exacerbation in FEV_1 and FVC are recovered partly from the seventh day. However, after one month, only 75% of the patients had returned to baseline, and after three months, 7% had not recovered to pre-exacerbation levels [4, 5, 6, 9].

During an exacerbation, if the patients present with hypercapnic respiratory failure, they have a higher probability of hospital readmission rate and mortality. The most common cause of death in patients with COPD is respiratory failure [5].

The strongest predictors of mortality are age, right ventricular hypertrophy, ischemic heart disease, chronic renal failure, and reduced FEV_1 [5].

The Role of COPD Subtypes and Comorbidities

When mentioning COPD both in stable status and during an exacerbation, it is essential to consider comorbidities and subtypes that significantly influence the prognosis. These diseases may appear independent from COPD or related in terms of shared risk factors. Sometimes the differential diagnosis between COPD and these comorbidities can be difficult, being essential a high clinical suspicion. It is crucial to diagnose these hidden pathologies to have adequate treatment and lessen the potential consequences of quality of life, morbidity, and mortality.

Combined Pulmonary Fibrosis and Emphysema (CPFE)

This association was first described as a syndrome by Cottin et al., in 2005 and is characterized by heavy smoking history, exercise hypoxemia, and dyspnoea, followed by disruptive cough and recurrent exacerbations [10, 11].

The diagnosis of the CPFE syndrome is based on high-resolution computed tomography (HRCT) imaging which shows the coexistence of emphysema (mainly in the upper lobes) and pulmonary fibrosis (including subpleural reticular opacities, honeycomb images, and traction bronchiectasis) in the lower lobes [10, 11].

The emphysematous lesions include the presence of either diffuse (centrilobular and bullous) emphysema or paraseptal emphysema with predominance in the subpleural areas. The usual interstitial pneumonia (UIP) is the most commonly reported finding on the fibrotic lesions, followed by fibrotic non-specific interstitial pneumonia (f-NSIP) [10, 11].

Most CPFE patients maintain preserved spirometric values and static lung volumes regarding pulmonary function tests. This results from balancing the restrictive effects of pulmonary fibrosis and the hyperinflation caused by emphysematous lesions. Therefore, the increased traction caused by pulmonary fibrosis prevents the elastic recoil of the lungs caused by emphysema and supports the small airways, preventing the airway collapse and preserving the forced expiratory volume in one second (FEV_1). On the other hand, there is a substantial reduction of the diffusion capacity of carbon monoxide (DLCO), which is associated with pulmonary hypertension, with consequent severely diminished gas exchange. This occurs due to the reduced vascular surface area and pulmonary capillary blood volume caused by fibrotic and emphysematous lesions. Resting and especially exercise hypoxemia is the most frequent change, whereas hypercapnia usually occurs lastly. The blood gas analysis of CPFE is usually more similar to IPF than to COPD. However, in the presence of advanced COPD, gas exchange abnormalities usually result in hypoxemia and hypercapnia [10, 11].

In terms of epidemiology, the prevalence of this pathology is still not precisely determined. It is estimated that 8 to 50% of patients with IPF present emphysema, and 4 to 8% of patients with emphysema have pulmonary fibrosis. CPFE seems to occur more often in males with a heavy smoking history after the sixth decade of life [10, 11].

Relating to the pathogenesis of CPFE, it is not clear if the emphysematous and fibrotic lesions progress independently or if one results from the other. However, cigarette smoking is a common aspect and a major etiologic risk factor. Other triggers may include environmental exposure, connective tissue disease, and genetic predisposition [10, 11].

Concerning the prognosis, pulmonary arterial hypertension (PAH) is a much more common complication present in CPFE (prevalence of 50-90%) than in COPD (50%) and IPF (30-45%). Most CPFE patients have moderate to severe PAH, which can result from hypoxic pulmonary vasoconstriction and reduced capillary beds due to the combination of pulmonary fibrosis and emphysema, chronic inflammation, and vascular remodeling. Identifying this entity is important because it is associated with a poor prognosis. There is also an increased risk of lung cancer [10, 11].

Patients with CPFE also suffer acute exacerbations, which can be attributed to the emphysematous or fibrotic component of CPFE. It is crucial to distinguish because each exacerbation has a characteristic clinical progression, outcome, and treatment [10, 11].

The emphysematous exacerbation can be defined according to COPD guidelines. It is an acute worsening of respiratory symptoms, usually requiring hospitalization, with airflow obstruction and ventilatory hypercapnic pump failure. Radiologically it may show an array of alterations like airway wall thickening, consolidations, mucous impaction, atelectasis, and mediastinal adenopathy. Studies show that COPD-like exacerbations have better outcomes, requiring less invasive therapy, including invasive mechanical ventilation and ECMO, compared to fibrotic ones [10, 11].

On the other hand, there could be an exacerbation with a more fibrotic component, which is similar to an IPF exacerbation. It is characterized by acute respiratory deterioration leading to hypoxic respiratory failure. Radiologically there is a change in baseline imaging varying from the presence of ground-glass opacities, interlobular septal thickening, or new consolidations on a background pattern consistent with UIP that is not fully explained by cardiac failure or fluid overload [10, 11].

Regarding prevalence, CPFE patients are less likely to experience an acute exacerbation compared to IPF. This can be a consequence of the balance created between both components, as emphysema contributes to the preservation of lung volumes, making these patients less prone to alveolar collapse and recurrent atelectatic lung injury. Even within the CPFE patients, the ones with the emphysematous predominance were the less likely to experience an exacerbation [10, 11].

Chronic Obstructive Pulmonary Disease and Asthma

Recently, the term asthma and COPD overlap (ACO) is no longer recommended and instead highlights the individuality of both disorders. Even so, COPD and asthma can still coexist in an individual patient, even though diagnosing both pathologies can be difficult because of their common traits and clinical features [1].

One should consider this possibility when asthmatic patients, particularly smokers and some patients with severe asthma, have increased neutrophils, are less responsive to corticosteroids, and have an accelerated decline in lung function, which are characteristics of

COPD. On the other hand, some COPD patients may have wheezing, some reversibility to bronchodilators, a better response to corticosteroids, increased eosinophilia in sputum, and an increased FeNO, which are characteristic features of asthma [12].

To help with the diagnosis, a thorough clinical and personal history is essential, along with a pulmonary function exam, blood analysis, and radiology [1, 12].

If in the presence of both pathologies, management should primarily follow the asthma guidelines without disregarding the COPD recommendations [1, 12].

Despite the difficulty, it is essential to identify these patients and evaluate their long-term evolution to confirm the diagnosis. The prevalence of COPD and asthma is unknown, varying according to the criteria and the study used. It varies widely in studies, from 0.3 to 5.0% in the general population, from 3.2 to 51.4% in patients with asthma, and from 12.6 to 55.7% in patients with COPD [12].

Studies show that patients with COPD and asthma have poorer clinical outcomes than patients with just one condition. They have more severe respiratory symptoms, worse quality of life and lung function, more use of lung medication, a higher risk of severe exacerbation and hospitalization, and a higher mortality rate than patients with either disease alone [12, 13].

It was also shown that high blood eosinophil count was the only helpful index for distinguishing responders from no responders to corticosteroid treatment. Patients with COPD and asthma had a significantly decreased risk of an exacerbation if following asthma management guidelines [12, 13].

Chronic Obstructive Pulmonary Disease and Obstructive Sleep Apnoea

It is estimated that 10-15% of the patients with COPD also have obstructive sleep apnoea (OSA). Patients with both conditions have a worse prognosis when compared with either disease alone. Furthermore, during sleep, these patients have more frequent oxygen desaturation episodes and more sleep time with hypoxemia and hypercapnia than patients with only OSA [14, 15].

Additionally, COPD-OSA patients have more profound hypoxemia during apnoeic events and cardiac arrhythmias and are more likely to develop daytime pulmonary hypertension. Subsequently, these patients with a greater than expected sleep disorder have considerably more risk of morbidity and mortality, with worse quality of life, especially poor sleep quality. Among these patients, the ones with worse lung functions and poorer adherence to continuous positive airway pressure (CPAP) have a higher probability of exacerbations [14, 15].

Furthermore, COPD severe acidotic exacerbations occurring in patients with coexistent OSA and requiring NIV may be a challenge for the clinicians in terms of achievement of a good synchronism between patient and ventilator.

Conclusion

COPD is a chronic disease, however, during its natural course, patients may suffer from COPD exacerbations, with consequent lower quality of life and higher morbidity and mortality rates. These exacerbations are triggered most frequently by airway infections (viral and/or bacterial) and air pollution. During COPD exacerbations, ventilation (especially the expiratory time) is impaired, preventing end-expiratory lung volume from achieving natural relaxation values at the end of a tidal expiration, leading to lung overinflation.

Key Points

- Many patients suffer from COPD exacerbations, resulting in lower quality of life and increased morbidity and mortality rates.
- Some risk factors identified are bronchiectasis, eosinophilia, and prior exacerbations.
- The most prevalent triggers are airway infections (viruses and bacteria) and air pollution.
- Airway inflammation, expiratory flow limitation, reduced lung recoil pressure, and small airway obstruction are typically present.
- In COPD, ventilation is compromised, preventing end-expiratory lung volume from achieving natural relaxation volume at the end of a tidal expiration, leading to lung overinflation, which worsens during exacerbations.

References

[1] The Global Initiative for Chronic Obstructive Lung Disease (GOLD). Global Strategy for the Diagnosis, Management, and Prevention of Chronic Obstructive Pulmonary Disease: 2022 Report. *The Lancet Respiratory Medicine*, 10(2), E20.

[2] Ko F., Chan K., Hui D., Goddard J., Shaw J., Reid D., Ian A. Yang. Acute exacerbation of COPD. *Respirology* 2016;21(7):1152-65.

[3] Fishman A., Grippi M., Elias J., Fishman J., Kotloff R., Pack A., Robert M. Senior, Mark D. Siegel. *Fishman's Pulmonary Diseases and Disorders*. New York: The McGraw-Hill Education; 2015.

[4] Tsoumakidou M., Siafakas N. Novel insights into the etiology and pathophysiology of increased airway inflammation during COPD exacerbations. *Respir Res* 2006;7(1).

[5] Papi A., Luppi F., Franco F., Fabbri L. Pathophysiology of Exacerbations of Chronic Obstructive Pulmonary Disease. *Proc Am Thorac Soc* 2006;3(3);245-51.

[6] O'Donnell D., Parker C. COPD exacerbations - 3: Pathophysiology. *Thorax* 2006;61(4):354-361.

[7] Sapey E., Stockley A. COPD exacerbations - 2: Aetiology. *Thorax* 2006; 61(3): 250-8.

[8] Viniol C., Vogelmeier C. Exacerbations of COPD. *Eur Respir Rev* 2018;27(147):170103.

[9] Demoule A., Brochard L., Dres M., Heunks L., Jubran A., Laghi F., Armand Mekontso-Dessap, Stefano Nava, Lamia Ouanes-Besbes, Oscar Peñuelas, Lise Piquilloud, Theodoros Vassilakopoulos, Jordi Mancebo. How to ventilate obstructive and asthmatic patients. *Intensive Care Med* 2020;46(12):2436-49.

[10] Hage R., Gautschi F., Steinack C., Schuurmans M. Combined Pulmonary Fibrosis and Emphysema (CPFE) Clinical Features and Management. *Int J Chron Obstruct Pulmon Dis* 2021; Volume 16:167-77.

[11] Zantah M., Dotan Y., Dass C., Zhao H., Marchetti N., Criner G. Acute exacerbations of COPD versus IPF in patients with combined pulmonary fibrosis and emphysema. *Respir Res* 2020;21(1).

[12] Hosseini M., Almasi-Hashiani A., Sepidarkish M., Maroufizadeh S. Global prevalence of asthma-COPD overlap (ACO) in the general population: a systematic review and meta-analysis. *Respir Res* 2019;20(1).

[13] Menezes A., Montes de Oca M., Pérez-Padilla R., Nadeau G., Wehrmeister F., Lopez-Varela M., Adriana Muiño, José Roberto B. Jardim, Gonzalo Valdivia, Carlos Tálamo, PLATINO Team. Increased

Risk of Exacerbation and Hospitalization in Subjects With an Overlap Phenotype. *Chest* 2014; 145(2):297-304.

[14] Jaoude P., El-Solh A. Predictive factors for COPD exacerbations and mortality in patients with overlap syndrome. *Clin Respir J* 2019 Oct;13(10):643-51.

[15] Soler X., Gaio E., Powell F., Ramsdell J., Loredo J. Malhotra A., Andrew L. Ries, High Prevalence of Obstructive Sleep Apnea in Patients with Moderate to Severe Chronic Obstructive Pulmonary Disease. *Ann Am Thorac Soc* 2015;12(8):1219-25.

Chapter 22

Recognition and Consequences of COPD Exacerbation

Jithin K. Sreedharan[1,*]
and Keerthi N. Satheesan[2,†]
[1]Department of Respiratory Care,
Prince Sultan Military College of Health Sciences,
Dammam, Saudi Arabia
[2]Royal Service Medical College of Nursing and Health Sciences,
Bahrain Defense Force, Bahrain

Abstract

Chronic obstructive pulmonary disease (COPD) is the most common chronic lung disease in the world. Exacerbations of COPD determine disease-related morbidity, mortality, resource burden, and healthcare expenditures. Acute exacerbation care requirements extend from impulsive primary care visits to the emergency room to inpatient or intensive care admission, causing associated health burdens and mounting costs in COPD management. Recognition of COPD exacerbation in its emerging stages could potentially aid to prevent the rapid decline in lung function, perhaps the critical consequences if acted upon.

Keywords: chronic obstructive pulmonary disease, acute exacerbation, lung function

Introduction

Chronic obstructive pulmonary disease (COPD) is a serious public health issue worldwide. COPD is the leading risk of death globally, accounting for 3.23 million deaths in 2019. More than 80% of these deaths occurred in low- and middle-income nations [1]. Risk factors other than smoking account for a significant part of the COPD burden. The prevalence of COPD is directly related to indoor, outdoor, and occupational pollution and smoking. Exposure to these risk factors is estimated to contribute a significant part to the increasing global burden of COPD. COPD is a common, preventable, and treatable disease that is characterized by

* Corresponding Author's Email: jithinksree@gmail.com
† Corresponding Author's Email: jithinksree@psmchs.edu.sa.

In: Chronic Obstructive Pulmonary Disease
Editor: Jaber S. Alqahtani
ISBN: 979-8-88697-333-4

persistent respiratory symptoms and airflow restriction that is due to airway and/ or alveolar aberrations generally affected by significant exposure to toxic elements or gases and predisposed by host factors as well as abnormal lung development. The chronic airflow limitation is caused by parenchymal destruction and small airway diseases and is measured by spirometry to evaluate lung function [2].

Anatomical and Physiological Changes in COPD

The response of airway protective mechanisms to inhaled toxins are increased in COPD which leads to the destruction of lung tissue, and impairment of normal defense mechanism which restrict the disruption of repairing mechanisms. Inflammatory and structural changes in the airway increase with the severity of the disease and remain even after the cessation of the cause of COPD. The imbalance between proteases and antiproteases and oxidative stress in the lungs are the two major processes involved in the pathogenesis of COPD. The physiological abnormalities that result from the pathological changes are hypersecretion of mucus, ciliary dysfunction, airflow limitation, and hyperinflation which leads to gas exchange abnormalities, pulmonary hypertension, and other systemic effects. The hypersecretion of mucus and ciliary dysfunction is due to squamous metaplasia, increase in goblet cell count, and enlargement of bronchial submucosal glands which leads to abnormal mucociliary clearance and results in expectoration difficulty. Small conducting airways that are < 2 mm are more prone to airflow obstruction which is the consequence of airway remodeling (inflammation and narrowing) and the presence of exudates in small airways. Destruction of alveolar walls (loss of elastic recoil) and loss of alveolar support also contribute to airflow obstruction which will progressively trap air during expiration, and progress into hyperinflation. The imbalance between ventilation and perfusion observed in COPD is due to the anatomical changes, which is the major mechanism for abnormal gas exchange. Pulmonary hypertension is associated with pulmonary arterial constriction, endothelial dysfunction, pulmonary artery remodeling, and damage to the pulmonary capillary bed caused by abnormal ventilation-perfusion ratios [3].

Exacerbation of COPD

An exacerbation of COPD (ECOPD) is defined as a sudden deterioration of respiratory symptoms followed by a variable degree of physiological characteristics [4]. An exacerbation can be a sudden worsening of existing respiratory symptoms like cough, sputum production, and shortness of breath which are associated with an increase in mucus production, airway inflammation, and significant gas trapping and might require therapeutical support. Exacerbation has a negative influence on patients' health status, hospitalization and readmission rates, and disease progression. These factors contribute to increased dyspnea which is the prominent symptom of COPD exacerbation [2].

Triggers/Risk Factors

One of the major triggers of COPD exacerbation is viral and bacterial respiratory infections. The common organisms include haemophilus influenza, streptococcus pneumonia, mycoplasma pneumonia, klebsiella pneumonia, Escherichia coli, etc. The risk factors strongly associated with frequent exacerbations include prior exacerbations, dyspnea, reduced lung function, depression, poor quality of life, and female gender [2]. The risk of COPD exacerbations is higher with exposure to certain environmental and chemical elements. The non-chemical triggers are seasonal variations, weather changes, acute illness, and physical activity, whereas chemical exposures to car and truck exhaust and scented laundry products are associated with higher exacerbation occurrence. Exposure to air pollution can significantly increase the risk of exacerbation. According to the TIOSPIR trial, seasonal changes have a great impact on COPD exacerbations. Exacerbation rates are higher in winter compared with the summer season. COPD Patients with cardiovascular diseases, bronchiectasis, gastroesophageal reflux disease, pulmonary embolism, diabetes mellitus, obstructive sleep apnea syndromes, skeletal muscle weakness, and chronic kidney diseases are at high risk for developing exacerbation [5].

Classification (GOLD Classification and Rome Proposal)

COPD is a highly heterogeneous disease condition with a wide range of clinical manifestations in both stable and acute states. Prevention of exacerbation is focused primarily on the phenotype of the stable disease condition. The Global Initiative for Chronic Obstructive Lung Disease (GOLD) classified COPD exacerbation as mild, moderate, and severe according to the treatment and requirement of hospitalization. A mild COPD exacerbation is characterized by deterioration of symptoms that can be treated with only short-acting bronchodilators (SABA). Antibiotics and oral corticosteroids are required to treat a moderate COPD exacerbation. Severe exacerbations of COPD necessitate hospitalization and emergency department visits, which are mostly associated with acute respiratory failure, which can be life-threatening [4]. Although this healthcare utilization definition is useful in clinical studies, its reliance is limited to factors like access to health care, and the social and financial situation of the patient other than underlying pathophysiological conditions. It has limitations as patient illness severity should be a composite of underlying disease severity, frequency, and presence of co-morbidities. According to the patient's reported symptom changes, the severity level is altered.

This definition of exacerbation of COPD has several flaws that negatively impact clinical and healthcare outcomes. The shortcoming of the current definition includes 1) It is primarily based on the subjective perception of a patient's worsening respiratory symptoms, which varies from one patient to other [6]. The other conditions like cardiac events, pneumonia, and pulmonary embolism can mimic the symptoms of ECOPD [4]. 2) It does not establish the relation between symptoms to measurable pathophysiological factors that could characterize the exacerbation event itself. 3) The severity classification can vary subjectively with the variations in healthcare system availability and difference in practitioners [7]. All these limitations are overcome by integrating current evidence and accessible technology capable of measuring laboratory and clinical variables that can act as a primary indicator of exacerbation severity. The Rome proposal defines exacerbation as the occurrence of dyspnea episodes, cough, and sputum production that worsen over 14 days, accompanied by tachypnea and/ or tachycardia with increased local and systematic inflammation caused by airway inflammation, pollution, and other airway injuries along with severity classification. The diagnostic approach evaluates whether the event is life-threatening and requires adequate treatment. It also incorporates detailed clinical examination for evidence of COPD and other possible respiratory/ non-respiratory diseases, assessment of symptoms and signs, severity evaluation using appropriate investigations and establishes the cause of the event [8].

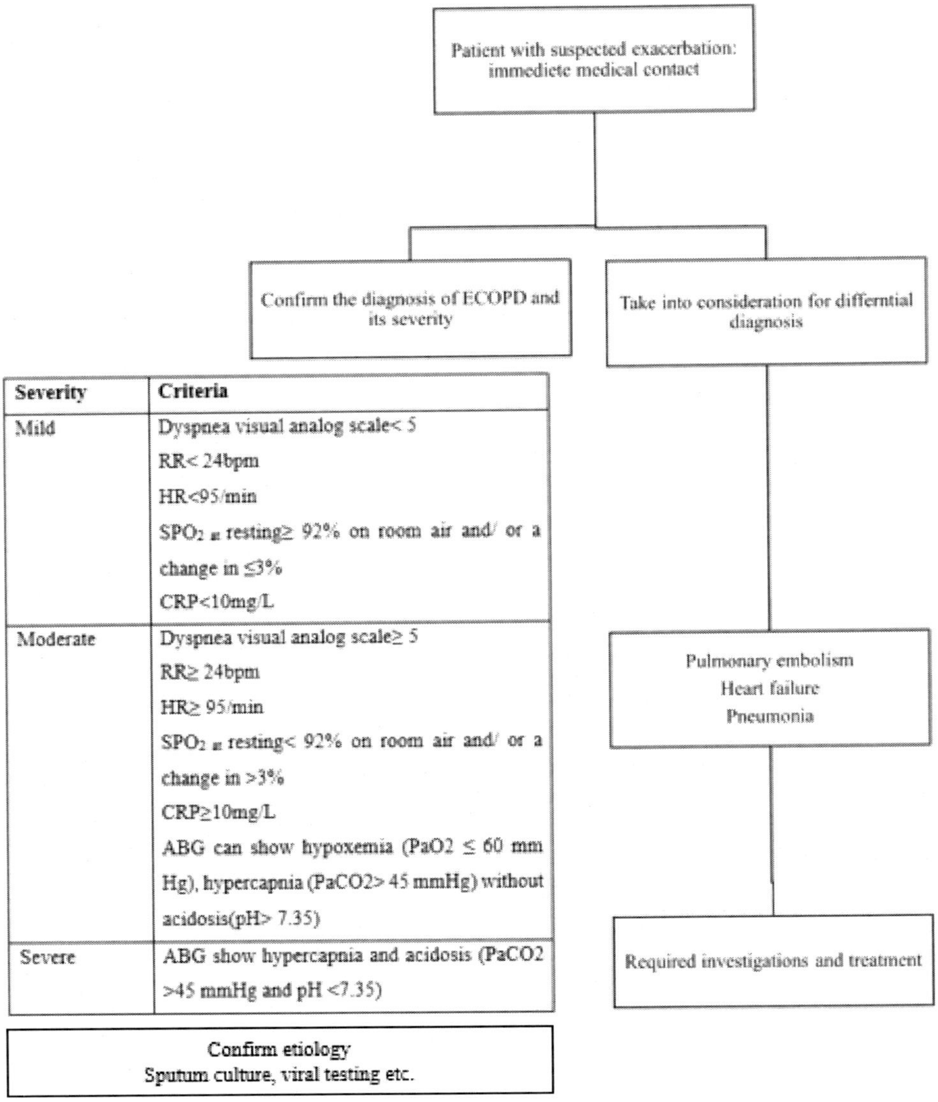

Figure 1. *Rome proposal:* Diagnostic approach to a patient suspected of ECOPD (8).

Why Early Recognition of Exacerbation Is Important

COPD patients should be educated to recognize exacerbation signs early. If patients can identify the early warning signs of exacerbation by themselves, they will be able to manage and prevent acute worsening of symptoms. If reported early, the majority of exacerbations can be managed with the bronchodilator, and oral corticosteroids on an outpatient basis. Unreported exacerbations may lead to worsening symptoms and to poor outcomes. Inability to recognize the symptom is the most common reason for the poor untimely reporting in most cases. Long-term effects of unreported exacerbations include declined lung function, hospitalization, and mortality [9]. Remote patient monitoring (RPM) can be used to improve patient involvement and to identify symptomatic changes at the earliest, allowing the physician to initiate proactive interventions to avoid poor health outcomes. Early identification of COPD exacerbations is possible with RPM and accessible by physicians to implement interventions without delay [10]. Healthcare workers play a major role in caring for, assisting, and providing guidance about observable patterns, warning symptoms, prodromal signs, and major risk factors to live with diagnosed COPD [11].

Exacerbation Recognition Tools

Patient diary cards are valid measures of exacerbation signs and symptoms. The advantages of this approach include standardized data, decreased recall bias, and the ability to identify events and assess resolution based on a pre-defined scoring algorithm. Breathlessness, cough, sputum, chest symptoms, difficulty to expectorate sputum, fatigued or weak, sleep disturbances, and feeling anxious about the condition are assessed in the Exacerbation of chronic pulmonary disease tool (EXACT) diary. The four major respiratory domains (breathlessness, cough, sputum, and chest symptoms) are rated on a five- or six-point ordinal scale, with the summed total score expressed in a 0- 100 scale, with the higher score indicating more severe exacerbation. EXACT is an effective tool for evaluating severity in an outpatient setting when the event was reviewed by healthcare utilization and London COPD cohort diary cards. EXACT scores indicate the severity by exacerbation duration, lung function, and systemic inflammation [12].

The Acute COPD Exacerbation Prediction Tool (ACCEPT) is a tool that can predict the rate and severity of COPD exacerbation on an individual level. ACCEPT identifies a personalized risk level for each patient, allowing clinicians to alter treatment plans to the specific needs of patients. ACCEPT is a model that incorporates simple, easily available clinical and demographic data to predict the risk and severity of exacerbation over a 12-month period, allowing personalized management for COPD patients. ACCEPT uses an individual history of exacerbation to predict future risk of exacerbation. This tool is geographically generalizable because external cohort validation includes data from 12 different nations. ACCEPT can estimate the number of exacerbations within the given period, the time for the next exacerbation, and the risk of occurrence of a specific number of both severe and non-severe exacerbations up to one year. It provides accurate predictions that allow clinicians to appropriately risk stratify two patients with the same history of exacerbation. A few of the limitations of ACCEPT don't include patients with mild (GOLD 1) severity, thus doesn't estimate predictions in this subgroup, and it has insufficient data on vaccination, biomarkers, comorbidities, and socioeconomic status of COPD patients [13].

One of the newest tools developed for the recognition of exacerbation is COPD Exacerbation Recognition Tool (CERT). The primary purpose of the development of CERT is to promote exacerbation reporting. CERT is not a diagnostic tool or set criteria for determining the presence of exacerbation. It is designed to detect signs and symptoms that are suggestive of exacerbation, thus it is more like a case-finding tool than a diagnostic tool [14].

Consequences of COPD Exacerbation

Impact on Symptom Duration

COPD exacerbations that last for a prolonged time increase the risk of future incidents and deteriorate health status. A prolonged exacerbation period in COPD patients is associated with an increased risk of the next episode, a worse health state, and unusual exacerbation duration. Prolonged exacerbations are related to causing a greater inflammatory burden which makes the next episode more likely, thus longer exacerbation duration is associated with a greater risk of development of another episode. The faster lung function decline in patients who experience frequent exacerbations compared with few or zero exacerbations is due to a delay in lung function recovery following an episode of exacerbation [15]. All these findings emphasize the significance of detecting COPD exacerbation and providing early treatment may help to reduce symptoms and lung function deterioration.

Impact on Lung Function

Exacerbations have a negative impact on lung function. Patients with frequent exacerbations are shown to decline faster (about 25%) compared with infrequent exacerbations [15]. Patients who had experienced one or more exacerbations had a greater decline in FEV_1 and delayed recovery in peak expiratory flow (PEF) than patients who had recovered from exacerbations. Exacerbations accompanied by a sore throat and cold-like symptoms are more likely to cause impairment in lung function and, as an impact contributes to disease progression. The progression of COPD is influenced by eosinophilic inflammation of the airways, in patients who are not on inhaled corticosteroids. A patient who has multiple exacerbations and high blood eosinophil count, who is not on ICS therapy may be subject to a faster decline in lung function [16].

Impact of Co-Morbidities on COPD

The presence of comorbidities along with COPD is a pervasive problem and it is associated with a substantial risk of mortality and as well as poor patient outcomes. The presence of different comorbidities contributes to hospitalization risk, length of hospital stays, and mortality. Anemia has been identified as a risk factor for long-term oxygen dependency in COPD patients. Lower hemoglobin level causes a reduction in the oxygen content of the blood. Decreased total oxygen content and limiting lung reserve gradually increase V/Q mismatch and contribute to hypoxia. The coexistence of obstructive sleep apnea (OSA) and COPD, defined as "overlap syndrome" has been associated with a range of negative outcomes. Overlap syndromes are related to intermediate cardiovascular outcomes, economic burden, and mortality. Obesity has been related to various outcomes like deteriorating health status, poor quality of life, and dyspnea. The burden of obesity on COPD is associated with lower lung volume and functional residual capacity also due to the presence of expiratory tracheal collapse in obese patients. HIV/ AIDS is a chronic disease, it coexists with COPD in about 10-16% [17].

After adjusting for traditional risk factors of COPD like smoking, drug use, and socioeconomic status, HIV appears to be an important risk factor for the development of COPD disease. The prevalence of COPD in patients with lung cancer is 50% [18]. There are several possible mechanisms for increased lung cancer risk and mortality in COPD patients. Evidence suggests that lung cancer and COPD share similar genetic loci, according to genome-wide association studies. Additionally, the significant prevalence and impact of these comorbidities on COPD and its outcomes should not be overlooked.

Systemic Consequences of COPD

COPD is a disease commonly accompanied by the development of extrapulmonary diseases. These systemic manifestations including cardiovascular diseases, osteoporosis, skeletal muscle dysfunction, and cachexia play a significant role in decreased quality of life and higher mortality in COPD patients. Studies suggest that even minor reductions in lung function increase the risk of coronary events, ventricular arrhythmias, and cardiovascular mortality. A 10% reduction in FEV_1 increases the risk of cardiovascular events by 30% in COPD patients. The presence of a higher level of circulating thrombotic factors VII and VIII also increase the risk of cardiovascular diseases. The mechanism of the development of cachexia in COPD patients is multifactorial and is associated with decreased functional capacity, poor health, and higher mortality. Different causes of cachexia in COPD patients include imbalance and protein degradation and replacement· presence of cytokines and chemokines, and presence of human growth hormone, steroids, glucocorticoids, and catecholamines which promote catabolism [19].

Although the pathways relating to COPD and these systemic manifestations are not clear, the local and systemic inflammation, oxidative stress, and changes in neuro-humeral states are some of the most likely underlying pathways through which these extrapulmonary complications are caused. All these extrapulmonary manifestations should be treated aggressively once diagnosed, as they contribute to the overall morbidity and mortality of patients with COPD. While diagnosing COPD, physicians should be aware of these extra-pulmonary manifestations and to determine these co-morbidities, detailed history, physical examination, and appropriate investigations are required.

Impact on Mental Health

COPD patients have a higher incidence of developing psychological disorders such as anxiety and depression compared with the general population. Three of the variables in mental health are identified as the presence of mental disorder, psychological distress, and consumption of psychiatric medication. All these independent variables were present in patients with COPD and are associated with higher mental morbidity. Women with COPD were found to have poor self-perceived health. With the three variables identified, higher usage of health services is associated with poor mental health. COPD patients who are active have reduced psychological discomfort, and alcohol consumption appears to reduce the intake of psychotropic medicines, whereas smoking increases the chance of poor mental health [20].

Impact on Cognitive Function

COPD is associated with neuronal damage due to hypoxia and altered cerebral metabolisms. Evidence suggests that the presence of c- reactive proteins is associated with a decline in cognitive function either through the neurotoxic effect or due to cerebral atherosclerosis. Studies found that individuals with COPD should be always monitored for cognitive impairment on regular basis, as various levels of dysfunction might affect self-management, adherence, and personal independence. Impaired cognitive function will adversely affect the prognosis of COPD itself. Poor cognitive function impairs the patient's capacity to plan and do tasks, gradually patients will experience difficulty in taking decisions on their treatment and medical care which eventually leads to non-adherence to medications and self-care [21].

The Economic Impact of COPD

COPD exacerbations have a higher economic burden due to hospitalizations and relapse. Exacerbations are the most expensive component of COPD treatment. Hospitalizations due to exacerbation account for about 58% of the overall cost, followed by 32.2% for pharmaceutical acquisitions [22]. The severity of COPD, frequency of exacerbation, and symptoms were found to generally increase direct costs. The number of past exacerbations, as well as the presence and type of comorbidities, were the major factors identified as the predictors of economic burden in moderate-very-severe COPD. It emphasizes the significance of the management of comorbidities along with optimal COPD treatment to reduce health resource utilization and associated costs.

Impact on Physical Activity/Exercise Performance

COPD patients experience loss of muscle mass particularly in the thighs and upper arms. Loss of skeletal muscle mass is the primary cause of skeletal muscle dysfunction in COPD patients. As the disease progresses, the patient loses exercise endurance and develops dyspnea and fatigue on with minimal exertion. These changes in COPD are related to increased apoptosis, oxidative stress, inflammatory changes, and lactic acidosis. With disease progression, patients become breathless on minimal exertion and adopt a sedentary lifestyle. This leads to deconditioning and disuse, and muscles progressively become weaker, atrophic, and have decreased ability to withstand physical and oxidative stress. Physical and functional impairment like muscle strength and postural stability decreases with hospitalizations due to exacerbation; deterioration increases between discharge and follow-up in these subjects. Exercise capacity and muscular strength were observed to decline with mild COPD exacerbations and lower levels of physical activity were associated with an increased risk of subsequent exacerbations and mortality. Implementing a pulmonary rehabilitation program would be interesting for these individuals to reduce their physical and functional impairment due to COPD [23].

Impact on Health-Related Quality of Life/Long Term Impact

Exacerbation of COPD has an impact on a variety of aspects of a patient's quality of life. Patients who had frequent exacerbations (more than 3times per year) had considerably lower quality of life than patients who had fewer exacerbations (<3 times per year). Patients with COPD have a lower quality of life, which deteriorates significantly as the disease progresses. A significant increase in St George's Respiratory Questionnaire for COPD (SGRQ-C) is associated with increasing severity of COPD. The quality of life of a COPD patient with symptoms and reduced mental health is also affected by a higher smoking index. A decrease in FEV_1 or the incidence of at least one severe exacerbation is associated with significant deterioration in disease-specific Health-Related Quality of Life (HRQoL) [24].

Impact on Mortality

Severe acute exacerbation of COPD has an adverse prognostic impact on mortality and increases with the frequency of severe exacerbations which require hospital admissions. There is a higher crude mortality risk of 2.94- fold in exacerbations requiring hospital admissions compared with those without requiring admission. Reducing the number and severity of COPD exacerbations should be considered as the leading objective in COPD management [25].

Conclusion

Exacerbations epitomize an important event in the usual history of COPD patients and are linked with substantial morbidity and mortality. Moreover, it has a significant socio-economic impact and deleterious consequences on patients' lung function, quality of life, and exercise performance. Nevertheless, considerable advancement is observed in the understanding of the etiology of exacerbations in COPD, much still needs to be learned. Improving physician and patient recognition, patient education, and increasing awareness of the impact of COPD exacerbations and the need for reporting are key to curtailing detrimental effects. More research, preferably cohort studies are required about the prevalence, incidence, and natural history of various phenotypes of COPD and exacerbations, and their economic encumbrance on societies.

Key Points

- COPD Exacerbation is a serious event that affect COPD patients.
- Although much progress has been made in understanding the etiology of COPD exacerbations, there is still more to be discovered.
- Patients' quality of life and exercise performance are adversely affected by COPD exacerbations, which has a considerable socioeconomic effect.

- In order to reduce the negative impacts of COPD exacerbations, healthcare professionals must be better recognized, educated, and informed of the severity of the illness and the importance of reporting it.
- More study is needed on the prevalence, incidence, natural history, and economic burden of COPD phenotypes and exacerbations.

References

[1] World Health Organization (WHO). (2020). *The Top 10 Causes of Death*. https://www.who.int/news-room/fact-sheets/detail/the-top-10-causes-of-death.

[2] GOLD. (2022). *Global Strategy for Prevention, Diagnosis and Management of COPD*.

[3] MacNee, W. (2006). ABC of chronic obstructive pulmonary disease Pathology, pathogenesis, and pathophysiology. *BMJ Open*, *69332*(3), 1202–1204. https://doi.org/10.5586/asbp.2000.026.

[4] Wedzicha, J. A., & Seemungal, T. A. (2007). COPD exacerbations: defining their cause and prevention. *Lancet*, *370*(9589), 786–796. https://doi.org/10.1016/S0140-6736(07)61382-8.

[5] Hogea, S. P., Tudorache, E., Fildan, A. P., Fira-Mladinescu, O., Marc, M., & Oancea, C. (2020). Risk factors of chronic obstructive pulmonary disease exacerbations. *Clinical Respiratory Journal*, *14*(3), 183–197. https://doi.org/10.1111/crj.13129.

[6] Scioscia, G., Blanco, I., Arismendi, E., Burgos, F., Gistau, C., Foschino Barbaro, M. P., Celli, B., O'Donnell, D. E., & Agustí, A. (2017). Different dyspnoea perception in COPD patients with frequent and infrequent exacerbations. *Thorax*, *72*(2), 117–121. https://doi.org/10.1136/thoraxjnl-2016-208332.

[7] Effing, T. W., Kerstjens, H. A. M., Monninkhof, E. M., Van Der Valk, P. D. L. P. M., Wouters, E. F. M., Postma, D. S., Zielhuis, G. A., & Van Der Palen, J. (2009). Definitions of exacerbations: Does it really matter in clinical trials on COPD? *Chest*, *136*(3), 918–923. https://doi.org/10.1378/chest.08-1680.

[8] Celli, B. R., Fabbri, L. M., Aaron, S. D., Agusti, A., Brook, R., Criner, G. J., Franssen, F. M. E., Humbert, M., Hurst, J. R., O'Donnell, D., Pantoni, L., Papi, A., Rodriguez-Roisin, R., Sethi, S., Torres, A., Vogelmeier, C. F., & Wedzicha, J. A. (2021). An updated definition and severity classification of chronic obstructive pulmonary disease exacerbations: The rome proposal. *American Journal of Respiratory and Critical Care Medicine*, *204*(11), 1251–1258. https://doi.org/10.1164/rccm.202108-1819PP.

[9] Langsetmo, L., Platt, R. W., Ernst, P., & Bourbeau, J. (2008). Underreporting Exacerbation of Chronic Obstructive Pulmonary Disease in a Longitudinal Cohort. *American Journal of Respiratory and Critical Care Medicine*, *177*(14), 396–401. https://doi.org/10.1164/rccm.200708-1290OC.

[10] Polsky MB, Moraveji N. Early identification and treatment of COPD exacerbation using remote monitoring. *Respiratory Medicine Case Reports*. 2021 Jan 1; 34:101475.

[11] Chatreewatanakul, B., Othaganont, P., & Hickman, R. L. (2022). Early symptom recognition and symptom management among exacerbation COPD patients: A qualitative study. *Applied Nursing Research*, *63*, 1–12. https://doi.org/10.1016/j.apnr.2021.151522.

[12] Leidy, N. K., Wilcox, T. K., Jones, P. W., Jones, P., Roberts, L., Powers, J. H., Sethi, S., Donohue, J., Eremenco, S., Erickson, P., Martinez, F., Patrick, D., Rennard, S., Rodriguez-Roisin, R., & Schünemann, H. (2011). Standardizing measurement of chronic obstructive pulmonary disease exacerbations: Reliability and validity of a patient-reported diary. *American Journal of Respiratory and Critical Care Medicine*, *183*(3), 323–329. https://doi.org/10.1164/rccm.201005-0762OC.

[13] Adibi, A., Sin, D. D., Safari, A., Johnson, K. M., Aaron, S. D., FitzGerald, J. M., & Sadatsafavi, M. (2020). The Acute COPD Exacerbation Prediction Tool (ACCEPT): a modelling study. *The Lancet Respiratory Medicine*, *8*(10), 1–9. https://doi.org/10.1016/S2213-2600(19)30397-2.

[14] Jones, P. W., Wang, C., Chen, P., Chen, L., Wang, D., Xia, J., Yang, Y., Wang, Y., & Ma, Q. (2022). The Development of a COPD Exacerbation Recognition Tool (CERT) to Help Patients Recognize When to Seek Medical Advice. *International Journal of Chronic Obstructive Pulmonary Disease*, *17*, 213–222.

[15] Donaldson, G. C., Law, M., Kowlessar, B., Singh, R., Brill, S. E., Allinson, J. P., & Wedzicha, J. A. (2015). Impact of prolonged exacerbation recovery in chronic obstructive pulmonary disease. *American Journal of Respiratory and Critical Care Medicine*, *192*(8), 943–950. https://doi.org/10.1164/rccm.201412-2269OC.

[16] Ora, J., Laveneziana, P., Ofir, D., Deesomchok, A., Webb, K. A., & O'Donnell, D. E. (2009). Combined effects of obesity and chronic obstructive pulmonary disease on dyspnea and exercise tolerance. *American Journal of Respiratory and Critical Care Medicine*, *180*(10), 964–971. https://doi.org/10.1164/rccm.200904-0530OC.

[17] Crothers, K., Butt, A. A., Gibert, C. L., Rodriguez-Barradas, M. C., Crystal, S., & Justice, A. C. (2006). Increased COPD among HIV-positive compared to HIV-negative veterans. *Chest*, *130*(5), 1326–1333. https://doi.org/10.1378/chest.130.5.1326.

[18] Young, R. P., Hopkins, R. J., Christmas, T., Black, P. N., Metcalf, P., & Gamble, G. D. (2008). COPD prevalence is increased in lung cancer, independent of age, sex and smoking history. *European Respiratory Journal*, *34*(2), 380–386. https://doi.org/10.1183/09031936.00144208.

[19] Wing SS, Goldberg AL. Glucocorticoids activate the ATP-ubiquitin-dependent proteolytic system in skeletal muscle during fasting. *American Journal of Physiology-Endocrinology and Metabolism*. 1993 Apr 1;264(4):E668-76.

[20] Dahlén I, Janson C. Anxiety and depression are related to the outcome of emergency treatment in patients with obstructive pulmonary disease. *Chest*. 2002 Nov 1;122(5):1633-7.

[21] Miravitlles, M., Murio, C., Guerrero, T., & Gisbert, R. (2002). Pharmacoeconomic evaluation of acute exacerbations of chronic bronchitis and COPD. *Chest*, *121*(5), 1449–1455. https://doi.org/10.1378/chest.121.5.1449.

[22] Smith D, Lovell J, Weller C, Kennedy B, Winbolt M, Young C, Ibrahim J. A systematic review of medication non-adherence in persons with dementia or cognitive impairment. *PloS one*. 2017 Feb 6;12(2):e0170651.

[23] Torres-Sánchez, I., Cabrera-Martos, I., Díaz-Pelegrina, A., Valenza-Demet, G., Moreno-Ramírez, M. P., & Valenza, M. C. (2017). Physical and functional impairment during and after hospitalization in subjects with severe COPD exacerbation. *Respiratory Care*, *62*(2), 209–214. https://doi.org/10.4187/respcare.04597.

[24] Stöber, A., Lutter, J. I., Schwarzkopf, L., Kirsch, F., Schramm, A., Vogelmeier, C. F., & Leidl, R. (2021). Impact of lung function and exacerbations on health-related quality of life in copd patients within one year: Real-world analysis based on claims data. *International Journal of COPD*, *16*(August), 2637–2651. https://doi.org/10.2147/COPD.S313711.

[25] Soler-Cataluña, J. J., Martínez-García, M. Á., Román Sánchez, P., Salcedo, E., Navarro, M., & Ochando, R. (2005). Severe acute exacerbations and mortality in patients with chronic obstructive pulmonary disease. *Thorax*, *60*(11), 925–931. https://doi.org/10.1136/thx.2005.040527.

Chapter 23

Management of Exacerbations

Valeria Maione[1,*], MD, Miguel Guia[1,2,3], MD, Raffaele Scala[4], MD and Paula Pinto[1,2,3], MD, PhD

[1]Thorax Department,
Centro Hospitalar Universitário Lisboa Norte, Lisbon, Portugal
[2]Sleep and Non-Invasive Ventilation Unit,
Centro Hospitalar Universitário Lisboa Norte, Lisbon, Portugal
[3]Instituto de Saúde Ambiental (ISAMB),
Faculty of Medicine, Lisbon University, Lisbon, Portugal
[4]Pulmonology and Respiratory Intensive Care Unit,
S. Donato Hospital, Arezzo, Italy

Abstract

Chronic Obstructive Pulmonary Disease (COPD) exacerbations are frequently underdiagnosed as a significant part of patients do not seek medical attention to treat their symptoms. When medical intervention is required, it is crucial to define a plan and start treatment as soon as possible.

We should always start with assessing severity and defining the most appropriate treatment setting to decide whether the patient should be admitted to the hospital or if an ambulatory treatment is possible.

To delineate a good treatment strategy, it is important to determine the presence or absence of respiratory failure and infection and the coexistence of comorbidities. An appropriate antibiotic therapy considering local resistance patterns is required when an infection is suspected. In the presence of respiratory failure, the gas exchange must be guaranteed through the use of supplementary oxygen or high flow nasal therapy or ventilatory support, invasive or not invasive. The hallmark of treatment in every patient with an acute exacerbation of COPD is bronchodilators and systemic corticosteroids, as they help alleviate symptoms, shorten recovery time, and improve lung function (FEV_1) and hypoxemia and reduce the risk of early relapse, treatment failure, and length of hospital stay. After an exacerbation is appropriately managed, a suitable discharge plan should be prepared. This will depend on the severity of the exacerbation but should generally include reclassification of the patient according to the GOLD criteria, optimization of pharmacological treatment and reassessment of inhaler technique, and management of comorbidities. After discharge and during follow-up, it is also essential to reinforce smoking cessation and plan influenza and pneumococcal vaccination. Finally, end-of-life

* Corresponding Author's Email: valeriamaione276@gmail.com.

In: Chronic Obstructive Pulmonary Disease
Editor: Jaber S. Alqahtani
ISBN: 979-8-88697-333-4

shared decisions should be faced with patients and familiars after resolving the exacerbated status, especially in subjects with advanced COPD.

Keywords: COPD, exacerbation, ventilation, lung function, corticosteroids

Introduction

There is no unequivocal definition of a Chronic Obstructive Pulmonary Disease (COPD) exacerbation, but common features of all definitions are: worsening of baseline cough and dyspnoea and change in sputum production or characteristics. The most used definition is an acute worsening of respiratory symptoms that results in additional therapy. Independently from the definition we adopt, the critical point is to recognize the exacerbations and start proper treatment. Always remind those other comorbidities frequently associated with COPD that may also worsen respiratory symptoms, especially when decompensated, simulating a COPD exacerbation (ECOPD). Thus, it is crucial to assess and exclude other diagnoses before starting treatment for ECOPD, such as pneumonia, pneumothorax, pleural effusion, pulmonary embolism, pulmonary edema due to cardiac-related conditions, and cardiac arrhythmias. For this purpose, it can be necessary to perform some exams, such as chest radiograph or ultrasound, D-dimer and Doppler sonogram of lower extremities, chest tomography, and cardiac tests (EKG, cardiac enzymes, cardiac ultrasound).

Appropriate management of COPD exacerbations represents a clinical challenge. In order to guide therapy, it is essential to identify the underlying cause; however, in about one-third of severe exacerbations of COPD, a cause cannot be identified. The most common triggers are viral respiratory infections, especially rhinovirus and bacterial infections, and it is known that some environmental factors can initiate or amplify the event, such as cold and air pollution [1, 2].

As important as acute management of COPD exacerbation, it is also essential to define a good discharge plan to prevent future exacerbations, as it is known that a previous exacerbation is the leading risk factor for future ones, implying acceleration of the long-term decline of lung function.

An appropriate discharge plan should generally include reclassification of the patient according to GOLD criteria, optimization of pharmacological therapy, management of comorbidities, patient (or caregiver) education on the correct use of inhaled therapy, and ambulatory revaluation by a Pulmonology clinician, smoking cessation and respiratory rehabilitation program.

End-of-life decision-making issues should be included in the management plan of COPD patients after a severe acute exacerbation, especially in end-stage disease.

The treatment goals of ECOPD are to minimize the negative effect of the current event and prevent the occurrence of new exacerbations.

Assess Severity

It is recognized that many exacerbations do not come to medical attention nor are reported to healthcare professionals because frequently, the patient underestimates the symptoms.

However, they still may have a negative impact on health and do not receive appropriate treatment in the acute phase and after, causing a decline in lung function over time.

When a patient is referred to medical observation, the severity of the exacerbation should always be assessed, and the event should be classified as mild when treated only with short-acting bronchodilators – SABD, moderate, which need to be treated with systemic corticosteroids and antibiotics on top of SABD, or severe, which require hospitalization.

Unfortunately, this severity range is currently only specified after the event, and until now, no prospective classification of severity has been validated, and no analytic parameter threshold has been defined in order to assess the severity of the event prior to treatment.

Despite the absence of a specific parameter to classify the exacerbation, there are some clinical and instrumental elements that should be evaluated, such as breathlessness, cough or sputum, new limitation of daily activities, use of accessory respiratory muscles, paradoxical chest wall movements, cyanosis, peripheral oxygen saturation level, hemodynamic instability, and deteriorated mental status. All these clinical elements may guide the clinician in therapeutic choices and help him define the treatment setting. The coexistence of multiple non-pulmonary comorbidities must be considered in the choice of the setting for the management of acute ECOPD; for example, if an exacerbated patient develops acute multiple organ dysfunction, admission to an intensive care unit (ICU) or respiratory high dependency unit is suggested.

If the patient is being examined in a hospital setting, arterial blood gases and chest radiography should be performed, as well as whole blood count and basic biochemical tests, as they can give the clinicians more elements to guide their decision. In cases where the use of antibiotics is not clear, measuring procalcitonin blood level may guide the initiation of therapy since it has been suggested as a more specific marker for bacterial infections.

If an infectious etiology is suspected (in a patient presenting fever or mucopurulent sputum, for example), blood cultures and sputum cultures are recommended before starting any antibiotic treatment. In cases where the use of antibiotics is not clear, measuring procalcitonin blood level may guide the initiation of therapy since it has been suggested as a more specific marker for bacterial infections..

In cases with previous bacterial isolations, especially in patients with pulmonary structural changes, they should guide the choice of antibiotic as a multi-resistant organism may be responsible for respiratory tract colonization.

Define the Setting of Treatment

Once the severity of the exacerbation has been assessed, an appropriate setting of treatment should be defined. Depending on the severity of the exacerbation or of the underlying disease, the patient can be managed as an outpatient (more than 80% of the cases) when clinically stable or inpatient, when needing monitoring and specific therapies that can only be delivered in a hospital setting. In this group of patients, it is crucial to identify those needing intensive or intermediate care unit admission as soon as possible.

Regarding pharmacological treatment and place of treatment, if exacerbations are mild and non-infectious, they may be treated at home with an increase in the dosage of maintenance bronchodilators.

Moderate exacerbations require treatment with systemic corticosteroids and antibiotics. These should be treated as outpatients as these exacerbations do not require hospitalization unless it is for socioeconomic reasons.

In the case of patients who had a severe exacerbation requiring hospitalization, they should be reclassified, and after-discharge therapy should be reviewed.

The GOLD 2022 guidelines suggest the following classification, depending on the presence of respiratory failure:

- *No respiratory failure*: respiratory rate 20-30 bpm, no use of accessory respiratory muscles, no changes in mental status, hypoxemia improved with supplemental oxygen with FiO_2 24-35%, no increase in $PaCO_2$.
- *Nonlife-threatening acute respiratory failure*: respiratory rate >30bpm, use of accessory respiratory muscles, no change in mental status, hypoxemia improved with supplemental oxygen FiO_2 >35%, $PaCO_2$ 50-60mmHg or increased compared with baseline.
- *Life-threatening acute respiratory failure*: respiratory rate >30bpm, use of accessory respiratory muscles, acute change in mental status, hypoxemia not improved with supplemental oxygen or requiring FiO_2 >40%, $PaCO_2$ >60mmHg, or increased compared with baseline, or acidosis.

Depending on the access to local resources, the patient's home support, and the presence of severe comorbidities, we can consider different settings of treatment.

For what concerns respiratory failure, we define the following settings of treatment:

- Patients with no respiratory failure can be treated in a medical ward or at home when possible.
- In case of acute respiratory failure, it is mandatory to treat the patient in a hospital setting. We should remember that failure to respond to initial medical treatment, presence of severe comorbidities, and insufficient home support are indications of admission to the hospital.
- In those hospitals with semi-intensive care units, admission to these units can be considered when Non-Invasive Ventilation (NIV) is needed, requiring close monitoring.

  Admission to an Intensive Care Unit (ICU) should be considered when facing a life-threatening acute respiratory failure and, depending on local resources, in patients with changes in mental status (confusion, lethargy, coma), persistent or worsening hypoxemia, and severe/worsening respiratory acidosis (pH<7.25) despite supplemental oxygen and non-invasive ventilation [3].

  Other criteria for Intensive Care Unit admission should also be applied, such as hemodynamic instability with the need for vasopressors, multi-organ failure, or the need for invasive mechanical ventilation.

Long-term prognosis following hospitalization for ECOPD is poor, with a mortality rate of about 50% in five-year following the event. Factors independently associated with poor outcomes include older age, lower body mass index, comorbidities (cardiovascular disease or lung cancer), previous hospitalizations for ECOPD, clinical severity of the exacerbation, and need for long-term oxygen therapy at discharge. Patients with a higher prevalence and severity of respiratory symptoms, poorer quality of life, worse lung function, lower exercise capacity, lower lung density, and thickened bronchial walls on CT-scan are also at increased risk for higher mortality following an ECOPD.

Some COPD patients are particularly susceptible to frequent exacerbations (two or more per year), and these patients have been shown to have worse health status and morbidity than patients with less frequent exacerbations.

The strongest predictor of a patient's future exacerbation frequency remains the number of exacerbations they have had in the prior year [1, 2].

Pharmacological Treatments

The three pillars of ECOPD pharmacological treatment are bronchodilators, corticosteroids, and antibiotics that manage to control acute phase symptoms, as well as prevent accelerated progression of the disease. A graphical representation of ECOPD management is shown in figure 1.

It is mandatory to start appropriate treatment as soon as possible to avoid disease progression, which is even more likely if recovery from the exacerbation is slow.

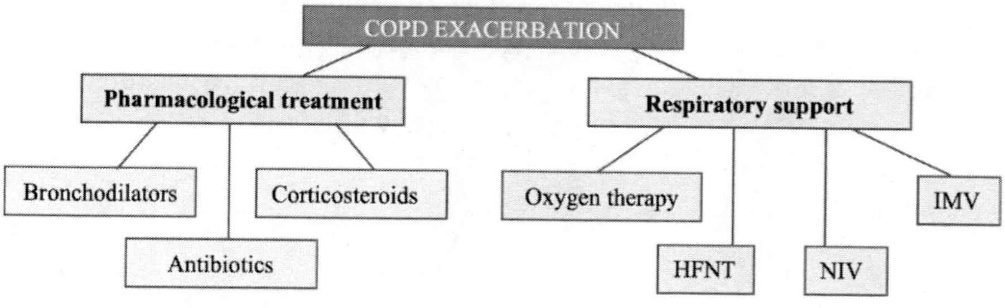

Figure 1. Management of ECOPD.

Bronchodilators

Short-acting inhaled β2 agonists (SABAs) with or without short-acting muscarinic antagonists (SAMAs) remain the basis for the treatment of symptoms and airflow obstruction during ECOPD and should always be the initial treatment in the acute phase in any of the formulations available (pressure metered-dose inhaler, nebulization, etc.).

Although there is no study evaluating the use of long-acting bronchodilators during an exacerbation, it is recommended to continue the treatment during the exacerbation if the patient was already using it or starting as soon as the patient is in a more stable condition.

For those cases treated as an outpatient that were not previously medicated with long-acting bronchodilators, it is important to remember that close revaluation is not always possible, and the patient should be provided with long-term therapy after the use of SABAs and/or SAMAs during the initial phase. Thus, it is crucial to properly identify and medicate these patients when observing them at home or in the primary care/emergency room before discharging them. As for other agents, intravenous methylxanthines have been largely used in the past years, but nowadays, these medications are not recommended due to their significant side effects [1, 2].

Corticosteroids

The role of systemic corticosteroids during ECOPD has been widely studied, and there is evidence that they shorten recovery time, improve lung function (FEV_1) and hypoxemia, and may reduce the risk of early relapse, treatment failure, and length of hospital stay.

Thus, a short course of systemic corticosteroids is suggested during exacerbation.

The 2022 update to the GOLD strategy document recommends treatment with oral prednisone 40 mg per day for five days without any reference to the treatment setting, suggesting that a short course of systemic corticosteroids should be done in hospitalized patients as well as in outpatients.

More extended administration is not recommended because of the increased risk of complications, such as pneumonia, sepsis, and death, and because of the reduced beneficial effect in addition to shorter courses [4, 5].

No difference in efficacy has been demonstrated between oral and intravenous administration. On the other hand, intravenous use of corticosteroids is associated with a more significant percentage of complications and adverse effects; thus, oral administration should always be preferred to intravenous one, if possible, according to the patient's status.

Phenotypic identification of responders to oral corticosteroids is an area of research that should be explored. Some data suggest that patients with an elevated blood eosinophil count will respond more to oral corticosteroids than patients with a low blood eosinophil count, but further investigation should be done to define whether it can be used as a biomarker and to establish a threshold [5].

Antibiotics

Another controversial point is the use of antibiotics to treat an exacerbation. Although it is well known that almost 50% of ECOPD are due to bacterial infections, there is no consensus on the indications to start antibiotic treatment [6].

Many guidelines (GOLD, NHS) recommend antibiotics for patients who present an increase in dyspnoea, sputum volume, and sputum purulence. However, when purulence of sputum is present, only another symptom is necessary or for exacerbations severe enough to require mechanical ventilation (invasive or non-invasive).

This conviction is based on many studies indicating the purulence of sputum as the clinical sign with the highest sensitivity and specificity for bacterial infection. In a study conducted by Stockley et al., it was demonstrated that the presence of purulent sputum was 94.4% sensitive and 77.0% specific for high bacterial load, while all patients who produced white (mucoid) sputum during the acute exacerbation improved without antibiotic therapy [7].

Some biomarkers have been suggested as helpful in optimizing antibiotic treatment, such as C-reactive protein (CRP) or procalcitonin.

In patients with exacerbation and elevated CRP levels (>50 mg/L), a significantly higher rate of clinical success for antibiotic treatment was demonstrated, suggesting an important role of this biomarker that could help avoid unnecessary use of antibiotic therapy that can lead to adverse effects and development of bacterial resistance [8]. For all patients, the choice of antibiotic should be guided by the local bacterial resistance pattern, the microbiology story of the patient, and other risk factors, like the presence of underlying structural lung disease (such as bronchiectasis) or an immunocompromised state.

Usually, initial empirical treatment is aminopenicillin with clavulanic acid, a macrolide, or a tetracycline, but local bacterial resistance patterns should always be kept in mind when choosing empirical antibiotic treatment.

In patients with severe exacerbations and those with prior therapy with antibiotics and oral corticosteroids, broader spectrum antibiotics are recommended, and in the presence of underlying structural lung disease, such as bronchiectasis, antibiotics targeting Pseudomonas species should be considered.

Although the most effective duration of treatment is still to be defined, the recommended length of antibiotic therapy is usually 5–7 days, but treatment duration will depend on the antibiotic used [6, 9].

When antibiotic treatment is established, sputum should be sent for culture, as resistant pathogens not sensitive to the above-mentioned antibiotics may be present.

Adjunct Therapies

It could be necessary to establish other therapies, depending on the patient's clinical condition.

An appropriate fluid balance and use of diuretics can be indicated, especially if the patient suffers from chronic heart failure, a condition that is frequently decompensated during ECOPD.

Anticoagulants and other prophylactic measures should be considered in hospitalized patients to prevent the risk of deep vein thrombosis and pulmonary embolism.

Among COPD patients hospitalized with a suspected exacerbation, up to 5.9% were found to have a pulmonary embolism. [1] [6]

Treatment and stabilization of other comorbidities and nutritional aspects are also crucial for a better outcome.

At all times, healthcare professionals should enforce the need for smoking cessation.

Respiratory Support

When COPD exacerbation is severe enough to produce respiratory failure, conventional oxygen therapy, high flow nasal therapy (HFNT), or ventilatory support should be considered.

Evaluating the most appropriate form of respiratory support is crucial to avoid collateral effects such as hypercapnia or unnecessary measures that can be uncomfortable for the patient.

Oxygen

Conventional oxygen therapy is of beneficial value in ECOPD as patients are often hypoxemic, and targeted oxygen therapy should be delivered, aiming for peripheral saturation levels of

88%–92%, especially in patients with hypercapnia. In these patients, hyperoxia has been linked with poor outcomes, and the use of uncontrolled oxygen therapy in the prehospital setting is associated with worsening respiratory acidosis and an increased risk of death.

Once the oxygen therapy is started, arterial blood gases should be monitored to avoid CO_2 retention or worsening of acidosis, and appropriate measures should be taken as soon as a worsening of the clinical condition is detected.

HFNT

High Flow Nasal Therapy delivers a humidified and heated air-oxygen mixture up to a flow of 80 L/min. In patients with hypoxemic respiratory failure, it is associated with reduced work of breathing, improved gas exchange, improved lung volume, and dynamic compliance [10].

This form of oxygen delivery has also been associated with ventilation improvement and reduction of hypercapnia in acute exacerbations due to dead space washout. However, it is essential to monitor arterial blood gases accurately and check for early evidence of hypercapnia, primarily when a high inspired fraction of oxygen is used.

Therefore, in mild-to-moderate respiratory acidosis cases, HFNT might be an alternative to NIV in exacerbated COPD patients who do not tolerate or reject NIV [10, 11].

HFNT might also be a valid alternative to conventional oxygen therapy during breaks of NIV or to facilitate NIV discontinuation [12].

Although promising, the evidence of use of HFNT in ECOPD is still poor, and more extensive studies need to be conducted before a formal indication of using this technique in acute respiratory failure with hypercapnia.

Non-Invasive Ventilation (NIV)

A major advance in the treatment of ECOPD has been the implementation of non-invasive positive pressure ventilation (NIPPV or NIV). NIV has been shown to improve acute respiratory acidosis, decrease respiratory rate and work of breathing, and reduce the severity of breathlessness, need for intubation, and length of hospital stay.

Proposed indications to initiate NIV during ECOPD are:

- Respiratory acidosis ($PaCO_2 \geq 45$mmHg and arterial pH ≤ 7.35)
- Severe dyspnea with clinical signs of respiratory muscle fatigue and increased work of breathing, such as the use of respiratory accessory muscles, paradoxical motion of the abdomen, or retraction of the intercostal spaces
- Persistent hypoxemia despite supplemental oxygen therapy and medical therapy

Choice of modality strictly depends on the comorbidities of the patient and the type of respiratory failure. In fact, if hypoxia is isolated, continuous positive airway pressure (CPAP) can be used, whereas if hypercapnia is also present, bi-level ventilation is preferred, as well as in case of respiratory muscle fatigue or to reach for the comfort of the patient.

In terms of respiratory system mechanics, COPD is characterized by the development of dynamic hyperinflation, implying that alveolar pressure remains positive during the expiration, which leads to the development of auto-positive end-expiratory pressure (auto-PEEP). The presence of dynamic hyperinflation and auto-PEEP should be considered if the expiratory flow does not cease at end-expiration.

In COPD, auto-PEEP is primarily caused by expiratory flow limitation due to small airway collapse that increases airway resistance. Especially during exacerbations, respiratory rate increases, and expiratory time shortens.

In patients triggering their ventilator, initiation of inspiratory flow requires inspiratory force to overcome auto-PEEP, which translates into an increased inspiratory effort during the triggering phase. Ultimately, this increased effort may fail to trigger the ventilator, leading to ineffective triggering, one of the most frequent dyssynchronies.

Dynamic hyperinflation worsens the increase in right ventricular impedance (afterload effect), while large negative intrathoracic pressure swings increase the venous return to the right ventricle (preload effect). Both favor direct ventricular interaction with a left-ward shift of the septum [3]. The inspiratory flow rates and inspiratory to expiratory time ratios should be adjusted to provide a prolonged duration of expiration to minimize dynamic hyperinflation (auto-PEEP), preferring an inspiratory-expiratory ratio of 1:3. When auto-PEEP is detected, attention should be paid to adjust EPAP properly, which should be titrated to correspond to 75-80% of intrinsic-PEEP.

Other indications and contraindications of NIV also apply in ECOPD, such as level of consciousness and hemodynamic stability, among others.

Invasive Mechanical Ventilation (IMV)

If contraindications are present or if NIV is inadequate, patients may require intubation and invasive support.

However, an important consideration to avoid hyperinflation, barotrauma, and volutrauma should be implemented. This result can be achieved by adequately sedating the intubated patient and implementing controlled hypoventilation awaiting the effects of other treatments to reduce airway obstruction.

Despite advances in NIV, invasive mechanical ventilation is still important in a subgroup of patients, and rapidly selecting appropriate candidates is crucial.

In patients with COPD, weaning can be difficult, and when extubation fails, NIV can be introduced to help prevent reintubation and reduce mortality [2, 3, 13].

ECOPD has functional consequences with persistent peripheral muscle weakness, loss of fitness, and decline in outdoor activities, making these patients more likely to become sedentary and require pulmonary rehabilitation. This is especially important in patients undergoing sedation and invasive mechanical ventilation.

Novel approaches in the management of respiratory failure due to ECOPD include helium-oxygen mixture (Heliox) and extracorporeal carbon dioxide removal (ECCO2R).

Therapy at Discharge

After an exacerbation is appropriately managed, a suitable discharge plan should be prepared. This will depend on the severity of the exacerbation, but should generally include reclassification of the patient according to the GOLD criteria, optimization of pharmacological treatment and reassessing inhaler technique, management of comorbidities, referral to a Pulmonology Consultation, and integration of smoking cessation and pulmonary rehabilitation program [2, 13].

An example of follow-up recommendations is proposed in figure 2.

It is important to reassess GOLD class to define appropriate pharmacological treatment, especially for those patients already very symptomatic, in whom we may consider introducing inhaled corticosteroid, depending on peripheral eosinophil level (if more than 300 eosinophils/uL, or 100 eosinophils/uL in a patient with ≥2 moderate exacerbations or one hospitalization).

In patients still exacerbating despite triple therapy or those treated with LABA/LAMA with eosinophil level< 100/uL, roflumilast or azithromycin can be considered. Roflumilast should be used in patients with chronic bronchitis phenotype, FEV_1 <50%, and azithromycin can be used in former smokers.

The remaining pharmacological therapy should follow GOLD indications for stable patients [14].

Discharge

- Reassess GOLD class
- Review maintenance therapy and inhaler technique
- Assess need for continuing oxygen therapy
- Explain withdrawal of acute phase medication (corticosteroids, short-acting bronchodilators, antibiotics, etc.)
- Reenforce smoking cessation

1-4 weeks

- Review inhaler technique
- Reassess need for long-term oxygen
- Document symptoms (CAT or mMRC) and prognosis (i.e. BODE)
- Reenforce smoking cessation
- Plan anti-pneumococcal and Influenzae vaccination

12-16 weeks

- Review inhaler technique
- Reassess need for long-term oxygen
- Measure lung function (spirometry)
- CT scan (when indicated)
- Reenforce smoking cessation

Figure 2. Follow-up recommendations.

GOLD 2022 guidelines recommend revaluating the patient at 1-4 weeks and later at 12-16 weeks after hospital discharge, but the plan needs to be adapted to local resources. In the early follow-up (within one month after hospital discharge), it is essential to review the plan and confirm therapy and inhalator technique; in the additional follow-up (at three months), it is crucial to reassess symptoms (CAT or mMRC) and prognosis (ex. BODE score), evaluate lung function and arterial blood gases to reassess the need for long-term oxygen. At every revaluation, it is important to reassess and review the correct use of inhaled therapy with the patient and caregiver.

In patients with frequent exacerbations, a CT scan could be helpful in documenting bronchiectasis and emphysema.

Appropriate control and management of other comorbidities are also important to help reduce cough, dyspnea, and intolerance to physical activity due to other diseases (p.e. cardiac, obesity, peripheral venous insufficiency) and reduce global mortality.

After discharge and during follow-up, it is always important to reinforce smoking cessation, as it is the intervention with the greatest capacity to influence the natural history of COPD, as well as plan influenza and pneumococcal vaccination.

Even though significant advances have been made in preventing new exacerbations, they remain the most important indicator of poor prognosis in COPD patients.

They are highly heterogeneous events with considerable variation in underlying causes and biological processes.

Survival after an episode of acute respiratory failure for COPD patients with hypercapnia is about 50% at two years after discharge with about half of the patients being readmitted to the hospital within six months [2, 6, 15].

Conclusion

Exacerbations may be mitigated clinically by early detection and prompt treatment, improving health-related quality of life and reducing the likelihood of hospital admission. The detrimental consequences of the existing morbidity and mortality caused by exacerbations will be reduced to the greatest extent possible if patient and physician comprehension of the causes of COPD exacerbations and the benefits of early treatment are improved.

Key Points

- Many exacerbations do not come to medical attention nor are reported to healthcare professionals because frequently, the patient underestimates the symptoms, but they still may have a negative impact on health and do not receive appropriate treatment in the acute phase and after causing a decline of lung function over time.
- Mild and non-infectious exacerbations can be treated at home with an increase in the dosage of maintenance bronchodilators; moderate exacerbations require treatment with systemic corticosteroids and antibiotics and should be treated as outpatients if these exacerbations do not require hospitalization for clinical or socioeconomic reasons; severe exacerbations should be admitted to hospital and treated in the most appropriate setting.

- Survival after an episode of acute respiratory failure for COPD patients with hypercapnia is about 50% at two years after discharge, with about half of the patients being readmitted to the hospital within six months.
- The strongest predictor of a patient's future exacerbation is the number of exacerbations they have had in the prior year.
- The pillars of ECOPD pharmacological treatment are bronchodilators and corticosteroids that are known to shorten recovery time, improve lung function and hypoxemia, and may reduce the risk of early relapse, treatment failure, and length of hospital stay. Antibiotic treatment is also crucial when an infection is suspected.

References

[1] MacLeod M, Papi A, Contoli M, Beghé B, Celli BR, Wedzicha JA, Fabbri LM. Chronic obstructive pulmonary disease exacerbation fundamentals: Diagnosis, treatment, prevention and disease impact. *Respirology,* 2021 Jun; 26(6):532-51.

[2] Reis AJ, Alves C, Furtado S, Ferreira J, Drummond M, Robalo-Cordeiro C. (2018). COPD exacerbations: Management and hospital discharge. *Pulmonology,* 24(6), 345-50.

[3] Demoule A, Brocharde L, Dres M, Heunks L, Jubran A, Laghi F, Mekontso-Dessap A, Nava S, Ouanes-Besbes L, Peñuelas O, Piquilloud L, Vassilakopoulos T, Mancebo J. How to ventilate obstructive and asthmatic patients. *Intensive Care Med,* 2020 Dec; 46(12):2436-49.

[4] Bafadhel M, McKenna S, Terry S, Mistry V, Pancholi M, Venge P, Lomas DA, Barer MR, Johnston SL, Pavord ID, and Brightling CE. Blood eosinophils to direct corticosteroid treatment of exacerbations of chronic obstructive pulmonary disease: A randomized placebo-controlled trial. *Int J Chron Obstruct Pulmon Dis,* 2016 Feb 19; 11 Spec Iss (Spec Iss):21-30.

[5] Walters JAE, Tan DJ, D. J., White CJ, Gibson PG, Wood-Baker R., Walters EH. (2014). Systemic corticosteroids for acute exacerbations of chronic obstructive pulmonary disease. *Cochrane Database Syst Rev,* 2014 Sep 1; (9).

[6] «National Institute for Health and Care Excellence (NICE) Clinical Guideline, Management of chronic obstructive pulmonary disease in adults in primary and secondary care updated, 2010.

[7] Stockley RA, O'Brien C, Pye A, Hill SL. Relationship of sputum color to nature and outpatient management of acute exacerbations of COPD. *Chest,* 2000 Jun; 117(6):1638-45.

[8] Daniels JM, Schoorl M, Snijders D, Knol DL, Lutter R, Jansen HM, Boersma WG. Procalcitonin vs C-reactive protein as predictive markers of response to antibiotic therapy in acute exacerbations of COPD. *Chest,* 2010 Nov; 138(5):1108-15.

[9] Wedzicha JA, Miravitlles M, Hurst JR, Calverley PM, Albert RK, Anzueto A, Criner GJ, Papi A, Rabe KF, Rigau D, Sliwinski P, Tonia T, Vestbo J, Wilson KC, Krishnan JA (ATS co-chair). Management of COPD exacerbations: A European respiratory society/American thoracic society guideline. *Eur Respir J,* 2017 Mar 15; 49(3):1600791.

[10] Fraser JF, Spooner AJ, Dunster KR, Anstey CM, Corley A. Nasal high flow oxygen therapy in patients with COPD reduces respiratory rate and tissue carbon dioxide while increasing tidal and end-expiratory lung volumes: A randomised crossover trial. *Thorax,* 2016 Aug; 71(8):759-61.

[11] Bräunlich J, Dellweg D, Bastian A, Budweiser S, Randerath W, Triché D, Bachmann M, Kähler C, Bayarassou AH, Mäder I, Geiseler J, Köhler N, Petroff D, Wirtz H. Nasal high-flow versus noninvasive ventilation in patients with chronic hypercapnic COPD. *Int J Chron Obstruct Pulmon Dis,* 2019 Jul 5; 14:1411-21.

[12] Pisani L, Astuto M, Prediletto I, Longhini F. High flow through nasal cannula in exacerbated COPD patients: A systematic review. *Pulmonology,* Nov-Dec 2019; 25(6):348-54.

[13] Qureshi H, Sharafkhaneh A, Hanania NA. (2014). Chronic obstructive pulmonary disease exacerbations: Latest evidence and clinical implications. *Ther Adv Chronic Dis,* 2014 Sep; 5(5):212-27.

[14] Galli JA, Krahnke JS, Mamary AJ, Shenoy K, Zhao H and Criner GJ. (2014). Home non-invasive ventilation use following acute hypercapnic respiratory failure in COPD. *Respir Med,* 2014 May; 108(5):722-8.

[15] Pavord ID, Jones PW, Burgel PR and Rabe KF. (2016). Exacerbations of COPD. *International Journal of Chronic Obstructive Pulmonary Disease,* 11(Spec Iss), 21.

Chapter 24

Role of Pulmonary Rehabilitation and COPD Exacerbations

Alessandro Domingues Heubel, Naiara Tais Leonardi and Renata Gonçalves Mendes*

Department of Physical Therapy,
Federal University of São Carlos (UFSCar),
São Carlos, Brazil

Abstract

Pulmonary rehabilitation (PR), including physical exercise as its main component, is an evidence-based strategy in the management of stable chronic obstructive pulmonary disease (COPD). However, in acute exacerbation of COPD (AECOPD), the indication of an exercise-based PR program is not a consensus, although growing evidence shows that the intervention is safe and leads to benefits in exercise capacity and health-related quality of life. In addition, the lack of practical guidance makes it a challenge to deliver PR during AECOPD, especially for hospitalized patients with severe symptoms. Similarly, to avoid the deleterious effects of immobility and physical inactivity, it is imperative to keep the patient active during hospitalization, as well as to establish safety criteria to mobilize this patient. However, in this context, there are some key questions to answer: 1) How to assess safety before mobilizing the hospitalized AECOPD patient? 2) What instruments and tests should be used to evaluate AECOPD inpatients before and after a PR program? 3) What does the evidence show about exercise prescription (type, frequency and intensity) as part of the PR program for this population? Considering this background and in light of scientific evidence, this chapter aims to address the role of exercise-based PR during AECOPD.

Keywords: chronic obstructive pulmonary disease, exacerbation, physical inactivity, rehabilitation, exercise therapy

Introduction

Pulmonary rehabilitation (PR) is defined as "a comprehensive intervention based on a thorough patient assessment followed by patient-tailored therapies that include, but are not limited to,

---

* Corresponding Author's Email: renatamendes@ufscar.br.

In: Chronic Obstructive Pulmonary Disease
Editor: Jaber S. Alqahtani
ISBN: 979-8-88697-333-4

exercise training, education, and behavior change, designed to improve the physical and psychological condition of people with chronic respiratory disease (CRD) and promote the long-term adherence to health-enhancing behaviors" [1]. The benefits of PR in patients with stable chronic obstructive pulmonary disease (COPD) are well established: it improves exercise capacity, muscle strength, functional capacity and health-related quality of life; it reduces symptoms, hospitalizations and unscheduled healthcare visits; and enhances self-management and self-efficacy [1]. Given these positive effects, it seems logical and reasonable to consider PR as a management strategy for acute exacerbation of COPD (AECOPD). However, current knowledge points to a lack of clinical consensus on the indication of PR during the peri-exacerbation phase.

In 2017, the last European Respiratory Society (ERS)/American Thoracic Society (ATS) guideline made a conditional recommendation against the initiation of PR during hospitalization and a conditional recommendation in favor of starting PR within 3 weeks after hospital discharge [2]. However, these recommendations were supported by a low level of evidence, particularly by a study that found higher 1-year mortality among AECOPD inpatients who received early PR [3]. The mentioned study has some limitations that make it difficult to establish a direct link between early PR and mortality outcome. Thus, given this low-quality evidence supporting the recommendation against PR during hospitalization, the position of the ERS/ATS Task Force was harshly criticized and questioned by the main PR authorities around the world [4].

Indeed, delivering a PR for AECOPD patients is a challenge and must be addressed cautiously, especially when the PR program includes exercise training for hospitalized patients with severe symptoms. Recently, a high-quality systematic review, in which most studies were conducted in an inpatient setting, demonstrated that exercise-based PR during AECOPD is a safe approach, leading to more significant positive effects on exercise capacity and health-related quality of life [5]. In this chapter, considering this background on the role of exercise-based PR in severe AECOPD, we set out to address important aspects that include: (1) consequences of the AECOPD and rationale for an exercise-based PR program; (2) recommendations on safety parameters for mobilizing AECOPD inpatients; (3) evaluation of this patient in a hospital ward setting; and (4) evidence of exercise-based PR for hospitalized AECOPD patients.

Consequences of AECOPD and Rationale for Exercise-Based Pulmonary Rehabilitation

AECOPD is characterized as an acute worsening of respiratory symptoms that requires additional treatment. Dyspnea is recognized as the key symptom of AECOPD, as a result of increased airway inflammation, marked gas trapping, and lung hyperinflation. Other symptoms include fatigue, increased sputum purulence and volume, as well as increased coughing and wheezing. The consequences of these clinical characteristics depend on the severity of AECOPD, but often have a profound negative impact on the patient's health status, which can lead to disease progression and increased rates of hospitalization, morbidity and mortality [2].

As a result of increased respiratory symptoms, AECOPD patients commonly experience a substantial decrease in physical activity levels. In an interview-based survey, almost 90% of the patients reported that AECOPD had a significant influence on their activities of daily living, and almost 50% completely stopped all activities [6]. These findings were also corroborated by a global survey that revealed that most COPD patients felt that exacerbations prevented them from making plans for the future and affected daily activities such as sleeping, speaking, and walking [7].

In fact, simple daily tasks such as climbing stairs and walking become extremely unpleasant experiences for AECOPD patients, especially for those hospitalized with severe symptoms. This marked activity limitation in AECOPD inpatients has already been demonstrated by studies with objective measurements using accelerometers. For example, Pitta et al., showed that AECOPD hospitalized patients spent only 7% of their time on weight-bearing activities on the second day of hospital admission, and only increased 2% by hospital discharge [8]. These findings corroborate another observational study in which the authors found that inpatients with AECOPD spent 87% of their time lying down or sitting during hospitalization [9].

This significant decrease in physical activity may lead to devastating impairments for AECOPD patients, trapping them in a vicious cycle of deconditioning, exercise intolerance and increased symptoms (Figure 1). This cycle is also negatively influenced by skeletal muscle dysfunction, which is mainly the result of immobility and disuse atrophy, but also has other possible contributing factors such as systemic inflammation, blood gas abnormalities, oxidative stress, corticosteroids, increased resting metabolic rate and suppressed appetite [10].

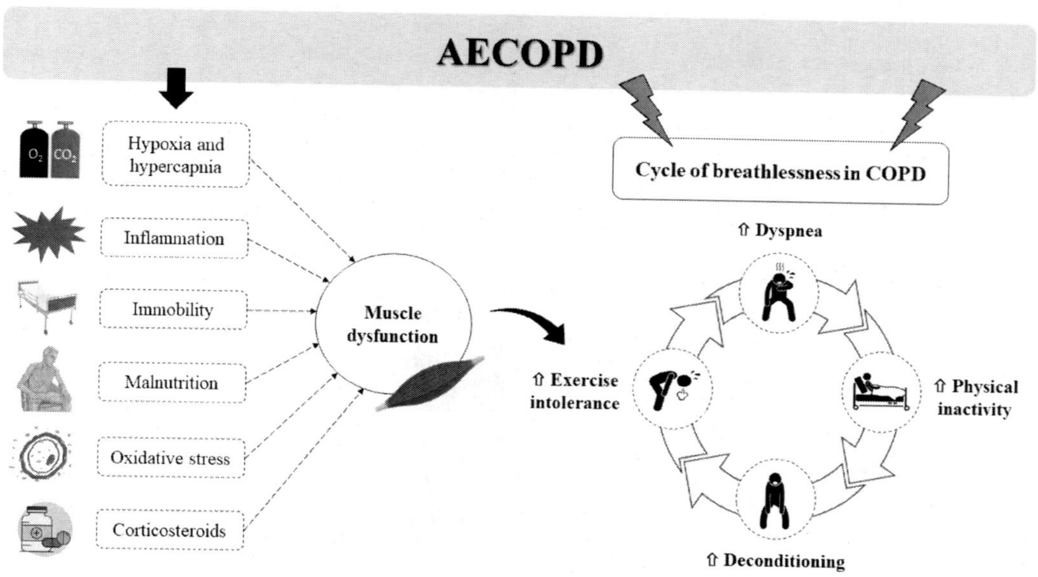

Figure 1. Impacts of AECOPD and muscle dysfunction on the cycle of symptoms and physical inactivity.

Given these multiple negative consequences of AECOPD in decreased physical activity levels, the clinical rationale for early intervention is precisely to counteract the vicious cycle and keep the patient physically active during the time course of exacerbation. Exercise training is a potential therapeutic strategy to attenuate the detrimental effects of exacerbation, including skeletal muscle dysfunction and exercise intolerance [10]. Although it has been speculated that exercise training during AECOPD could increase systemic inflammation and muscle oxidative stress, this concern has been refuted by some studies [11, 12], with evidence that exercise may still up-regulate the anabolic milieu in the skeletal muscle [12].

Despite that, exercise prescription in this context should be addressed with caution and individually. Exercise modality, volume and intensity should take into account the patient's clinical condition and the degree of dyspnea and fatigue [10]. In hospitalized AECOPD patients, exercise training may be more challenging, as the clinical condition tends to be more severe, in which acute respiratory failure or multiple comorbidities often coexist with the possibility of decompensation. Therefore, it is essential to establish safety parameters for patient mobilization based on a careful assessment.

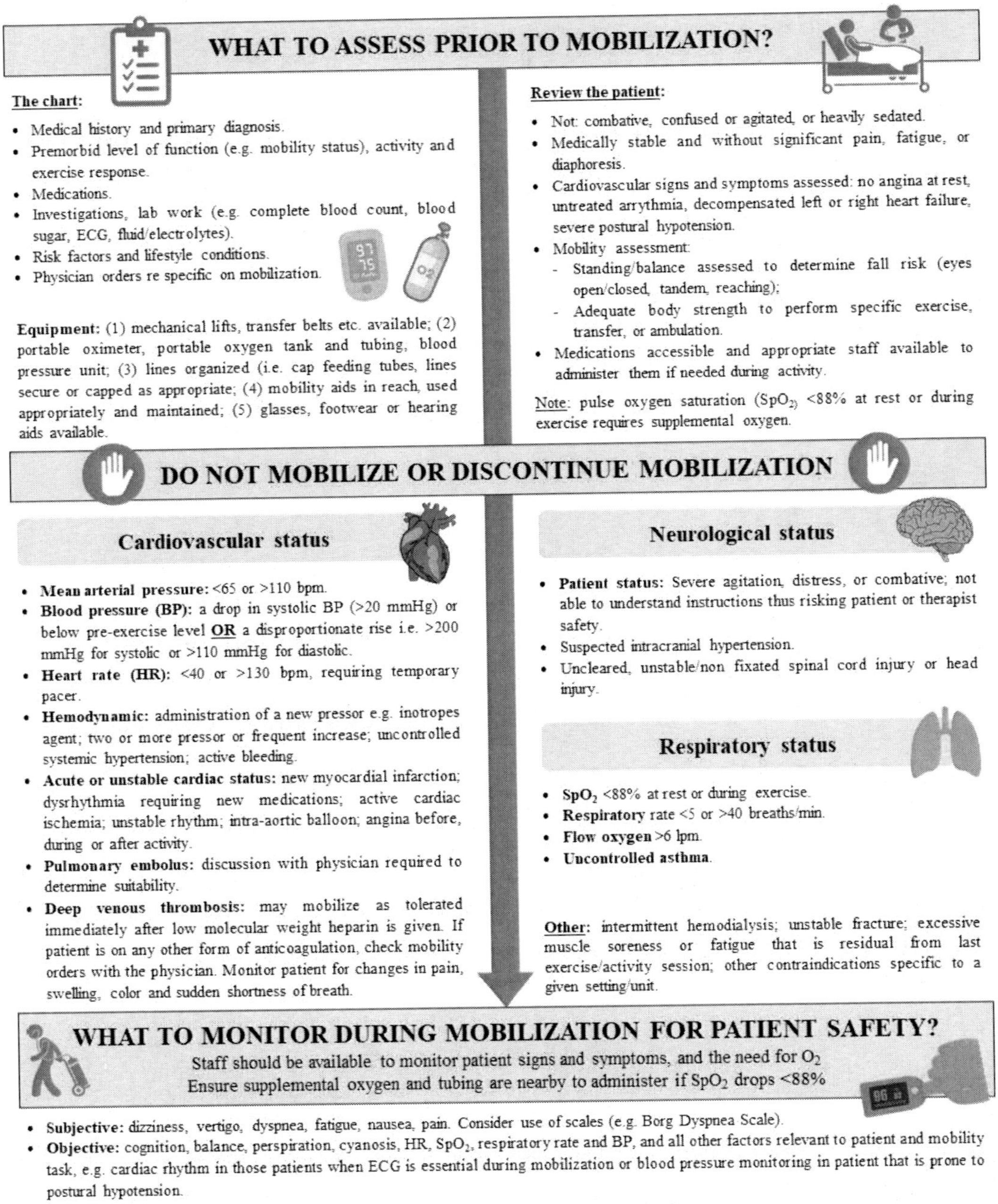

Figure 2. Compilation of SAFEMOB and AECOPD-Mob clinical decision-making tools.

Recommendations on Safety Parameters for Mobilizing AECOPD Patients

Improving the mobility of hospitalized AECOPD patients is a priority of care. However, the therapist must be aware of the patient's clinical condition before mobilization. Thus, a previous detailed anamnesis and physical examination are necessary. Imaging exams and laboratory tests, including arterial blood gases, complete blood count, and inflammatory markers, can help identify underlying clinical conditions that should be considered in the clinical decision to mobilize or not the patient. Additionally, integration and participation of the physician and multidisciplinary team in the continuous assessment to initiate in-hospital rehabilitation program is mandatory.

One of the main difficulties in implementing therapeutic exercise is the lack of specific guidelines to guide the safety criteria for mobilization of AECOPD patients in a hospital setting. In 2009, a task force from the Physiotherapy Association of British Columbia developed the SAFEMOB project, a decision-making tool to guide physical therapy clinicians in making evidence-informed decisions relevant to the safe mobilization of patients in acute care settings [13]. Later, in 2016, these recommendations were specially adapted for AECOPD patients, in a document entitled Mobilization in Acute Exacerbations of Chronic Obstructive Pulmonary Disease (AECOPD-Mob), which was developed from the findings of a systematic review and a Delphi process with multiple health care disciplines and patients/families [13, 14]. This document is based on four steps of recommendations: (1) what to assess prior to mobilization; (2) when not to mobilize; (3) what to monitor during mobilization; and (4) how to mobilize and progress. Figure 2 shows an adaptation of recommendations 1 to 3, from a compilation of the SAFEMOB and AECOPD-Mob tools, aiming to apply them in hospitalized patients in a ward setting. Although the AECOPD-Mob tool does not replace the clinician's clinical reasoning skills and interprofessional collaboration [14], it may be useful and feasible for applications in a clinical and hospital setting to help healthcare providers guide safe mobilization of AECOPD patients.

Evaluation of AECOPD Patient in a Hospital Ward Setting

In an exercise-based program for AECOPD inpatients, all of them must be evaluated at the beginning and at the end to prescribe individualized exercise training and verify the results obtained from the intervention. Preferably, assessments should focus on limitations resulting from the consequences of AECOPD, including increased symptoms of dyspnea and fatigue, exercise intolerance, peripheral and respiratory muscle weakness, loss of balance with increased risk of falls, decreased functional status, activities and health-related quality of life [10, 15]. Based on previous studies, Figure 3 points to suggestions for instruments to assess AECOPD patients during hospitalization.

Physical performance assessments, and especially exercise tests, must be carefully selected, taking into account the safety of patient mobilization. The 6-minute walk test (6MWT) is an example of a submaximal exercise test that is well tolerated and safe for evaluating AECOPD patients, including those hospitalized. Although it was not the focus of the study, we recently published experiences from our laboratory showing that 6MWT is feasible and safe when applied within 24 to 48 hours of hospital admission [16] (Figure 4). Other studies [11,

12, 17-22] on AECOPD inpatients have also applied 6MWT to assess exercise capacity, without any adverse events reported during the test.

Patient limitation	Instruments for assessment	References
Symptoms	• Borg scale • Visual analogue scale • Modified Medical Research Council dyspnea scale	[17,18-21,24,25]
Exercise intolerance	• 3-min walk test • 6-min walk test • 30-sec sit-to-stand test	[11,12,15,17-25]
Muscle weakness	• Handgrip strength test • Peak muscle force with hand-held dynamometer • Manovacuometer (maximal respiratory pressures)	[11,12,15,21,23,24]
Loss of balance	• Berg balance scale* • Short Physical Performance Battery* • One-leg stance test	[15]
⇩ Quality of life	• Saint George Respiratory Questionnaire • Chronic Respiratory Disease Questionnaire • COPD Assessment Test	[11,17,18,22]
⇩ Functional status and activity	• Short Form Health Status Survey (SF-36) • London Chest Activity of Daily Living • Accelerometers or monitor of physical activity	[8,9,11,15,17,25]

Figure 3. Patient limitations and instruments to assess AECOPD patients.
**Tests suggested by the authors.*

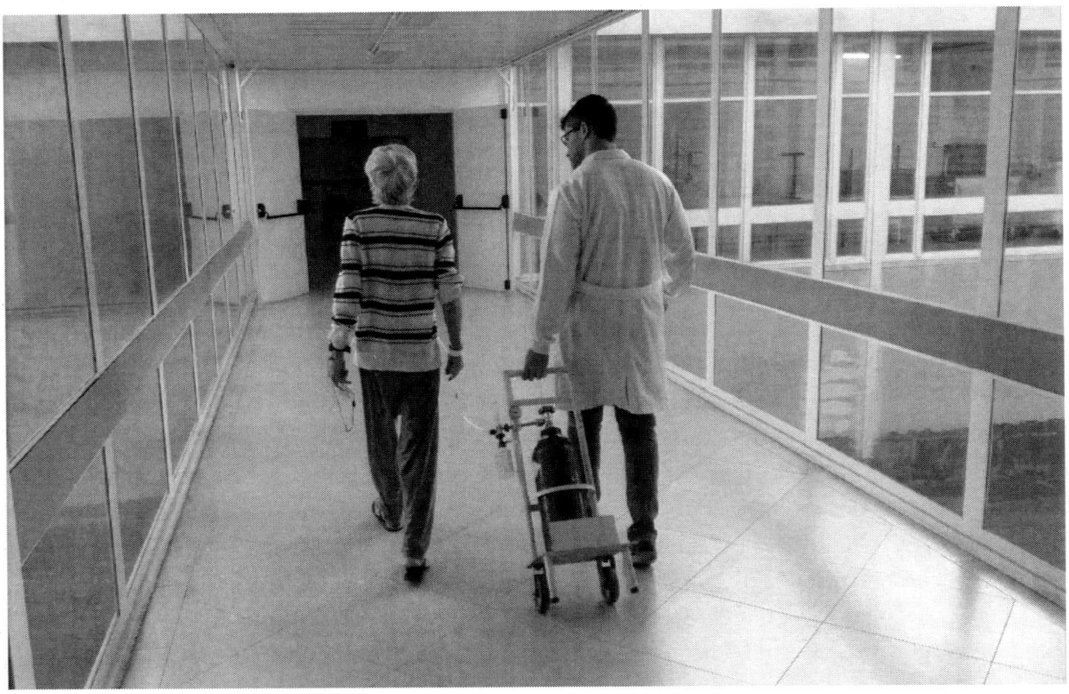

Source: Laboratory of Cardiopulmonary Physiotherapy, UFSCar.

Figure 4. Six-minute walk test in AECOPD patient hospitalized at the University Hospital of the Federal University of São Carlos (UFSCar).

Other exercise tests may offer advantages and disadvantages. For example, patients with severe symptoms may have difficulty sustaining a 6-minute exercise test. In this case, shorter tests (e.g., 3-minute walk test) may be an alternative to reduce cardiorespiratory burden [23]. In addition, self-paced tests (e.g., 3 and 6MWT) have the advantage of being more comfortable, possibly with better tolerance. However, the performance of this type of test may vary according to patient motivation, which is often negatively altered during AECOPD [6, 7]. Moreover, it is important to consider the location where the test will be performed. In a hospital setting, physical space is often limited, which makes walking tests difficult. Thus, chair stand tests [15, 24, 25] may be more appropriate. In addition, the choice of the test must always be individualized, considering the patient's clinical condition and the measurement properties of the assessment tool. Finally, it is mandatory that patients are closely monitored during testing, paying attention to the criteria for safety and exercise interruption.

Evidence of Exercise-Based Pulmonary Rehabilitation for AECOPD Inpatients

Although exercise training is widely consolidated as a management strategy in stable COPD, its early prescription during AECOPD remains a challenge. This becomes even more challenging in patients with severe symptoms who often require hospitalization. In this context, evidence has already shown that exercise-based rehabilitation during hospital stay offers beneficial effects, such as improved symptoms, exercise capacity, muscle strength, functionality and quality of life [11, 12, 15, 17-25]. However, the differences between the training programs used throughout the studies make it difficult to reach a consensus on the best clinical practices. These heterogeneous characteristics include mainly the time to start the intervention, the exercise modalities, and the volume and intensity of the training.

Regarding the evidence, Table 1 shows the prescription of exercise-based PR for hospitalized AECOPD patients according to twelve randomized controlled trials [11, 12, 15, 17-25]. From this set of studies, some characteristics of training were predominant. For example, most started the exercise program from day 2-3 of admission [14, 15, 18, 21, 23-25] and lasted until hospital discharge [15, 17, 18, 21, 23-25]. Regarding the modalities, aerobic training was the most used [15, 17-25], commonly prescribed as walking [17-23] or cycling [15, 21, 24, 25]. Mostly, intensity was determined based on an initial exercise test (e.g., 75% of the distance walked in the 6MWT) or according to the patient's subjective perception, using a fatigue or dyspnea score <6 on the modified Borg scale [19, 24]. Resistance training was also applied alone [11, 12] or combined with aerobic training [17, 18, 23]. The forms of resistance application were varied: own body weight [18], free weights [11, 12, 17, 18] and elastic bands [23, 25]. The intensity of the resistance exercise, when reported, was determined based on the 1-repetition maximum test, using mostly a load ≥70% [11, 12, 23]. The training frequency was prescribed predominantly in 1-2 sessions per day [11, 12, 17, 18, 20-25], with a total duration of 30-45 minutes per session [17, 18, 21, 22, 23, 24, 25]. Few studies have used adjunct therapeutic resources, such as inspiratory muscle training [21] and neuromuscular electrical stimulation [24, 25].

Table 1. Randomized controlled trials involving early exercise-based pulmonary rehabilitation with AECOPD hospitalized patients

Study (year)	Timing ⏱	Intervention groups	Duration of intervention	Frequency, duration and exercise intensity	Outcome measures	Effect of intervention [positive (☺) or no effect (😐)]	Adverse events
Eaton et al., (2009) [17]	As soon as medical appropriate.	• CG: usual care. • IG: usual care + walking exercise + upper and lower limb strengthening exercises.	Until discharge with follow-up.	• 1 session/day. • ≥30min/day. • Intensity not stated. Progression: no.	• 6MWT. • BODE index. • Chronic respiratory questionnaire. • SF-36 questionnaire. • Hospital anxiety and depression scale. • Hospital readmission at 3 months.	• Exercise capacity: 😐 • Impact of disease: 😐 • HRQoL: 😐, except for fatigue (☺) and physical function (☺). • Anxiety: ☺ • Depression: 😐 • Readmission rate: 😐	No.
He et al., (2015) [18]	From the 2nd day of admission.	• CG: usual care. • IG: education + breathing retraining + exercise training (walking exercise + upper limb endurance + strength exercises with free weights or the subject's own body weight).	Until discharge.	• 2 sessions/day. • 30 min/session. • Aerobic: walking at 60% of peak work rate in 6MWT and dyspnea between 3-5 at modified Borg. • Strength: 1-3 sets of 10 repetitions, and dyspnea between 3-5 at modified Borg. Progression: yes.	• 6MWT. • BODE index. • COPD assessment test. • Activity of Daily Living Dyspnea scale. • Modified Borg scale. • mMRC dyspnea scale. • Chronic respiratory questionnaire.	• Exercise capacity: ☺ • Impact of disease: ☺ • Symptoms: ☺ • HRQoL: ☺	No.
Kirsten et al., (1998) [19]	6-8 days after admission.	• CG: usual care. • IG: usual care + walking exercise.	10 days.	• 5 sessions/day. • Duration not stated. • At least 75% of treadmill walking distance. Progression: yes.	• 6MWT. • Oxygen uptake. • FEV_1 • Inspiratory capacity. • Modified Borg scale.	• Exercise capacity: ☺ • Lung function: 😐 • Symptoms: ☺	Not reported.
Liao et al., (2015) [20]	Not stated.	• CG: usual care and health education. • IG: education, sputum clearance treatments, pursed lip breathing, upper-limb exercise with deep breathing, walking exercise.	4 days.	• 2 sessions/day. • 10min/session. • Intensity not stated. Progression: not reported.	• 6MWT; • Visual analog scale. • Modified Borg scale.	• Exercise capacity: ☺ • Dyspnea: ☺ • Cough: ☺ • Sputum expectoration: ☺	Not reported.

Study (year)	Timing ⊕	Intervention groups	Duration of intervention	Frequency, duration and exercise intensity	Outcome measures	Effect of intervention [positive (☺) or no effect (😐)]	Adverse events
Nava (1998) [21]	3-5 days after admission.	• CG: standard medical care + basic ambulation program. • IG: passive mobilization + early ambulation + respiratory and lower skeletal muscle training + lower extremity training on a treadmill.	Until discharge.	• 2 sessions/day. • 30-45 min/session. • IMT: 50% of MIP. • Cycling: 15W, and dyspnea <6 at modified Borg. • Climb a flight of 25 stairs at least 5 times. • Walking at 70% of the load achieved on the incremental pre-exercise test. Progression: yes.	• 6MWT. • FEV_1. • MIP. • Visual analog scale. • Hospital stay. • Deaths.	• Exercise capacity: ☺ • Lung function: 😐 • Inspiratory muscle strength: ☺ • Dyspnea: ☺ • Length of hospital stay: 😐 • Mortality: 😐	No.
Song et al., (2014) [22]	The day before discharge.	• CG: usual care. • IG: education + breathing exercises + walking exercise.	Not stated.	• 2 sessions during hospital stay. • 45 min/session. • Walking: 10-min-per-toleration. Progression: no.	• 6MWT. • Peak expiratory flow. • St. George's respiratory questionnaire;	• Exercise capacity: 😐 • Lung function: 😐 • HRQoL: ☺	Not reported.
Tang et al., (2012) [23]	From the 2nd day of admission.	• CG: usual care + physical therapy, including sputum clearance techniques, mobility assessments, and functional training required for safe discharge. • IG: usual care + standard physical therapy treatment + aerobic and resistance exercises.	Until discharge.	• 2 sessions/day. • Total of ~30 min/session. • Walking exercise: 40% or 70% of 3-minute walk test (7.5 min/session). • Resistance exercise with elastic bands: 2 sets, 20-25 repetitions (40% 1-RM) or 8-10 repetitions (70% 1-RM) of hip abductors, lunges, simulated lifting and chest press. Progression: yes.	• 3-minute walk test. • Hand-held dynamometry. • Barthel index. • FEV_1. • Hospital stay.	• Exercise capacity: 😐 • Muscle strength: 😐 • Functional capacity: 😐 • Lung function: 😐 • Length of hospital stay: 😐	Yes. One serious (arrhythmia). 12 other minor adverse events.
Torres-Sánchez et al., (2017) [15]	From the 2nd day of admission.	• CG: std medical care. • IG: std medical care + exercise using a pedal exerciser.	Until discharge.	• Frequency and duration of session not stated. • Dyspnea and fatigue levels <6 at modified Borg. Progression: yes.	• 30-sec sit-to-stand test. • Handheld dynamometry. • One-leg stance test. • Monitor of physical activity. • Hospital stay.	• Exercise capacity: 😐 • Muscle strength: ☺ • Balance: ☺ • Physical activity level: ☺ • Length of hospital stay: 😐	No.

Table 1. (Continued)

Study (year)	Timing ⊕	Intervention groups	Duration of intervention	Frequency, duration and exercise intensity	Outcome measures	Effect of intervention [positive (☺) or no effect (😐)]	Adverse events
Lopez-Lopez et al., (2019) [24]	From the 2nd day of admission.	• CG: std medical care. • IG: std care + one or twice per day of cycling exercise combined with NMES.	Until discharge.	• 1 or 2 sessions/day. • 30 min/session. • Dyspnea and fatigue levels <6 at modified Borg. Progression: yes.	• Handheld dynamometry. • 5-times sit-to-stand. • Modified Borg scale. • Visual analog scale. • Days of hospital stay.	• Quadriceps strength: ☺ • Lower limb function: ☺ • Symptoms: ☺ • Length of hospital stay: 😐 Note: the group that received intervention twice a day had a better response.	No.
Lopez Lopez et al., (2018) [25]	From the 2nd day of admission.	• CG: std medical treatment. • IG: Usual care + NMES with pedaling exercise on a cycle ergometer. Usual care + NMES adding lower-limb elastic band resistance exercises.	Until discharge.	• 1 session/day. • 30 min/session. • Intensity not stated. Progression: no.	• 5-times sit-to-stand. • London Chest Activity of Daily Living. • Modified Borg scale. • Fatigue Severity Scale. • Days of hospital stay.	• Exercise capacity: ☺ • Functionality: ☺ • Dyspnea: 😐 • Fatigue: ☺ • Length of hospital stay: 😐	Not reported.
Borges and Carvalho (2014) [11]	From the third day of admission.	• CG: usual care. • IG: usual care + resistance training (shoulder flexion and abduction, elbow flexion, knee extension and flexion, hip flexion).	Not stated.	• 1 session/day. • Duration not stated. • ≥80% of 1-RM; symptoms <7 at modified Borg. Progression: yes.	• 6MWT. • St. George's respiratory questionnaire • Handheld dynamometry. • Inflammatory markers. • Monitor of physical activity.	• Exercise capacity: ☺ • HRQoL: 😐 • Lower-limb muscle strength: ☺ • Systemic inflammation: 😐 • Physical activity level: 😐	No.
Troosters et al., (2010) [12]	Since admission.	• CG: usual care. • IG: usual care + quadriceps resistance training on a knee-extension chair.	7 days.	• 1 session/day. • 3 sets of 8 repetitions. • 70% of 1-RM. Progression: yes.	• 6MWT. • Maximal voluntary quadriceps force; • Inflammatory, anabolic and catabolic markers. • Hospital readmission.	• Exercise capacity: ☺ • Quadriceps muscle force: ☺ • Anabolism markers: ☺ • Systemic inflammation: 😐 • Readmission rate after 6 months: 😐	No.

Abbreviations: COPD, Chronic obstructive pulmonary disease; FEV_1, forced expiratory volume in the first second; CG, control group; IG, intervention group, 6MWT, 6-minute walk test; BODE, index which integrates body mass index, FEV_1, dyspnea and 6MWT; SF-36, 36-Item Short Form Health Survey; SpO_2, pulse oxygen saturation; HRQoL, health-related quality of life; 1-RM, one-repetition maximum; IMT, inspiratory muscle training; MIP, maximal inspiratory pressure; NMES: neuromuscular electrical stimulation; ☺ (happy green emoticon), positive effect of the intervention; 😐, neutral yellow emoticon, no effect of the intervention.

Regarding exercise safety for AECOPD inpatients, only one study [23] reported the occurrence of adverse events. The single serious event reported was cardiac arrhythmia during walking exercise, however, the patient already had a previous history of atrial fibrillation, and the event was completely resolved within one hour. In the same study, 12 other minor adverse events (associated with changes in vital signs) were also recorded, but which quantitatively did not differ from the control group. Therefore, the current body of evidence suggests the feasibility and safety of early exercise-based rehabilitation for AEDPOC patients, which is also supported by a recent systematic review [5]. However, future studies are needed to determine optimal timings to start the intervention, the total duration of the intervention, the duration and frequency of sessions, and the intensity for exercise prescription [5].

Conclusion

Evidence suggests feasibility and safety of early exercise-based rehabilitation for AECOPD patients, however, there is no ideal recommendation in terms of best time to start rehabilitation sessions, frequency of sessions, and exercise prescription. Operational concerns should include the patient's clinical condition, contraindications, and criteria for exercise interruption.

Key Points

- Current evidence points to the great benefits of PR in AECOPD patients, especially in exercise capacity and health-related quality of life.
- An exercise-based PR program is safe and feasible during AECOPD, even among hospitalized patients.
- Operational concerns should include safety parameters for patient mobilization, paying special attention to the patient's clinical condition, contraindications and criteria for exercise interruption.
- The choice of assessment tool should be individualized, with evidence showing that walking tests are well tolerated.
- Aerobic and resistance exercise seem to be the most prescribed modalities, but there is still no consensus on the intensity, duration and frequency of sessions.

References

[1] Spruit M. A., Singh S. J., Garvey C., ZuWallack R., Nici L., Rochester C, Kylie Hill, Anne E. Holland, Suzanne C. Lareau, William D. C. Man, Fabio Pitta, Louise Sewell, Jonathan Raskin, Jean Bourbeau, Rebecca Crouch, Frits M. E. Franssen, Richard Casaburi, Jan H. Vercoulen, Ioannis Vogiatzis, Rik Gosselink, Enrico M. Clini, Tanja W. Effing, François Maltais, Job van der Palen, Thierry Troosters, Daisy J. A. Janssen, Eileen Collins, Judith Garcia-Aymerich, Dina Brooks, Bonnie F. Fahy, Milo A. Puhan, Martine Hoogendoorn, Rachel Garrod, Annemie M. W. J. Schols, Brian Carlin, Roberto Benzo, Paula Meek, Mike Morgan, Maureen P. M. H. Rutten-van Mölken, Andrew L. Ries, Barry Make, Roger S. Goldstein, Claire A. Dowson, Jan L. Brozek, Claudio F. Donner, Emiel F. M. Wouters, ATS/ERS Task Force on Pulmonary Rehabilitation. An official American Thoracic Society/European Respiratory

Society statement: key concepts and advances in pulmonary rehabilitation. *Am J Respir Crit Care* Med 2013;188:13-64.

[2] Wedzicha J. A., Miravitlles M., Hurst J. R., Calverley P. M., Albert R. K., Anzueto A., Gerard J. Criner, Alberto Papi, Klaus F. Rabe, David Rigau, Pawel Sliwinski, Thomy Tonia, Jørgen Vestbo, Kevin C. Wilson, Jerry A. Krishnan (ATS co-chair). Management of COPD exacerbations: a European Respiratory Society/American Thoracic Society guideline. *Eur Respir J* 2017;49:1600791.

[3] Greening N. J., Williams J. E., Hussain S. F., Harvey-Dunstan T. C., Bankart M. J., Chaplin E. J., E. Vincent, Rudo Chimera, M. Morgan, Sally J. Singh, M. Steiner. An early rehabilitation intervention to enhance recovery during hospital admission for an exacerbation of chronic respiratory disease: randomised controlled trial. *BMJ* 2014;349:g4315.

[4] Spruit M. A., Singh S. J., Rochester C. L., Greening N. J., Franssen F. M. E., Pitta F., Thierry Troosters, Claire Nolan, Ioannis Vogiatzis, Enrico M. Clini, William D. C. Man, Chris Burtin, Roger S. Goldstein, Lowie E. G. W. Vanfleteren, Klaus Kenn, Linda Nici, Daisy J. A. Janssen, Richard Casaburi, Takanobu Shioya, Chris Garvey, Brian W. Carlin, Richard L. ZuWallack, Michael Steiner, Emiel F. M. Wouters, Milo A. Puhan. Pulmonary rehabilitation for patients with COPD during and after an exacerbation-related hospitalisation: back to the future? *Eur Respir J* 2018;51:1701312.

[5] Machado A., Matos Silva P., Afreixo V., Caneiras C., Burtin C., Marques A. Design of pulmonary rehabilitation programmes during acute exacerbations of COPD: a systematic review and network meta-analysis. *Eur Respir Rev* 2020;29:200039.

[6] Kessler R., Ståhl E., Vogelmeier C., Haughney J., Trudeau E., Löfdahl C. G., Martyn R. Partridge. Patient understanding, detection, and experience of COPD exacerbations: an observational, interview-based study. *Chest* 2006;130:133-42.

[7] Barnes N., Calverley P. M., Kaplan A., Rabe K. F. Chronic obstructive pulmonary disease and exacerbations: patient insights from the global Hidden Depths of COPD survey. *BMC Pulm Med* 2013;13:54.

[8] Pitta F., Troosters T., Probst V. S., Spruit M. A., Decramer M., Gosselink R. Physical activity and hospitalization for exacerbation of COPD. *Chest* 2006;129:536-44.

[9] Borges R. C., Carvalho C. R. Physical activity in daily life in Brazilian COPD patients during and after exacerbation. *COPD* 2012;9:596-602.

[10] Burtin C., Decramer M., Gosselink R., Janssens W., Troosters T. Rehabilitation and acute exacerbations. *Eur Respir J* 2011;38:702-12.

[11] Borges R. C., Carvalho C. R. Impact of resistance training in chronic obstructive pulmonary disease patients during periods of acute exacerbation. *Arch Phys Med Rehabil* 2014;95:1638-45.

[12] Troosters T., Probst V. S., Crul T., Pitta F., Gayan-Ramirez G., Decramer M., Rik Gosselink. Resistance training prevents deterioration in quadriceps muscle function during acute exacerbations of chronic obstructive pulmonary disease. *Am J Respir Crit Care Med* 2010;181:1072-7.

[13] Camp P. G., Reid W. D., Chung F., Kirkham A., Brooks D., Goodridge D., Darcy D. Marciniuk, Alison M. Hoens. Clinical Decision-Making Tool for Safe and Effective Prescription of Exercise in Acute Exacerbations of Chronic Obstructive Pulmonary Disease: Results From an Interdisciplinary Delphi Survey and Focus Groups. *Phys Ther* 2015;95:1387-96.

[14] Camp P. G., Benari O., Dechman G., Kirkham A., Campbell K., Black A., Frank Chung, Preeya Dajee, Amy Ellis, Alison M. Hoens, Rosalyn Jones, Beena Parappilly, Chiara Singh, Philip Sweeney, Ellen Woo. Implementation of an Acute Care COPD Exacerbation Patient Mobilization Tool. A Mixed-Methods Study. *ATS Sch* 2021;2:249-64.

[15] Torres-Sánchez I., Valenza M. C., Cabrera-Martos I., López-Torres I., Benítez-Feliponi Á., Conde-Valero A. Effects of an Exercise Intervention in Frail Older Patients with Chronic Obstructive Pulmonary Disease Hospitalized due to an Exacerbation: A Randomized Controlled Trial. *COPD* 2017;14:37-42.

[16] Kabbach E. Z., Heubel A. D., da Luz Goulart C., Di Lorenzo V. A. P., Phillips S. A., Borghi-Silva A., Renata Gonçalves Mendes. Association of exercise capacity and endothelial function in patients with severe exacerbations of chronic obstructive pulmonary disease. *Sci Rep* 2021;11:461.

[17] Eaton T., Young P., Fergusson W., Moodie L., Zeng I., O'Kane F, Nichola Good, Leanne Rhodes, Phillippa Poole, John Kolbe. Does early pulmonary rehabilitation reduce acute health-care utilization in

COPD patients admitted with an exacerbation? A randomized controlled study. *Respirology* 2009;14:230-8.

[18] He M., Yu S., Wang L., Lv H., Qiu Z. Efficiency and safety of pulmonary rehabilitation in acute exacerbation of chronic obstructive pulmonary disease. *Med Sci Monit* 2015;21:806-12.

[19] Kirsten D. K., Taube C., Lehnigk B., Jörres R. A., Magnussen H. Exercise training improves recovery in patients with COPD after an acute exacerbation. *Respir Med* 1998;92:1191-8.

[20] Liao L. Y., Chen K. M., Chung W. S., Chien J. Y. Efficacy of a respiratory rehabilitation exercise training package in hospitalized elderly patients with acute exacerbation of COPD: a randomized control trial. *Int J Chron Obstruct Pulmon Dis* 2015;10:1703-9.

[21] Nava S. Rehabilitation of patients admitted to a respiratory intensive care unit. *Arch Phys Med Rehabil* 1998;79:849-54.

[22] Song H. Y., Yong S. J., Hur H. K. Effectiveness of a brief self-care support intervention for pulmonary rehabilitation among the elderly patients with chronic obstructive pulmonary disease in Korea. *Rehabil Nurs* 2014;39:147-56.

[23] Tang C. Y., Blackstock F. C., Clarence M., Taylor N. F. Early rehabilitation exercise program for inpatients during an acute exacerbation of chronic obstructive pulmonary disease: a randomized controlled trial. *J Cardiopulm Rehabil Prev* 2012;32:163-9.

[24] Lopez-Lopez L., Torres-Sanchez I., Rodriguez-Torres J., Cabrera-Martos I., Cahalin L. P., Valenza M. C. Randomized feasibility study of twice a day functional electrostimulation in patients with severe chronic obstructive pulmonary disease hospitalized for acute exacerbation. *Physiother Theory Pract* 2019;37:1360-7.

[25] Lopez Lopez L., Granados Santiago M., Donaire Galindo M., Torres Sanchez I., Ortiz Rubio A., Valenza M. C. Efficacy of combined electrostimulation in patients with acute exacerbation of COPD: randomised clinical trial. *Med Clin (Barc)* 2018;151:323-8.

Chapter 25

Self-Management of Acute Exacerbation of COPD: Conventional vs. Telehealth Interventions

Hayat Mushcab[1,*], PhD,
Donna Alabdulbaqi[2], MD, PhD
and Abdulmuhsin Babsail[3], MD
[1]Johns Hopkins Aramco Healthcare,
Research Office, Dhahran, Eastern Province, Saudi Arabia
[2]Saudi Electronic University,
Public Health Department, Dammam, Eastern Province, Saudi Arabia
[3]Johns Hopkins Aramco Healthcare,
Population Health Department, Dhahran, Eastern Province, Saudi Arabia

Abstract

Acute exacerbation in chronic obstructive pulmonary disease (COPD) is characterized by an acute deterioration in respiratory symptoms that negatively impacts the disease progression, quality of life, and mortality. Self-management interventions in chronic illness such as COPD are intended to help individuals to better self-manage their condition and prevent exacerbation events. These self-management interventions have varied throughout the years from conventional interventions where patients received educational material and coaching to best manage their condition on their own, to tele-monitoring where patients record their health data automatically and transmit it to a healthcare provider via the web. This approach is anticipated to help patients and their healthcare providers detect early symptoms of acute exacerbation and intervene as early as possible to avoid deterioration and hospitalization, however, the efficacy of these interventions is still undetermined.

In this paper, we reviewed the available evidence in the literature for conventional and telehealth interventions for self-management of acute exacerbation of COPD (AECOPD) to assess the clinical effectiveness of both approaches. We conducted a literature search on April 1st, 2022, using OVID Medline, PubMed, Cumulative Index to Nursing and Allied Health Literature (CINAHL), the Wiley Cochrane Library, and Google Scholar for articles published from January 2012 until April 2022. We included all study designs that investigated self-management interventions (conventional and telehealth) for AECOPD. Seven studies for the conventional intervention and eight study for the telehealth intervention met the criteria and were included in this review. We conclude that the

* Corresponding Author's E-mail: hayat.almushcab@jhah.com.

In: Chronic Obstructive Pulmonary Disease
Editor: Jaber S. Alqahtani
ISBN: 979-8-88697-333-4

consensus on which components of self-management interventions are still controversial. The telehealth intervention can be promising to achieve self-management of AECOPD, however the optimal solution requires integration of several elements along with the advanced technology such as personal skills, digital literacy, and availability of remote monitoring capabilities.

Introduction

Chronic obstructive pulmonary disease (COPD) is a common respiratory condition characterized by airflow limitation [1]. Approximately 10% of individuals aged 40 years or older have COPD, although the prevalence varies between countries and increases with age [1, 2, 3]. It is the fourth-ranked cause of death in the United States, causing death for more than 120,000 individuals yearly [4] and the third leading cause worldwide causing 3.23 million deaths in 2019 [5, 6]. As a consequence of its high prevalence and chronicity, COPD causes high resource utilization with frequent clinician office visits, frequent hospitalizations due to acute exacerbations, and the need for chronic therapy [7]. COPD causes persistent and progressive respiratory symptoms, including difficulty in breathing, cough and/or phlegm production [5]. It is a result of long-term exposure to harmful gases and particles combined with individual factors, including events which influence lung growth in childhood and genetics [5]. The main causes of COPD include tobacco exposure from active smoking or passive exposure to second-hand smoke [8, 5], occupational exposure to dust, fumes, or chemicals [8], and indoor air pollution such as biomass fuel (wood, animal dung, crop residue) or coal that is frequently used for cooking and heating in low- and middle-income countries with high levels of smoke exposure [8]. Medical history can also account for COPD including early life events such as poor growth in utero, prematurity, and frequent or severe respiratory infections in childhood that prevent maximum lung growth [8], Asthma in childhood, and a rare genetic condition called alpha-1 antitrypsin deficiency, which can cause COPD at a young age [8].

There is no cure for COPD, but early diagnosis and treatment are important to slow the progression of symptoms and reduce the risk of flare-ups [9]. COPD is suspected if a person presented with typical symptoms, then a spirometry test which measures the lungs' function is performed to confirm the diagnosis. However, the diagnosis is sometimes missed in low- and middle-income countries due to the unavailability of spirometry [10]. Several actions can be taken by people suffering from COPD to improve their overall health and help control their condition such as quitting smoking, exercise regularly, and receive vaccination against pneumonia, influenza, and against the most recent coronavirus SARS-CoV-2 [5]. Inhaled medication can be used to improve symptoms and reduce flare-ups. Flare-ups are often caused by a respiratory infection – people may be given an antibiotic or steroid tablets in addition to inhaled or nebulized treatment as needed [9]. However, information and education about the condition, the treatment and self-care must be provided to the patients to stay active and as healthy as possible [5].

Acute exacerbations are an important cause of mortality and morbidity in patients with COPD [11]. In 1996 a study of survival following hospital admission for acute exacerbations reported in-hospital mortality rate of 11%- and one-year mortality rate of 43% [12]. A more recent study reported in-hospital mortality at 8% with a 1-year mortality rate of 23% [13], confirming the prognostic importance of these episodes.

It is perhaps understandable that there is no standardized definition of an acute exacerbation of COPD (AECOPD) in research or in clinical practice. Exacerbation symptoms vary between individuals [14]. The most common being breathlessness, wheeze, chest tightness, increased cough, and increased sputum volume and purulence non-specific symptoms are also common (including fatigue and general malaise) [15]. However, no group of symptoms or measurements are diagnostic for an exacerbation.

The most referenced definition of AECOPD remains for Anthonisen et al. [16], which divided patients into three groups according to their symptomatology. Type 1 exacerbations were defined by the presence of increased breathlessness, sputum volume and sputum purulence; type 2 by the presence of two of these symptoms, and type 3 by the presence of one of these symptoms in addition to one of the following: an upper respiratory tract infection in the past 5 days, fever without other cause, increased wheezing or cough, or an increase in heart rate or respiratory rate by 20% compared with baseline readings. This definition was devised prospectively to analyze the effect of antibiotics on exacerbations and not to structure patient management [16]. More recent studies have adapted these criteria with varying degrees of success.

Exacerbations have a marked impact on the quality of life of patients. Frequent exacerbations (more than two per year) have been associated with more dyspnea and reduced exercise capacity [17], a greater decline in health status [18], and a greater likelihood of becoming housebound [19], than in patients with fewer acute episodes. It is expected that repeated exacerbations are associated with a faster decline in lung function. Published data suggest that 50–70% of exacerbations are due to respiratory infections [20], (including bacteria, atypical organisms and respiratory viruses), 10% are due to environmental pollution (depending on season and geographical placement) [21], and up to 30% are of unknown etiology [12]. Moreover, AECOPD appears to be related to heightened airway inflammation which leads to the composite of symptoms seen during these acute episodes. The evidence suggests that bacteria, viruses, and environmental pollution are the most important causes of exacerbations, and that purulent sputum is the key sign which differentiates between the former and latter two etiologies [22]. In addition, frequent exacerbations appear to be associated with worsening health outcomes, and efforts should focus on preventing these episodes or prompt effective treatment of each episode [22].

AECOPD are episodes of acute (typically days) symptom deterioration that punctuate the natural course of disease. Usually, AECOPD has a slower onset than asthma exacerbations. They contribute widely to poor outcomes, including decline in lung function [23], risk of cardiovascular events [24], poor quality of life [25], and death [26]. Most exacerbations develop symptoms over 2–3 days and will last 7–14 days; however, some may last longer or not recover to previous baseline [27]. After recovery, there is risk of early recurrence, and a subgroup of patients can enter a cycle of frequent exacerbations leading to further decline [28]. Developing effective and targeted means of treating these events, minimizing recurrence, and modifying future risk is a major focus in research and clinical care.

Self-management interventions have been used in variable chronic conditions such as diabetes, arthritis, heart diseases and respiratory diseases [29]. The concept of self-management is defined as "*the day-to-day management of chronic conditions by individuals over the course of an illness*" [30]. It includes managing the medical, behavioral, and emotional aspects of a chronic illness as well as the ability of problem solving, taking action, resource utilization and making partnerships with health care providers [30]. COPD self-management intends to enhance the wellbeing of patients and assist them to manage their condition through teaching them the skills they require to carry out their medical treatment and guide behavioral change [31]. It is essential that patients with COPD manage and respond properly to their frequently changing symptoms that are due to exacerbations and COPD progression [32]. Self-management interventions are heterogeneous and vary in their approach from merely providing a leaflet of information to taking more complex interventions such as delivering educational programs that may include an exercise program, nurse-based support, pulmonary rehabilitation, or telehealth interventions [32]. Smoking cessation, recognition and treatment of exacerbations, physical activity and exercise, nutritional advice, and dyspnea management are components that are specific to COPD self-management interventions [31]. Self-management programs for COPD should be tailored based on the severity of the disease, smoking status as well as the cognitive and physical limitations of the patient [31].

Telemedicine utilizes the advancement of technology to practice medicine and deliver patient care remotely by having the healthcare provider in one location and the patient at a distant [33]. On the other hand, Telehealth covers a broader range of health and educational services [34]. In the era of technology, healthcare providers and patients can use information technology and electronic communication means for diagnosis, examination, and medical assessments [35]. Telehealth is also used amongst healthcare providers to communicate for further consultations, train healthcare staff, attend scientific conferences, monitor a patient after recovery or hospital discharge remotely, or for health education purposes [35]. Telehealth allows healthcare providers to early detect exacerbation of COPD and provide an early medical intervention to avoid patient hospitalization; therefore, it improves patient's quality of life while reducing cost for the healthcare system [36]. Telehealth entails using telecommunication to make healthcare delivery more convenient and efficient to both healthcare providers and patients [34]. Tele-monitoring is one of the telehealth solutions and can be defined by having a system that collects patient's health outcomes, transmits these data to remote server where the healthcare provider will interpret them and provide feedback to the patient such as medication alteration, advice, or invite them to visit them in the clinic for a consultation if the patient needs immediate care [36]. Telemonitoring monitors the patient's vital signs, biological data such as oxygen saturation, symptoms, medication, and their daily physical activity [37]. However, there is limited evidence in the literature on the efficacy and effectiveness of telehealth solutions due to the lack of appropriate predictors for the early detection of AECOPD [38].

We use the term conventional in this review to distinguish between self-management interventions that use traditional methods such as provision of educational sessions and exercise programs from that use telecommunication and telehealth approach. The aspect of this review is to compare current conventional practices with telehealth and tele-monitoring self-management interventions in AECOPD management.

Methods

Search Strategy

A literature search was performed on April 1st, 2022, using OVID Medline, PubMed, Cumulative Index to Nursing and Allied Health Literature (CINAHL), the Wiley Cochrane

Library, and Google Scholar for articles published from January 2012 until April 2022. In addition, reference lists were also examined for any additional relevant studies reference list for any additional relevant studies that weren't identified in our database search. Suggested studies from Mendeley were also screened and relevant studies were included in this review. Abstract were reviewed by all authors, then full-text articles were obtained for those meeting the eligibility criteria. Disagreements were resolved by reaching consensus or by involving a third review author.

MeSH Terms

The search terms used in all databases for the conventional intervention were: (Self-management) AND (acute) AND (exacerbation) AND (copd OR chronic obstructive pulmonary disease). For the telehealth intervention the search terms were: (Telemedicine OR Telehealth OR Telecare OR Tele-monitoring OR Web-based OR Mobile Health OR mHealth) AND (Self-management) AND (Acute) AND (Exacerbation OR AECOPD) AND (Chronic Obstructive Pulmonary disease OR COPD)

Quality of Evidence

The quality of the body of evidence was assessed as high, moderate, low, or very low according to the Grading of Recommendation, Assessment, Development and Evaluation (GRADE) framework criteria. The following definitions of quality were used in grading the quality of evidence:

Table 1. Definition of quality rank assessment of the reviewed studies

High	The effect of the study reflects the actual effect and is very unlikely to change confidence in the estimate of effect.
Moderate	The effect of the study is close to the true effect, but it further research is likely to have an important impact on confidence in the estimate of effect and may change the estimated outcome.
Low	The true effect may differ significantly from the estimate and further research is important for the impact on confidence in the estimate and is likely to change it.
Very low	The true effect is likely to be substantially different from the estimated effect.

The criteria that were considered for the ranking included: randomized allocation, blinding, concealment, intention-to-treat (ITT), completion of trail, follow-up, consistency, and recommendation.

Inclusion/Exclusion Criteria

For the conventional self-management intervention, we included all studies that utilize any self-management intervention, ranging from educational programs to rehabilitation interventions. While for the telehealth solutions, we included studies that had transmission of participants' health data remotely to a server automatically for remote-monitoring or downloaded to personal computer for self-monitoring. Tele-monitoring had to have coordinated management and feedback system where the patient was able to communicate with the healthcare provider and vice versa.

We included randomized controlled trials (RCTs), quasi-randomized trials, pilot studies, and observational studies. Finally, we considered all papers published in the past decade, from January 1, 2012, until April 1, 2022.

We excluded papers that were published in languages other than English, tele-monitoring that included only tele-conferencing (phone calls) or had home visits from the healthcare provider (tele-nurse), not recording participant health data, study protocols, studies focused on COPD in general not AECOPD specifically, and studies that intended to test the solutions accuracy, reliability, and acceptability.

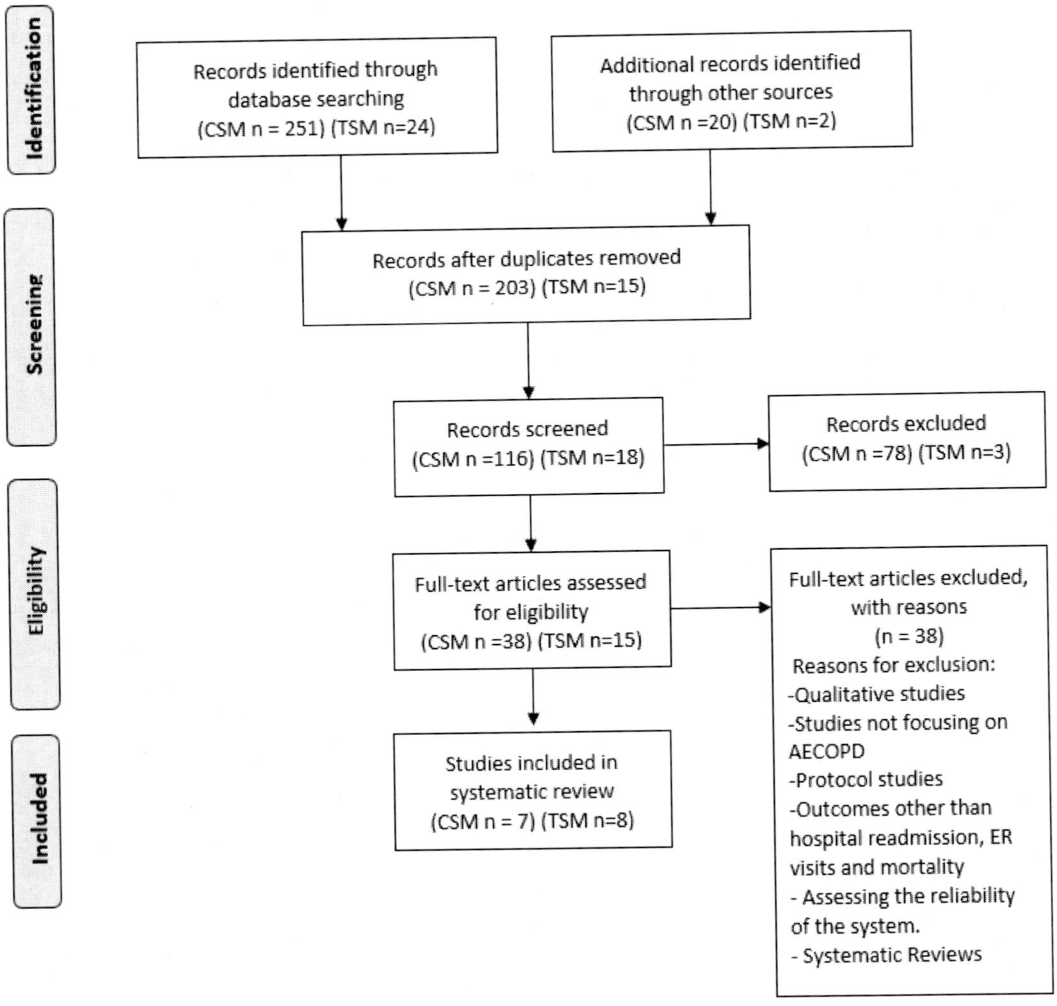

Figure 1. AECOPD conventional self-management (CSM) and telehealth self-management (TSM) interventions PRISMA.

Table 2. Summary table for all studies included in this review

Reference/year	Country	Study Design	Duration	Sample Size	Intervention	Conclusion
Conventional self-management interventions						
Wood-Baker et al, 2012	Australia	RCT	12 months	106	***Community nurse mentoring*** Home visits and telephone follow-ups were made by trained nurses to set an action plan with participants.	-Significant improvement in HRQoL and length of hospital stay in the intervention group. -No improvement in hospital admissions and mortality.
Bucknall et al, 2012	Scotland (UK)	RCT	12 months	464	***Training sessions and home visits by trained nurses*** Participants were trained to use a symptoms diary to monitor changes in sputum colour and breathlessness.	-No significant differences between groups in readmissions and mortality. -No significant differences between hospital anxiety and depression scores.
Greening et al, 2014	United Kingdom	RCT	12 months	389	***Early rehabilitation program utilizing SPACE (Self-management Program of Activity, Coping and Education)*** Participants received daily, supervised volitional (strength and aerobic training) and non-volitional (neuromuscular electrical stimulation) techniques by trained nurses and physiotherapists.	-No significant differences in hospital stay, readmissions and mortality.
Titova et al, 2015	Norway	RCT	24 months	172	***Integrated Care Intervention*** Participants received a COPD home model that utilized a call center, an interactive e-learning program and a post discharge individualized self-management plan as well as home visits by a specialist nurse	- Reduction in hospital readmissions and hospital stay in the intervention group. -Shorter survival time in the intervention group.
Benzo et al, 2019	United States	RCT	12 months	215	***Health coaching by a respiratory therapist*** Home visits were conducted to discuss the concepts of goal setting and action planning using motivational interviewing.	- Reduction in readmissions and emergency room visits. -Improvement in quality of life.
Aboumatar et al, 2020	United States	RCT	6 months	240	***Transition and long-term self-management support*** Participants received an individualized self-management support to take medications accurately, recognize the signs of exacerbations, stop smoking, adopt a healthy lifestyle, and recognize when to seek medical care.	-Improvement in HRQoL -A significant increase in COPD related hospitalizations and Emergency Department visits and mortality in the intervention group.
Hegelund et al, 2020	Denmark	RCT (pilot)	3 months	100	***Personalized action plan*** Participants received a personalized written action plan and a self-management dialogue of instructions utilizing a coaching and structured approach.	-Reduction in admissions and Hospital Depression Scores. -Improvement in CAT (COPD Assessment Test) scores.

Table 2. (Continued)

Reference/year	Country	Study Design	Duration	Sample Size	Intervention	Conclusion
Conventional self-management interventions						
Fernandez-Granero et al, (2015)	Spain	Observational pilot study	N = 16	6 months	The study aimed to evaluate the feasibility of using a respiratory sensor and machine learning for self-management of the condition among elderly patients, computerized analysis of respiratory sounds (CARS) and data mining for early detection of AECOPD remotely, thus, prompt treatment or prevention of AECOPD.	Home telehealth solution for monitoring respiratory sounds is positively beneficial for the early prediction of AECOPD on a day-to-day basis. Recording symptoms can facilitate treatment and support healthcare providers, patients, and the healthcare system as a whole.
Bourbeau et al, (2016)	France Germany Italy, and Spain	Multi-center parallel randomized controlled, open-label superiority trial	N = 159	2 years	The program includes extensive patient coaching by health care professionals to improve self-management, an e-health platform for reporting frequent health status updates, rapid intervention when necessary, and oxygen therapy monitoring. Comparator is the usual management as per the center's routine practice.	The COMET program has the potential to promote changes in improving home-based COPD management and patient health. The intervention showed significant reduction in acute care hospital admissions for exacerbation. It is expected that the program could reduce healthcare expenses, thus, its cost-effectiveness across different settings should provide an additional incentive to expand the program internationally.
Rubio et al, (2017)	Scotland (UK)	Observational study	N = 18	41 days	Participants in this study wore 4 BR monitors simultaneously in direct contact with the skin and a fifth for video-monitoring. Data then were downloaded from all devices to a personal computer in a database for each phase of the study for analysis.	Individual data showed various readings between patients. Gradual decrease in the mean of resting BR over time post exacerbation and BR remained stable throughout the whole period of the study. One patient was readmitted to the hospital and the monitor was able to capture an increase of BR and heart rate in the days prior hospitalization.
Deng et al, (2020)	China	Prospective observational study	N = 56	6 months	Each participant's care plan had had an individually tailored pathway to their condition. The pathway included risk evaluation, hierarchical management, follow-up, warnings, and compliance management. The patients used an app on their smart phones to record their daily health data	Pulmonary function did not significantly change with the implementation of this system, however, there was an improvement in COPD-specific quality of life and mental health assessments of participants.

Reference/year	Country	Study Design	Duration	Sample Size	Intervention	Conclusion
					cont. (medications and symptoms), and educational videos and text materials. In addition, patients were required to fill in their PEF score biweekly using a simple peak flow meter.	Patients' compliance was of a significant value and patients as well as healthcare providers thought the system was convenience to deliver and they were aware of the actions needed in different phases,
North et al, (2020)	UK	Feasibility randomized study	N = 41	6 months	Participants on the intervention arm had access to the application and required to enter their health data daily, as well as complete the COPD Assessment Tool (CAT) every four weeks.	The mean score of the CAT was lower in the intervention arm group compared to the TAU, which indicates a better control of the condition amongst the patients. The reduction was greater amongst participants in the myCOPD arm. The intervention is promising for better self-management of AECOPD
Stamenova et al, (2020)	Canada	3-arm randomized Controlled Trial	N = 122	6 months	The study compared the usual care to self-care and remote-monitoring care. The telehealth solution intervention arms had Bluetooth enabled device to monitor their oxygen saturation, blood pressure, temperature, weight, and symptoms. However, only patients in the remote-monitoring arm had a healthcare provider accessing their uploaded data and monitoring their vital signs and other symptoms.	Improvement was observed in all three groups with no significant difference on SGRQ activity or symptom scores, hospitalization, emergency department visits, or unplanned clinic visits.
Koff et al, (2021)	USA	Prospective quasi-randomized trial	N = 511	22 months	Proactive iCare consisted of a 9-month disease management program that included: (1) COPD education, (2) exacerbation education, (3) direct communication with study coordinators, and (4) remote home monitoring.	Proactive iCare achieves the goals of improving patient-centred outcomes and healthcare utilization when coupling remote monitoring to integrated care which increased the delivery of guideline-based care and by acting as an early-warning system for COPD exacerbations. The trial did not worsen mortality amongst patients with AECOPD.
Houchen-Wolloff et al, (2021)	UK	Single-center, nonrandomized feasibility study	N = 100	6 months	The aim of the SPACE program was to facilitate patients to better understand and manage their condition through education and home-based exercises. Participants were asked to complete the Bristol COPD Knowledge Questionnaire at baseline and after completing the study.	For patients who completed the study, completion rate of PR was double the previous audit estimates from the United Kingdom, disease knowledge improved, and the intervention was of value to patients.

Outcomes of Interest

In this review, we focused on hospitalization and re-admission of AECOPD, mortality, urgent and/or unplanned visits to the healthcare provider, length of stay, and patient's quality of life.

Results

A total of 15 studies are included in this review that met our criteria. Seven studies for the conventional self-management of AECOPD and eight for the telehealth self-management interventions (Table 2).

The conventional self-management interventions used in the included studies were: mentoring by community health nurses [39], supported self-management program delivered by trained nurses [40], an early rehabilitation programs [41], a COPD home-model [42], a transition plans [43], health coaching [44], and a personalized action plan [45]. The studies' outcomes varied between hospital readmissions, emergency room visits, length of hospital stay and health related quality of life. All conventional self-management intervention studies included in this review were RCTs and scored between moderate and strong using the GRADE criteria, as some of these studies did not mention the blinding and concealment process.

For the telehealth and home monitoring solutions, eight publications were found that met our criteria. These publications were evaluated according to the GRADE criteria. Out of the 8 studies, one randomized study was ranked strong [46], four were either feasibility-randomized or quasi-randomized trials that ranked moderate [47, 48, 49, 50], and three observational studies that were ranked low [38, 51, 52] (Figure 1).

Discussion

Currently, there is no cure for chronic obstructive pulmonary disease (COPD), thus, healthcare has leaned towards self-management strategies to slow the disease progression, reduce the frequency of acute exacerbation, improve patients' overall quality of life, and minimize hospitalization. Many randomized and observational studies were conducted to evaluate the conventional and advanced telehealth interventions for self-management of COPD, especially amongst patients following acute exacerbation. In this review we collate the available evidence from the past ten years on the effectiveness of both interventions in achieving the desired health and quality of life results.

Conventional Self-Management Intervention

In 2012 Wood-baker et al., conducted a controlled clinical trial in Australia aiming to examine the effects of a self-management program on the health-related quality of life and health care utilization in patients hospitalized for AECOPD [39]. A total of 106 participants who were recruited from hospital admissions were enrolled in this study. For a 12-month period, the intervention group received mentoring by community health nurses through multiple home visits and telephone call follow-ups were made to set an action plan and subsequently evaluate the participants' progress and reformulate the plan, if needed. Moreover, they were asked to record their cough, sputum, breathlessness, physical activity, and the use of medication in a daily diary [39]. The authors reported that there were significant improvements in the health-related quality of life aspects. However, there were no significant differences between the control and intervention groups with regards to hospital re-admissions where 62% and 67% of the participants in the intervention and control group were admitted, respectively. However, there was a reduction in the duration of hospital stay for intervention group. 23 participants died during the study for a variety of causes; 11 of them died due to respiratory causes [39]. The authors concluded that a mentor led program was effective in improving some aspects related to quality of life as well as the length of hospital admissions [39].

Another study published in 2012 by Bucknall et al. used a randomized study design to determine whether a supported self-management program influences hospital readmissions in patients with AECOPD in Glasgow, Scotland [40]. The aim of the intervention was to empower participants to be able to recognize and treat exacerbations independently through monitoring their symptoms, such monitoring the change of sputum color and breathlessness. 464 participants who were admitted to the hospital for an AECOPD were randomized to the study. The intervention group received training sessions and home visits from a trained nurse for a 12-month period, where they were trained to use a symptom diary to recognize exacerbations and subsequently start their self-management plan to either initiate treatment or seek medical advice [40]. The control group received the usual care. Bucknall et al. found that there was no significant difference in terms of readmissions or deaths between the intervention and the control groups as 48% of the intervention group and 47% of the control group were readmitted or died due to COPD within 12 months. This study also examined hospital anxiety and depression scores through administering questionnaires and found no significant difference between groups. The study concludes that the supported self-management program had no effect on hospital readmissions and death due to COPD [40].

Greening et al. conducted a prospective randomized controlled trial with 389 participants that were recruited between January 2010 and September 2011 from AECOPD admissions to three hospitals in the United Kingdom [41]. This study focused on early rehabilitation where the intervention group received a six-week rehabilitation program, within 48 hours of admission, aerobic, strength and non-volitional training as well as a self-management package that utilized the SPACE (Self-management Program of Activity, Coping and Education) manual [41]. The authors investigated the effect of early rehabilitation intervention on readmissions at 12 months, mortality, length of stay in hospital, physical performance, and health status. The results show that the length of hospital stay, and the hospital readmissions show no difference between groups where 60% of the participants were readmitted (75% of the admissions was due to a respiratory cause [41]. During the follow up period of 12 months, 21% of the participants died with higher mortality amongst participants in the intervention group. Therefore, the study concludes that early rehabilitation and self-management program did not reduce admissions or mortality [41].

In Norway, a single center prospective controlled clinical trial was conducted by Titova et al. to examine whether a COPD- Home model can effectively reduce hospital utilization of patients with COPD stage III and IV post discharge for AECOPD [42]. A total of 172 participants were allocated to a control group where they received the usual care, and an integrated care group where they received the COPD Home model. The COPD Home model entailed a call center run by specialist nurses to support patients through routine calls, an interactive e-learning program and a post discharge individualized self-management plan as well as home visits by a specialist nurse at set timings post discharge [42]. The self-management plan includes the tools required for the patient to monitor their symptoms and when to self-initiate treatment of prednisone and/or antibiotic accordingly. The results show that there was a 12.6% reduction in hospital admissions in the integrated care group during the first year of follow up and a 46.5% reduction during the second year of follow up when compared to admissions prior to the study taking place [8]. The study also reports that there is a reduction in the hospital days in the integrated care group in the two-year period of follow up. However, the survival time was shorter in the intervention group. The study concluded that COPD Home model is effective in reducing hospital utilization in patients with severe COPD and highlighted the need for individually tailored self-management programs [42].

A study was conducted by Aboumatar et al. to determine whether a hospital-based program that includes combined transition and long-term self-management support improves outcomes in hospitalized patients with AECOPD [43]. This study took place in the United States where a total of 240 participants were enrolled from March 2015 to May 2016. The study uses a single site, randomized clinical trial where the intervention group received a comprehensive three-month program whereas the control group received the usual care. Usual care included a 30-day follow-up after discharge to support patients to adhere to their discharge plan and remain in contact with outpatient care delivered by nurses trained to use standardized tools to support patients with COPD and their caregivers [43]. The purpose of the transition plan was to ensure that patients and their caregivers understand their post discharge care plan. Other aspects of the intervention included individualized self-management support to aid patients in taking their medications accurately, recognize the signs of exacerbations, stop smoking, adopt a healthy lifestyle, and recognize when to seek help as well as having access to community and treatment service [43]. The intervention's main aim was to improve the health-related Quality of Life (HRQAOL) outcomes and reduce emergency room visits. The results of this trial are somewhat surprising as it showed that there was a significant increase in COPD related hospitalizations and Emergency Department visits. There were 196 hospitalizations and 42 emergency room COPD visits. The study also reported 8 (6.7%) deaths in the intervention group and 7 (5.8%) deaths in the control group. The HRQOL outcomes showed significant differences between groups. The authors emphasize the need to be cautious about study interventions and the validity of their findings [43].

Benzo et al. utilized health coaching by a respiratory therapist or nurse as the intervention in their randomized controlled trial that took place in multiple sites in 2019 in the United States [44]. The study included 215 participants who were randomized into the study. The control group received the usual care. The intervention was delivered by health coaches through having weekly visits for the first three months and once per month after that, with patients post discharge. The visits discussed the concepts of goal setting and action planning through the use of motivational interviewing to empower the patient. To measure the outcomes, Benzo et al. used the Chronic Respiratory Disease Questionnaire mastery domain at 6- and 12-months follow-up [44]. The study concluded that their health coaching program was effective in reducing readmissions and emergency room visits and it showed an improvement in the quality of life for up to 12 months. Moreover, it improved the abilities of self-management. The authors recommend that to maintain the benefits of self-management to longer periods, some patients may require prolonged self-management support [44].

Hegelund et al. conducted a pilot study, in Denmark, that utilized a prospective, randomized, clinical, unblended trial to assess the effectiveness of a personalized action plan in reducing the number of readmissions and symptoms of anxiety and depression at 3-months follow-up [45]. The study had a total of 100 participants, who were discharged after an AECOPD, were randomly allocated to an intervention group where they received an action plan and the COPD Assessment Test (CAT), and a control group which received the usual care. Participants in the intervention group received a personalized written action plan and a self-management dialogue of instructions utilizing coaching and structured intervention. The personalized action plan was illustrated in an A4 sheet where the participant can write about their perceived condition and symptoms according to a colored map of green, yellow, and red [45]. The green step illustrated a stable condition, the yellow indicated increased symptoms and the red indicated being affected 'much more than the usual state'. Each colored zone provided suggestions for pharmacological and non-pharmacological actions that the patient should perform taking into consideration any changes in the sputum. The intervention also included inhaler technique correction, instructions on when to self-initiate treatment with antibiotics and steroids [45]. The results show that utilizing a tailored, personal action plan post discharge for AECOPD reduced readmissions, reduced HADS-depression and it showed significant improvements in the CAT scores. The authors suggest that in order to improve self-management support, patients should be introduced to their action plan during their admission for AECOPD and to receive a telephone or home visit follow up to complete the plan [45].

In 2015, two systematic reviews were published discussing self-management in COPD patients. The first one was published by Majothi et al. where they reviewed nine randomized controlled trials that compared patients who received a self-management intervention and those who received the usual care [53]. The interventions examined in this review varied between nursing based self-management whether at home or hospital, supported self-management and integrated care. The total sample size of all the RCTs in the review was 1466 participants who were followed up for a 2-12 monthperiod. The results show that there is no evidence of effect on hospital admissions or mortality hence the authors concluded that the evidence is not sufficient to support self-management for AECOPD [53]. The second systematic review was conducted by Maddocks et al. to assess the role of early pulmonary rehabilitation in the peri-acute and early post hospital discharge settings on reducing hospital readmissions [54]. The review searched for RCTs published between 1966 and 2014 and found nine RCTs that met their criteria. The included articles were reviewed to determine some of the modifiable risk factors for readmission by pulmonary rehabilitation which included health status, anxiety, physical activity, and exercise capacity [54]. The review concluded that early rehabilitation, especially exercise-based rehabilitation interventions reduce the risk of readmission and health care utilization. However, the authors call for further research of post discharge pulmonary rehabilitation [54].

Two years later, another systematic review published in 2017 included 22 RCTs that involved 3,854 participants with COPD published between 1995 and 2016 [55]. This paper reviewed studies of self-management intervention that included a written action plan for AECOPD and a collaborative process between the participants and their healthcare provider for feedback provision [55]. The trials reviewed by the authors in this review ranged from two months to 24 months with a diverse content of their self-management programs. The authors found that self-management interventions with AECOPD action plan that last for an average of

12 months had significantly lower risk for hospital readmission and significant beneficial effect on participants' health-related quality of life [55].

Another systematic review published in 2020 by Harrison et al. reviewed RCTs reporting self-management methods delivered during hospitalization or one month post an AECOPD [56]. The self-management interventions included action plans, educational material, and at least two of seven self-management skills such as: self-efficacy, problem solving, resource utilization, collaboration, emotional management, role management, and goal setting [56]. The authors found that self-management has a positive effect on knowledge and management of an AECOPD. However, the outcome measures of interventions that depend solely on the patients to self-manage their condition are still inconsistent and interventions delivered by healthcare providers that offer structured follow-ups are still necessary [56]. Shnaigat et al. also published a more recent systematic review in 2022 that suggested that patient activation can be used as a reliable tool for improving COPD self-management and clinical outcome, however, they found that this approach did not have a significant improvement on hospitalization, quality of life, and mental health [57].

Patients suffering from AECOPD are at risk of health deterioration and poor quality of life at any time. Involving these patients in managing their condition can help them have better control over their health and quality of living. However, these self-management interventions need a great amount of commitment from the patients and longer follow-ups from their healthcare providers to achieve ideal value of these programs.

Telehealth Self-Management Intervention

In 2012, The Medical Advisory Secretariat (MAS) in Canada conducted an evidence-based assessment of home telehealth technologies as part of the Ontario Health Technology Assessment Series for patients suffering from COPD aimed to provide informed recommendations regarding these solutions and services in Ontario [37]. This assessment concluded that telemonitoring solutions are placing patients towards decreased hospitalization and use of healthcare services, however, this conclusion needed further evidence and more randomized control trials of high quality to confirm it [37].

Fernandez-Granero et al. conducted an observational 6-month pilot study in 2015 on 16 participants with history of smoking and at least one hospital admission for exacerbation or two exacerbations treated with oral corticosteroids or antibiotics within the previous year [38]. The study aimed to evaluate the feasibility of using a respiratory sensor and machine learning for self-management of the condition among elderly patients, computerized analysis of respiratory sounds (CARS), and data mining for early detection of AECOPD remotely, thus, prompt treatment or prevention of AECOPD [38]. The authors took advantage of the availability of electronic stethoscopes and techniques of CARS and used it for improving the diagnosis of respiratory diseases like COPD. These advancements in technology allowed them to use Auscultation as a tool to listen to the patients' respiratory sounds for early detection and management of any worsening of the participants' condition [38]. The participants installed a home-based station and used a sensor to record their daily respiratory sounds over the 6 months. In addition, a microphone-based multifunctional sensor was also designed specifically for this study that allows easy data collection within a single user test on a daily basis [38]. During the study, 51 events of AECOPD were reported. Out of these 51 events, 18 cases who needed medical attention were associated with non-recovered exacerbations, thus, were not considered for this study, and the remaining 33 events corresponded to AECOPD. Out of the 33 events were caused by non-programmed medical interventions, while the remaining 8 were self-managed and treated with self-administered medication [38]. The authors concluded that the home telehealth solution for monitoring respiratory sounds is positively beneficial for the early prediction of AECOPD, and alongside with recording symptoms can facilitate treatment and support healthcare providers, patients, and the healthcare system as a whole [38].

In 2016, a multicenter randomized controlled trial called the COMET (COPD Patient Management European Trial) was conducted in four European countries that ran for up to 24 months for a total of 345 participants suffering from obstructive lung disease III/IV COPD [46]. In this study, the participants in the intervention group received four-at-home educational sessions before starting the program and a monthly session during the follow-up period. Participants in the control group received the standard care provided in their hospitals, while participants in the intervention group reported their symptoms via phone-based questionnaires weekly or when their condition is worsening. Their answers then were automatically transmitted to their electronic health data system (e-Health platform). The status of the participant's well-being, worsening condition, or an alarm is indicated by the system [46]. In the case of worsening or an alarming state of the participants, a standardized intervention will be trigger where it will ask the patient to perform self-measurements of pulse oximetry, spirometry, and body temperature, as well as a phone call from their case manager that will instruct the participant into taking action based on their individualized action plan [46]. The study exhibited a significant reduction (39.8%) in acute care hospitalization for exacerbation of COPD in the intervention group, 41% in emergency care, and 58.9% in unscheduled physician visits. The study concluded that using a home-based monitoring solution has the potential to promote self-management and improve the quality of life for patients with advanced COPD [46]. Following the COMET trial, another paper was published by the authors in 2018, comparing the results of the intervention group with the usual care and showed a significant reduction in acute care hospitalization days and mortality rate in severe COPD patients, however there was no significant improvement in the unplanned all-cause hospitalization days [58].

A study published in 2017 by Rubio et al. based on breathing rate (BR) as well using 2 different BR monitors that were validated with a 14-trial prior the study [51]. A total of 18 moderate-to-very severe COPD patients as defined by GOLD guidelines were recruited in a three-phase study during an episode of AECOPD to wear the monitors during their recovery period. Participants in this study wore 4 BR monitors simultaneously in direct contact with the skin and a fifth for video-monitoring [51]. Data was then downloaded from all devices to a personal computer in a database for each phase of the study for analysis. Although individual data showed various readings between patients, the study results showed a gradual decrease in the mean of resting BR over time post exacerbation and BR remained stable throughout the whole period of the study. One patient was readmitted to the hospital and the monitor was able to capture an increase of BR and heart rate in the days prior hospitalization, concluding that changes in the patient's condition and BR were accurately captured by these monitors [51].

A community-based observational prospective study was conducted in China between September 2017 and June 2018 by Deng et al. and published in 2020 [52]. In this study, a total of 56 participants were enrolled and instructed by the study team on how to install and use the mHealth solution as a phone application. Each participant's care plan had an individually tailored pathway to their condition. The pathway included risk evaluation, hierarchical management, follow-up, warnings, and compliance management [52]. The Peak Flow Measurement (PEF) was used in this study instead of the spirometry due to the lack of professional portable device support in Chinese remote area. PEF measures the air flowing out of lungs by measuring the maximum flow achieved during an expiration delivered with maximum force starting from full lung inhalation [59]. A PEF score less than 80% is a good indicator for detecting a case of COPD [52]. The COPD Assessment Tool (CAT) was also used to assess the impact of COPD on the participant's daily life. The mHealth solution included the patient's installed app to collect data, data then transmitted to a cloud server, and the healthcare provider station to retrieve the data from a web-based platform then interpret these data [52]. The app used smart phones to record patient's daily health data (medications and symptoms), and educational videos and text materials [52]. In addition, patients were required to fill in their PEF score biweekly using a simple peak flow meter. During the study, 459 warnings of acute exacerbation were detected by the system, however, only 110 events were confirmed as exacerbation of COPD by the healthcare provider. 64.5% of these exacerbations either visited the clinic or were hospitalized. The authors justified this high percentage of hospitalization due to the severity of COPD as more than 80% of the participants were placed on level 2 or higher on the Global Initiative for Chronic Obstructive Lung Disease (GOLD) criteria [52]. The study concluded that patients' compliance was of a significant value and patients as well as healthcare providers thought the system was convenience to deliver and they were aware of the actions needed in different phases, however, they suggested that the system could need improvement and a bigger trial is needed to have a stronger evidence-based results [52].

The RESCUE trial was published in 2020 by North et al. The trial was a feasibility randomized study that was conducted over 6 months for a total of 124 patients presented with exacerbation of COPD [49]. The study excluded patients who had other respiratory diseases such as asthma, sensitivity or allergy to saccharin, and lack of digital literacy. This led to a sample size of 41 participants who were randomized to the telehealth intervention arm (myCOPD) and to the Treatment as Usual (TAU) arm. The participants had a history of smoking and were reported as moderate to severe COPD. Participants on the intervention arm had access to the application and were required to enter their health data daily, as well as complete the COPD Assessment Tool (CAT) every four weeks [49]. Although the days of using myCOPD per week was continually declining in the number of users per week, the mean score of the CAT was lower in the intervention arm group compared to the TAU, which indicates a better control of the condition amongst the patients [49]. Moreover, fewer exacerbations were observed post intervention in both arms, however, the reduction was greater amongst participants in the myCOPD arm with only four readmissions compared to seven readmissions in the TAU [49]. The authors concluded that telehealth intervention can be promising for self-managing AECOPD and improved health, however, larger trials are required for greater evidence [49].

Another 3-arms RCT published in 2020 by Stamenova et al. [50] that included 122 participants. The usual care arm had 40 participants, while both remote-monitoring and self-monitoring arms had 41 participants. The telehealth solution intervention arms had Bluetooth enabled device to monitor their oxygen saturation, blood pressure, temperature, weight, and symptoms. However, only patients in the remote-monitoring arm had a healthcare provider accessing their uploaded data and monitoring their vital signs and other symptoms [50]. The study team used the Partners in Health (PIH) Scale, SGRQ, and BCKQ assessment tools. The authors reported improvement in all three arm groups with no significant difference on SGRQ activity or symptom scores, hospitalization, emergency department visits, or unplanned clinic visits [50]. The authors justified the results of their study due to lack of knowledge and structured educational components in the intervention groups, and the lack of integration of the action plan with the technology [50].

A recent prospective quasi-randomized clinical trial published in 2021 by Koff et al. concluded that remote monitoring can improve St George's Respiratory Questionnaire (SGRQ) significantly when compared to the standard care [47]. A total of 511 participants were enrolled in this study over a 22 month's period. Koff reported that the annual COPD-related urgent visits to the clinic were reduced by 76 visits per 100 participants. Moreover, smoking amongst participants was significantly decreased and improved symptoms, oxygen titration, as well as the body mass index-airway obstruction-dyspnea-exercise (BODE). Most importantly, the intervention helped identify unreported exacerbation and improved overall quality of life [47]. Out of 352 participants in the intervention group, 210 had COPD exacerbations during the study. The most common reported symptoms post exacerbation of COPD were increasing shortness of breath, decreased physical activity, lower oxygen saturation, and increased cough. 21% of the exacerbation-related reporting was self-reporter to their healthcare providers, 34% of these were reported to the intervention coordinator, and 45% were from the coordinator to the participants. Most of the exacerbation cases were treated with either oral corticosteroid, antibiotic, or short-acting bronchodilator alone. The results of this study suggested that introducing telehealth solution coupled with remote monitoring could improve health outcomes for patients with advanced COPD [47].

Another study published in 2021 by Houchen-Wolloff et al. assessed the feasibility and acceptability of a web-based program for COPD patients who were hospitalized due to acute exacerbation [48]. The intervention was called Self-management Program of Activity Coping and Education (SPACE) and it was coproduced in a 4-stage manual by healthcare professionals and patients. This program has shown improvement in symptoms, exercise tolerance, and quality of life amongst patients with AECOPD when compared to the standard care [48]. However, this program has been transitioned to a web-based format recently because of the ambition of healthcare services engaging with the new advancement of technology [48]. A total of 100 patients were recruited in the study with a mean age of 71, a history of smoking, and at least one comorbidity. At the end of the 6-month study, only 18% of participants had completed the web-based program. The study's primary outcome was the percentage of participants recruited and completing the Bristol COPD Knowledge Questionnaire (BCKQ), 42 participants returned the questionnaire with a 21% increase in the disease knowledge at 6 months. Patients participated in this study for several reasons, including: internal factors such as fear from experiencing another AECOPD, external factors such as the reassurance they received from the healthcare providers and family encouragement, some participants felt that their computer skills will allow them to engage properly in the program, the physical activity and exercise goal setting was found beneficial to all patients who reached stage 2 of the study, and the overall understanding of the disease has increased their knowledge via the educational material the program provided [48]. However, some of the participants found the program very complex and too steep for their skills [48]This could be due to the age group that was chosen for the study population. Overall, patients who engaged in the program felt confident and that it gave them focus and drive to take control of their health and reassess their condition perceptions. Which in return, some patients felt that the program helped them challenge themselves and positively change their health behaviors such as increasing their daily exercise and smoking cessation affirmation [48]. The authors concluded that digital self-management intervention is yet to be feasible for adoption following an AECOPD among COPD population. However, they found that with further refinement to such system, home-monitoring and web-based solutions may be a viable steppingstone for pulmonary rehabilitation, improving patients' knowledge, and positive behavioral changes with better identification of patients that will most likely benefit from such solution [48].

Telemedicine interventions are widely used for different chronic illnesses including COPD as a tool to improve access to healthcare with a great potential to decrease of healthcare provision cost and improve patients' quality of life with early detection of AECOPD and early medical intervention to prevent hospitalization. However, there are some barriers to adopting this technology such as digital literacy that prevailed as an issue to successfully implement telehealth in many healthcare settings.

Conclusion

The literature had high-quality evidence that showed moderate to great impact of rehabilitation on health-related quality of life and exercise capacity from participants after an acute exacerbation of COPD in both conventional and telehealth self-management interventions. However, the hospitalization and mortality results were still controversial in both interventions. This can be due to the complexity of the self-management program or the availability of regular educational material. Telehealth solutions can be promising in early detection of AECOPD, which will allow timely and proper actions taken from the patient for self-management and the healthcare providers, however, the parameters measured remotely such as pulse oximetry and spirometry can still be unreliable and more extensive trials are required to determine the best component integration within a telehealth solution for better self-management by the patient.

Key Points

- There is still no consensus on which components or intervention of self-management programs that are effective in leading to a positive outcome. The heterogeneity of interventions also hinders the comparability of the results.
- The impact of self-management interventions is often not sustained for a long period after the end of the intervention. Therefore, it may be worthwhile incorporating effective interventions in general care to ensure continuity.
- Self-management of AECOPD seems to be challenging as some patients find it difficult to recognize early exacerbations and subsequently start treatment appropriately, hence the high incidence of hospital readmissions.
- Telehealth solutions appear to have promising impact on self-management of AECOPD, however, it requires specific population with digital literacy which can limit elderly patients from using it.
- A comprehensive telehealth solution that integrates remote monitoring, continuous education, and advanced early detection of AECOP is yet to be achieved.

References

[1] GOLD, "*Global Strategy for the Diagnosis, Management and Prevention of Chronic Obstructive Pulmonary Disease: 2021 Report*," 2021. [Online]. Available: www.goldcopd.org. [Accessed 25 04 2022].

[2] Elgaddal, N. and E. A. Kramarow, "QuickStats: Percentage of Adults Aged ≥18 Years with Diagnosed Chronic Obstructive Pulmonary Disease, by Urbanization Level and Age Group — National Health Interview Survey, United States, 2019," *CDC*, 2019. [Online]. Available: https://www.cdc.gov/mmwr/volumes/70/wr/mm7026a3.htm. [Accessed 25 04 2022].

[3] Sullivan, J., V. Pravosud, D. M. Mannino, K. Siegel, R. Choate and T. Sullivan, "National and State Estimates of COPD Morbidity and Mortality — United States, 2014-2015," *Chronic Obstr Pulm Dis,* vol. 5, no. 4, p. 324–333, 2018.

[4] Kochanek, K. D., S. L. Murphy, J. Xu and E. Arias, "*Mortality in the United States, 2016. NCHS Data Brief 2017,*" National Center for Health Statistics, 12 2017. [Online]. Available: https://www.cdc.gov/nchs/products/databriefs/db293.htm#:~:text=Statistics%20System%2C%20Mortality.-,Summary,at%20birth%20decreased%200.1%20year. [Accessed 26 04 2022].

[5] WHO, "*Chronic obstructive pulmonary disease* (COPD)," World Health Organization, 21 06 2021. Available: https://www.who.int/news-room/fact-sheets/detail/chronic-obstructive-pulmonary-disease-(copd). [Accessed Online 26 04 2022].

[6] WHO, "*WHO Global Health Estimates*," World Health Organization, 2022. [Online]. Available: https://www.who.int/news-room/fact-sheets/detail/the-top-10-causes-of-death. [Accessed 26 04 2022].

[7] Buist, A. S., M. McBurnie, W. M. Vollmer, S. Gillespie, P. Burney, D. M. Mannino, A. M. Menezes, S. D. Sullivan, T. A. Lee, K. B. Weiss, R. L. Jensen, G. B. Marks, A. Gulsvik, E. Nizankowska-Mogilinicka and BOLD Collaborative Research Group, "International variation in the prevalence of COPD (the BOLD Study): a population-based prevalence study," *Lancet,* vol. 370, no. 9589, pp. 741-750, 2007.

[8] American Lung Association, "*COPD Causes and Risk Factors*," American Lung Association, 05 03 2021. [Online]. Available: https://www.lung.org/lung-health-diseases/lung-disease-lookup/copd/what-causes-copd. [Accessed 28 04 2022].

[9] NHS, "Treatment: Chronic obstructive pulmonary disease (COPD)," NHS, 20 09 2019. [Online]. Available: https://www.nhs.uk/conditions/chronic-obstructive-pulmonary-disease-copd/treatment/ [Accessed 28 04 2022].

[10] Siddharthan, T., A. C. Wosu, S. L. Pollard, S. Hossen, P. Alupo, T. Shade, R. Kalyesubula, S. Quaderi, R. A. Wise, J. R. Hurst, B. Kirenga and W. Checkley, "A Novel Case-Finding Instrument for Chronic Obstructive Pulmonary Disease in Low- and Middle-Income Country Settings," *Int J Chron Obstruct Pulmon Dis,* vol. 15, pp. 2769-2777, 2020.

[11] Sethi, S. and T. F. Murphy, "Bacterial infection in chronic obstructive pulmonary disease in 2000. A state-of-the-art review," *Clin Microbiol Rev,* vol. 14, no. 2, pp. 336-363, 2001.

[12] Connors Jr, A. F., N. V. Dawson, C. Thomas, F. E. Harrell Jr, N. Desbiens, W. J. Fulkerson, P. Kussin, P. Bellamy, L. Goldman and W. A. Knaus, "Outcomes following acute exacerbations of severe chronic obstructive lung disease. The SUPPORT investigators (Study to Understanding Prognosis and Preferences for Outcomes and Risks of Treatment," *Am J Respir Crit Care Med,* vol. 154, no. 4 Pt 1, pp. 959-967, 1996.

[13] Groenewegen, K. H., A. M. W. J. Schols and E. F. M. Wouters, "Mortality and mortality-related factors after hospitalisation for acute exacerbation of COPD," *Chest,* vol. 124, no. 2, pp. 459-467, 2003.

[14] Wedzicha, J. A. "The heterogeneity of chronic obstructive pulmonary disease," *Thorax,* vol. 55, no. 8, pp. 631-632, 2000.

[15] Pauwels, R. A., A. S. Buist, P. M. Calverley, C. R. Jenkins, S. S. Hurd and COLD Scientific Committee, "Global strategy for the diagnosis, management and prevention of chronic obstructive pulmonary disease. NHLBI/WHO Global Initiative for Chronic Obstructive Lung Disease (GOLD) workshop summary," *Am J Respir Crit Care Med,* vol. 163, no. 5, pp. 1256-1276, 2001.

[16] Anthonisen, N. R., J. Manfreda, C. P. Warren, E. S. Hershfield, G. K. Harding and N. A. Nelson, "Antibiotic therapy in exacerbations of chronic obstructive pulmonary disease," *Ann Intern Med,* vol. 106, no. 2, pp. 196-204, 1987.

[17] Hodgev, V. A., S. S. Kostianev, A. A. Torosian, I. B. Yanev and P. B. Mandoulova, "Long-term changes in dyspnea, lung function, and exercise capacity in COPD patients," *Folia Med (Plovdiv),* vol. 46, no. 3, pp. 12-17, 2004.

[18] Spencer, S., P. M. Calverley, P. S. Burge, P. W. Jones and I. S. i. O. L. D. ISOLDE Study Group., "Health status deterioration in patients with chronic obstructive pulmonary disease," *Am J Respir Crit Care Med,* vol. 163, no. 1, pp. 122-128, 2001.

[19] Dondaldson, G. C., T. M. Wilkinson, J. R. Hurst, W. R. Perera and J. A. Wedzicha, "Exacerbations and time spent outdoors in chronic obstructive pulmonary disease," *Am J Respir Crit Care Med,* vol. 171, no. 5, pp. 446-452, 2005.

[20] Ball, P. "Epidemiology and treatment of chronic bronchitis and its exacerbations," *Chest,* vol. 108, no. 2 Suppl, pp. 43S-52S, 1995.

[21] Sunyer, J., M. Saez, C. Murillo, J. Castellsague, F. Martinez and J. M. Anto, "Air pollution and emergency room admission for chronic obstructive pulmonary disease.," *Am J Epidemiol,* vol. 137, no. 7, pp. 701-705, 1993.

[22] Sapey, E. and R. A. Stockley, "COPD exacerbations · 2: Aetiology," *Thorax,* vol. 61, no. 3, pp. 250-258, 2006.

[23] Donaldson, G. C. T. A. R. Seemungal, A. Bhowmik and J. A. Wedzicha, "Relationship between exacerbation frequency and lung function decline in chronic obstructive pulmonary disease," *Thorax,* vol. 57, no. 10, pp. 847-852, 2002.

[24] Donaldson, G. C., J. R. Hurst, C. J. Smith, R. B. Hubbard and J. A. Wedzicha, "Increased risk of myocardial infarction and stroke following exacerbation of COPD," *Chest,* vol. 137, no. 5, pp. 1091-1097, 2010.

[25] Seemungal, T. A., G. C. Donaldson, E. A. Paul, J. C. Bestall, D. J. Jeffries and J. A. Wedzicha, "Effect of exacerbation on quality of life in patients with chronic obstructive pulmonary disease.," *Am J Respir Crit Care Med,* vol. 157, no. 5 Pt 1, pp. 1418-1422, 1998.

[26] Soler-Cataluna, J. J., M. A. Martinez-Garcia, P. R. Sanchez, E. Salcedo, M. Navarro and R. Ochando, "Severe acute exacerbations and mortality in patients with chronic obstructive pulmonary disease," *Thorax,* vol. 60, no. 11, pp. 925-931, 2005.

[27] Donaldson, G. C. and J. A. Wedzicha, "COPD exacerbations/1: Epidemiology," *Thorax,* vol. 61, no. 2, pp. 164-168, 2006.

[28] Papi, A., M. Contoli, B. Beghe, B. R. Celli, J. A. Wedzicha and L. M. Fabbri, "Chronic obstructive pulmonary disease exacerbation fundamentals: Diagnosis, treatment, prevention and disease impact," *Respirology,* vol. 26, pp. 532-551, 2021.

[29] Franek, J. "Self-Management Support Interventions for Persons With Chronic Disease: An Evidence-Based Analysis," *Ont Health Technol Assess Ser,* vol. 13, no. 9, pp. 1-60, 2013.

[30] Grady, P. A. and L. L. Gough, "Self-management: a comprehensive approach to management of chronic conditions," *Am J Public Health,* vol. 104, no. 8, pp. e25-31, 2014.

[31] Effing, T. W., J. Bourbeau, J. Vercoulen, A. J. Apter, D. Coultas, P. Meek, P. van der Valk, M. R. Partridge and J. van der Palen, "Self-management programmes for COPD: Moving forward," *Chron Respir Dis,* vol. 9, no. 1, pp. 27-35, 2012.

[32] Effing, T. W., J. H. Vercoulen, J. Bourbeau, J. Trappenburg, A. Lenferink, P. Cafarella, D. Coultas, P. Meek, P. van der Valk, E. W. M. A. Bischoff, C. Bucknall, N. A. Dewan, F. Early, V. Fan, P. Frith, D. J. A. Janssen, K. Mitchell, M. Morgan, L. Nici, I. Patel, H. Walters, K. L. Rice, S. Singh, R. Zuwallack, R. Benzo, R. Goldstein, M. R. Partridge and J. van der Palen, "Definition of a COPD self-management intervention: International Expert Group consensus," *Eur Respir J,* vol. 48, no. 1, pp. 46-54, 2016.

[33] AAFP, "What's the difference between telemedicine and telehealth?," American Academy of Family Physicians, 2022. [Online]. Available: https://www.aafp.org/news/media-center/kits/telemedicine-and-telehealth.html. [Accessed 07 04 2022].

[34] eVisit, "*Telehealth Solutions*," eVisit, 2022. [Online]. Available: https://evisit.com/resources/telehealth-solutions/. [Accessed 10 04 2022].

[35] MoH, "*Telemedicine*," Ministry of Health of Saudi Arabia, 30 03 2021. [Online]. Available: https://www.moh.gov.sa/en/Ministry/Information-and-services/Pages/Telemedicine.aspx. [Accessed 07 04 2022].

[36] NICE, "Self-management interventions, education and telehealth monitoring: Chronic obstructive pulmonary disease in over 16s: diagnosis and management: Evidence review C," in *NICE Guideline, No. 115*, London, National Institute for Health and Care Excellence (NICE), 2018.

[37] Franek, J. "*Home Telehealth for Patients With Chronic Obstructive Pulmonary Disease (COPD): An Evidence-Based Analysis*," Health Quality Ontario, Ontario, 2012.

[38] Fernandez-Granero, M. A., D. Sanchez-Morillo and A. Leon-Jimenez, "Computerised Analysis of Telemonitored Respiratory Sounds for Predicting Acute Exacerbations of COPD," *Sensors,* vol. 15, pp. 26978-26996, 2015.

[39] Wood-Baker, R., D. Reid, A. Robinson and E. H. Walters, "Clinical trial of community nurse mentoring to improve self-management in patients with chronic obstructive pulmonary disease," *Int J Chron Obstruct Pulmon Dis,* vol. 7, pp. 407-413, 2012.

[40] Bucknall, C. E., G. Miller, S. M. Lloyd, S. McCluskey, M. Cotton, R. D. Stevenson, P. Cotton and A. McConnachie, "Glasgow supported self-management trial (GSuST) for patients with moderate to severe COPD: Randomised controlled trial," *BMJ,* vol. 344, no. 7849, p. e1060, 2012.

[41] Greening, N. J., J. E. A. Williams, S. F. Hussain, T. C. Harvey-Dunstan, M. J. Bankart, E. J. Chaplin, E. E. Vincent, R. Chimera, M. D. Morgan, S. J. Singh and M. C. Steiner, "An early rehabilitation intervention to enhance recovery during hospital admission for an exacerbation of chronic respiratory disease: Randomised controlled trial," *BMJ,* vol. 349, p. g4315, 2014.

[42] Titova, E., S. Steinshamn, B. Indredavik and A. H. Henriksen, "Long term effects of an integrated care intervention on hospital utilization in patients with severe COPD: a single centre controlled study," *Respir Res,* vol. 16, no. 1, p. 8, 2015.

[43] Aboumatar, H., M. Naqibuddin, S. Chung, H. Chaudhry, S. W. Kim, J. Saunders, L. Bone, A. P. Gurses, A. Knowlton, P. Pronovost, N. Putcha, C. Rand, D. Roter, C. Sylvester, C. Thompson, J. L. Wolff, J. Hibbard and R. A. Wise, "Effect of a Hospital-Initiated Program Combining Transitional Care and Long-term Self-management Support on Outcomes of Patients Hospitalized with Chronic Obstructive Pulmonary Disease: A Randomized Clinical Trial," *JAMA,* vol. 322, no. 14, pp. 1371-1380, 2019.

[44] Benzo, R. and C. McEvoy, "Effect of health coaching delivered by a respiratory therapist or nurse on self-management abilities in severe COPD: Analysis of a large randomized study," *Respir Care,* vol. 64, no. 9, pp. 1065-1072, 2019.

[45] Hegelung, A., I. C. Andersen, M. N. Andersen and U. Bodtger, "The impact of a personalised action plan delivered at discharge to patients with COPD on readmissions: a pilot study," *Scand J Caring Sci,* vol. 34, no. 4, pp. 909-918, 2020.

[46] Bourbeau, J., P. Casan, S. Tognella, P. Haidl, J. B. Texereau and R. Kessler, "An international randomized study of a home-based self-management program for severe COPD: the COMET," *International Journal of COPD,* vol. 11, pp. 1447-1451, 2016.

[47] Koff, P. B., S. Min, T. Freitag, D. L. Diaz, S. S. James, N. F. Voelkel, D. J. Linderman, F. D. del Valle, J. K. Zakrajsek, R. K. Albert, T. M. Bull, A. Beck, T. J. Stelzner, D. P. Ritzwoller, C. M. Kveton, S. Carwin, M. Ghosh, R. L. Keith, J. M. Westfall and W. Vandivier, "Impact of Proactive Integrated Care on Chronic Obstructive Pulmonary Diseas," *Journal of the COPD Foundation,* vol. 8, no. 1, pp. 100-116, 2021.

[48] Houchen-Wolloff, L., M. Orme, A. Barradell, L. Clinch, E. Chaplin, N. Gardiner and S. J. Singh, "Web-Based Self-management Program (SPACE for COPD) for Individuals Hospitalized With an Acute Exacerbation of Chronic Obstructive Pulmonary Disease: Nonrandomized Feasibility Trial of Acceptability," *JMIR Mhealth and Uhealth,* vol. 9, no. 6, p. e21728, 2021.

[49] North, M., S. Bourne, B. Green, A. J. Chauhan, T. Brown, J. Winter, T. Jones, D. Neville, A. Blythin, A. Watson, M. Johnson, D. Culliford, J. Elkes, V. Cornelius and T. M. A. Wilkinson, "A randomised controlled feasibility trial of E-health application supported care vs usual care after exacerbation of COPD: the RESCUE trial," *NPJ Digit Med,* vol. 3, no. 1, p. 150, 2020.

[50] Stamenova, V., K. Liang, R. Yang, K. Engel, F. van Lieshout, E. Lalingo, A. Cheung, A. Erwood, M. Radina, A. Greenwald, P. Agarwal, A. Sidhu, R. Bhatia, J. Shaw, R. Shafai and O. Bhattacharyya,

"Technology-enabled self-management of chronic obstructive pulmonary disease with or without asynchronous remote monitoring: Randomized controlled trial," *J Med Internet Res,* vol. 22, no. 7, p. e18598, 2020.

[51] Rubio, N., R. A. Parker, E. M. Drost, H. Pinnock, C. J. Weir, J. Hanley, L. C. Mantoani, W. MacNee, B. McKinstry and R. A. Rabinovich, "Home monitoring of breathing rate in people with chronic obstructive pulmonary disease: observational study of feasibility, acceptability, and change after exacerbation," *Int J Chron Obstruct Pulmon Dis,* vol. 12, pp. 1221-1231, 2017.

[52] Deng, N., J. Chen, Y. Liu, S. Wei, S. Sheng, R. Lu, Z. Wang, J. Zhu, J. An, B. Wang, H. Lin, X. Wang, Y. Zhou, H. Duan and P. Ran, "Using Mobile Health Technology to Deliver a Community-Based Closed-Loop Management System for Chronic Obstructive Pulmonary Disease Patients in Remote Areas of China: Development and Prospective Observational Study," *JMIR mHealth and uHealth,* vol. 8, no. 11, p. e15978, 2020.

[53] Majothi, S., K. Jolly, N. R. Heneghan, M. J. Price, R. D. Riley, A. M. Turner, S. E. Bayliss, D. J. Moore, S. J. Singh, P. Adab, D. A. Fitzmaurice and R. E. Jordan, "Supported self-management for patients with copd who have recently been discharged from hospital: A systematic review and meta-analysis," *Int J Chron Obstruct Pulmon Dis,* vol. 10, pp. 852-867, 2015.

[54] Maddocks, M., S. S. C. Kon, S. J. Singh and W. D.-C. Man, "Rehabilitation following hospitalization in patients with COPD: Can it reduce readmissions?," *Respirology,* vol. 20, no. 3, pp. 395-404, 2015.

[55] Lenferink, A., M. Brusse-Keizer, P. D. van der Valk, P. A. Frith, M. Zwerink, E. M. Monninkhof, J. van der Palen and T. W. Effing, "Self-management interventions including action plans for exacerbations versus usual care in patients with chronic obstructive pulmonary disease," *Cochrane Database Syst Rev,* vol. 8, no. 8, p. CD011682, 2017.

[56] Harrison, S. L., T. Januadis-Ferreira, D. Brooks, L. Desveaux and R. S. Goldstein, "Self-Management Following an Acute Exacerbation of COPD: A Systematic Review," *Chest,* vol. 147, no. 3, pp. 646-661, 2020.

[57] Shnaigat, M., S. Downie and H. Hosseinzadeh, "Effectiveness of patient activation interventions on chronic obstructive pulmonary disease self-management outcomes: A systematic review," *Aust J Rural Health,* vol. 30, no. 1, pp. 8-21, 2022.

[58] Kessler, R., P. Casan-Clara, D. Koehler, S. Tognella, J. L. Viejo, R. W. Dal Negro, S. Diaz-Lobato, K. Reissing, J. M. Rodriguez-Moro, G. Devouassoux, J. Chavaillon, P. Botrus, J. Arnal, J. Ancochea, A. Bergeron-Lafaurie, C. De Abajo, W. J. Randerath, A. Bastian, C. G. Cornelissen, G. Nilius, J. B. Texereau and J. Bourbeau, "COMET: a multicomponent home-based disease-management programme versus routine care in severe COPD," *Eur Respir J,* vol. 51, p. 1701612, 2018.

[59] JHM, "*Peak Flow Measurement*," Johns Hopkins Medicine, 2022. [Online]. https://www.hopkinsmedicine.org/health/treatment-tests-and-therapies/peak-flow-measurement. [Accessed 20 04 2022].

Chapter 26

Digital Health Applications in COPD Management: Structural Roadmap for Successful Implementation

Saeed M. Alghamdi[1,2,*], PhD,
Keir E. J. Philip[1], MRCP,
Abdulelah M. Aldhahir[3], PhD
and Abdullah A. Alqarni[4], PhD
[1]National Heart and Lung Institute,
Imperial College London, London, UK
[2]Clinical Technology Department,
Faculty of Applied Medical Science,
Umm-Al Qura University, Makkah, Saudi Arabia
[3]Respiratory Therapy Department,
Faculty of Applied Medical Sciences,
Jazan University, Jazan, Saudi Arabia
[4]Department of Respiratory Therapy,
Faculty of Medical Rehabilitation Sciences,
King Abdulaziz University, Jeddah, Saudi Arabia

Abstract

The application of digital health approaches in chronic obstructive pulmonary disease (COPD) management is increasing, providing considerable opportunities in helping with symptom management, reduce health resource utilisation, and improve health status. Optimisation the accessibility and quality of digital health approaches in COPD management requires the identification and integration of context, mechanism, and intended outcome. Current digital health solutions in COPD care vary in terms of context of application, mechanisms of impact, and intended outcomes/impacts. Context refers to the intervention settings which the digital health solutions are proposed, the components of those solutions, and the populations targeted. Digital health mechanisms of impact are shaped by factors such as content, mode of delivery, strategy, intensity, and level of professional support. Additionally, the consideration of other factors, including patient engagement and co-creation, are required for effective intervention development. Optimisation of implementation has four central determinants and consideration, namely patient needs, familiarity with the technology, healthcare professional support, and data privacy. Current research suggests digital health solutions for COPD can be improve

* Corresponding Author's Email: alghamdi18@imperial.ac.uk.

In: Chronic Obstructive Pulmonary Disease
Editor: Jaber S. Alqahtani
ISBN: 979-8-88697-333-4

symptom management, detecting exacerbations, and improving physical activity and quality of life.

Keywords: digital health application, telehealth, COPD

Introduction

Chronic obstructive pulmonary disease (COPD) is a common progressive respiratory disease that is growing in prevalence worldwide. It is treatable and preventable, characterised by persistent airflow limitations predominantly caused by noxious gas exposures, including smoking and air pollution, leading to chronic inflammatory responses in the airways and the lungs [1]. The Global Initiative for Chronic Obstructive Lung Disease (GOLD) develops guidelines for COPD diagnosis, treatment, prevention, and management to assess the characteristics of COPD on a global scale and maximise available resources to support COPD care [1]. Existing digital health solutions for COPD have shown promise as behavioural and therapeutic interventions. A growing body of research supports various roles relating to self-management education, and the remote delivery of healthcare services, therefore helping individuals living with COPD manage their symptoms, reduce hospitalisations, and improve health status [2-5].

Digital Solutions in Health Services

Information and Communications Technology (ICT) is being increasingly used in clinical practice as a tool to aid in the assessment, monitoring, and treatment of COPD [6]. Due to its rapid emergence and expansion, ICT in the medical field is known by many different names and labels [6]. The terms 'digital health' and 'telehealth' have become the most common terminologies to describe this integration of ICT and healthcare services. These are currently the preferred terms because they capture the broad range of applications of using technology in healthcare delivery [7]. The term 'digital health' is broader, defined as "the use of digital technologies for health." Digital health is a broad concept that covering applications in planning, monitoring, assessment, diagnosis, education, and treatment [8]. *Tele* is a Greek word meaning "at a distance," so telehealth is the provision of healthcare at a distance [9, 10]. Telehealth is defined as the "use of electronic information and telecommunications technology to support long-distance clinical healthcare (including remote monitoring), health-related education for patients (including chronic patients) and professionals, public health, and health administration" [11]. Some ambiguity remains regarding terminology and interventions associated with digital health, with different terms being used interchangeably; alternative terms include telemonitoring, telerehabilitation, tele-homecare, teleconsultations, and tele-education [12]. Digital health has been used successfully in multiple healthcare disciplines, including cardio-respiratory disease management and the provision of home care or self-management for patients with chronic diseases such as COPD [11, 12]. Examples from the literature of the digital technologies and applications used for COPD care supplied in Figure 1.

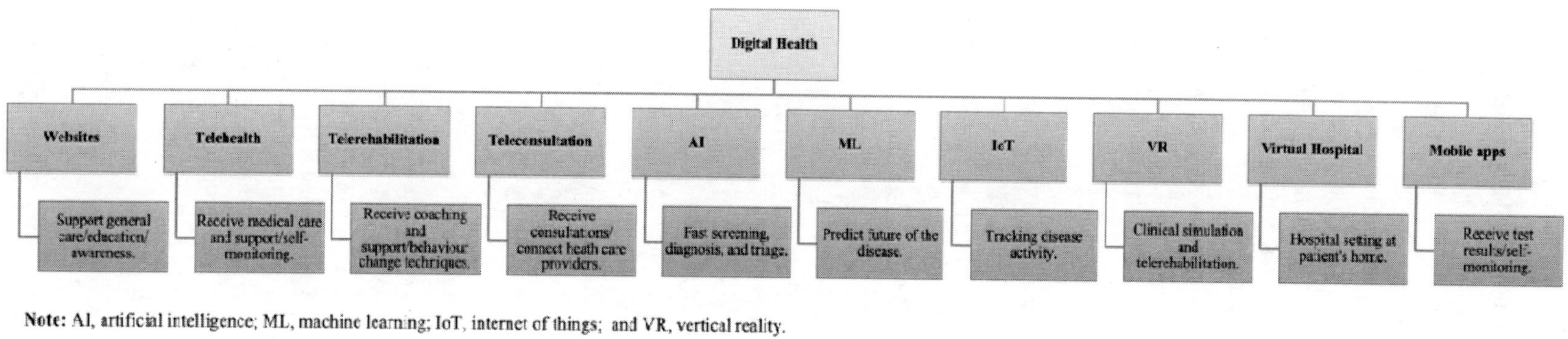

Note: AI, artificial intelligence; ML, machine learning; IoT, internet of things; and VR, vertical reality.

Figure 1. Examples of the digital technologies and applications that are used for COPD.

Optimising Digital Health Use in COPD Management

Digital health can be used in COPD care to improve the timeframe of therapeutic contact or as an alternative tool when access to care is not available [13]. Self-management is a core component of COPD management, which systematic reviews and meta-analyses show, can be supported by digital health solutions, especially for users with transport or economic limitations or geographical barriers through the use of remote delivery/telehealth applications [12, 14]. Reducing healthcare costs is another important consideration, where, digital health approaches could be used, potentially lowering costs while maintaining the quality of treatment in primary care clinics, decrease the pressure on special care clinics, deliver tailored care, and facilitate coordination of care among healthcare professionals [15]. Digital health applications can also facilitate educational opportunities for healthcare professionals, patients and caregivers [16]. Applications supporting self-management be particularly effective incorporating frequent reminders to users to practice behaviour that strengthens existing behaviours like self-monitoring and self-efficacy [17]. Further applications relate to telemonitoring which have the potential to facilitate early detection of COPD exacerbations, supporting prompt treatment aiming to reduce exacerbation severity and reduce emergency department attendances and hospital admissions [18].

Development and innovation in digital health are increasing rapidly [19]. However, effective integration and implementation within existing healthcare provision is required. Digital health is perhaps best considered as a potentially important element within the package we provide to healthcare users and the wider healthcare community, which could range from simple additional components such as pedometers, to complex interventions such as telerehabilitation.

In order to evaluate the functionality of digital health solutions in supporting disease management, three components must be considered: the context and content, the intended mechanism of action, and the intended outcomes or clinical impacts. However, one must also be aware that the specifics of these components is an area of ongoing discussion and clarification [20, 21].

Central to resolving this conflict is an understanding of the functionality of specific digital health solutions in COPD management [22, 23]. Functionality could be approached from a theoretical perspective when considering the associations between context, mechanisms, and outcomes of current digital health solutions for supporting disease management. In this way, conceptual frameworks can then be applied to identify and enhance the key elements and their connections.

This chapter discusses current evidence to consider in relation to leading a successful digital health solution in COPD management. Furthermore, we propose a guide for digital health application, specifically for improving disease management and self-management approaches. As such, we aim to facilitate the development and implementation of effective digital health interventions in COPD care, to achieve the targeted health outcomes.

Context of Digital Health Solutions

The context of digital health in COPD management includes three important factors: intervention settings, the process of intervention development, and identification of targeted populations.

Intervention Settings

The value of digital health applications in a range of intervention settings has potential benefits as described earlier in this chapter [24]. For example, in primary clinical settings, telehealth can facilitate communication between the healthcare professionals and patients and provide monitoring and assessment between clinical visits [25]. Such approaches have been found to be helpful in providing prompt feedback and enhancing exercise and treatment adherence [25].

As previously mentioned, telehealth can be used for health education and promotion of self-care. For example, Nield and Hoo [26] evaluated the acceptability and feasibility of real-time interactive voice and video calls via Skype for teaching breathing exercises and decreasing dyspnoea compared to usual care. The study results demonstrated that people who received the teaching via Skype experience less dyspnoea than with the usual care [27]. Tsai et al. evaluated the effects of remote coaching using digital health versus self-training without coaching in COPD, on physical activity levels [28]. The coaching in this study was provided by professionals as part of a telerehabilitation programme. The study found that exercise coaching using remote coaching helped COPD patients increase adherence and exercise capacity compared to self-coaching without remotely delivered coaching [28]. The aforementioned digital health solutions were described implementation in primary care settings. Secondary (and tertiary) care settings present other challenges that can be addressed using digital health solutions, including facilitating coordination of care between primary and secondary healthcare centres, and consultations with patients who do not live locally [29-32].

This coordination of care allows healthcare providers like specialists to assess patients and provide advice on the COPD action plan without travelling to the patient's area, or requiring the patients travel to the specialist centre [31, 32]. Mostly, this kind of digital health solution refers to teleconsultations [33]. Consideration of setting up and logistics requirements have become a necessary consideration for clinical COPD services, as an increasing proportion of providers are moving towards predominantly, or entirely, digital health provision. Drivers of this transition include infectious disease pandemics and outbreaks [34], and strategic plans to cut the burden of disease costs [35].

Digital Health Solutions Development

According to Consolidated Standards of Reporting Trials of Electronic and Mobile Health Applications and onLine TeleHealth (CONSORT-EHEALTH), telehealth interventions belong in one of three categories [36]. First, an educational tool to provide education and improve patient knowledge such as the "living well with COPD" resources or the "Asthma+Lung UK" Website and resources [37, 38]. Second, an electronic tool for communication and facilitating home monitoring and/or remote monitoring for individuals with COPD [39-41]. Third, comprehensive telehealth intervention to provide education, monitoring, assessment, and treatment to help the condition management, such as the virtual hospital [42, 43]. Development of digital health solutions in COPD must also consider patient engagement, which is found to be an overwhelmingly positive approach to optimise implementation [44].

COPD Populations

The GOLD guidelines were widely used in previous telehealth studies to identify and scale the severity of individuals with COPD as to who will get benefits from digital health solutions. As described earlier, COPD populations were classified according to airflow limitations, e.g., Force Expiratory Volume at 1 Second (FEV_1%) post-bronchodilators. The four GOLD grades are mild, moderate, severe, and very severe COPD [45]. So far, research suggests that a range of digital health solutions have been successfully applied for people with moderate to severe COPD, with predicted $FEV_1 < 50\%$, and patients who were recently hospitalised due to exacerbations [46, 47]. Further research exploring potential applications in other groups would provide useful additions to current research findings.

Mechanism

Digital health solutions for COPD are mostly multicomponent 'complex interventions,' however others are relatively simple or are non- interventional [48]. For example, certain telehealth tools only provide remote monitoring (telemonitoring) for COPD without any further interventions or even self-management or education [49, 50], while others provide a virtual hospital in the patient's home [3, 51]. The intended mechanism of impact delivered through digital health solutions broad, can be complex, and depends in part on the standard care and available resources. To describe the mechanisms through which digital health solutions aim to support COPD management, we must consider five important factors: content and format delivered by digital health solutions, modes of delivery and level of technology, strategy, professional support, and intensity of remote monitoring (including frequency and duration).

Content

Content of digital health solutions can be considered in two broad and overlapping categories. Firstly, the digitalization of existing evidence-based components of COPD care, and secondly, novel components of care made possible by digital health technologies. Evidence presents a wide range of variations in the content of digital health solutions that support COPD management [12, 21]. The variation in the content comes from the different perspectives on self-management support and/or different guidelines for managing COPD. For instance, self-management with COPD has been defined as the ability of individuals to master a broad range of tasks that include managing symptoms, physical activity, mental consequences, and lifestyle components while living with a chronic disease [52, 53]. This support flows through a continuous opening channel via digital health solutions and could include periodic home visits or calls to follow up with patients and give them feedback [54]. Studies show that the content of the self-management can be delivered via several digital health technologies, such as patient portals [55], secure webpages [56], internet platforms [57], special modems [58], videoconferences [59], clinical decision software [60], smartphone applications [61], professional call centres [62], and automated call centres [63]. In this context, all these technologies were facilitators for delivering the content and enhancing remote monitoring.

Based on the published work, studies of digital solutions that support disease management covered one or a combination of the following subjects: 1) symptoms management (i.e., breathlessness, medications, action plan), 2) physical activity (i.e., exercise training, maintaining a healthy lifestyle, energy-conserving technique), 3) psychological and health behaviours (smoking cessations, adherence, compliance, problem-solving, self-efficacy, stress and anxiety management) [57].

First, in symptom management using digital health solutions, the content was described in the literature as giving the patients instructions, advice, and recommendations on what actions must be taken to control symptoms, such as initiating a rescue pack of antibiotics or increasing the dose of the medication (i.e., Ventolin puffs), provide breathing exercises or techniques (i.e., pursed-lip breathing), and visits when to contact a health professional for further assessment [64-66]. Launching patient-professional communication or professional-professional communication to visualise and monitor symptoms, observe patient's behaviour toward suggested treatment and provide advice increased the patient's knowledge [64-66]. Health behaviours are at the core of self-management techniques and help both patients and professionals detect deterioration at an early stage. Digital solutions to track symptoms seemed effective in following up with patients who were recently discharged from the hospital [7, 43, 49].

The second frequently delivered content type is physical activity focused interventions via digital health. Physical activity interventions have been described as giving the patient instructions, advice, and recommendations on how to perform exercise and training [59, 67-69]. The exercises include one or a combination of the followings components: 1) structured physical exercise, 2) techniques for performing daily activities, 3) sitting exercises, 4) stretching and leg exercises, and 5) techniques to conserve energy. This content is mostly for stable COPD patients without recent exacerbations [59, 67-69].

The third content is mental health wellbeing support. Mental wellbeing support has been described [24-29] as giving the users instructions, advice, and recommendations on psychological support [27, 29, 70-73]. That psychological support could include one or a combination of the behaviour change techniques. The most common behaviour change techniques in digital health solutions with COPD were described in detail elsewhere [23]. Mostly mental health and wellbeing interventions delivered to the patient in person by the healthcare providers, when telemonitoring systems identified concerns. Healthcare providers then contacted the patients to provide appropriate mental health and wellbeing support, frequently including information, reassurance, guidance and relaxation advice [23].

In summary, digital health solutions for COPD management are heterogenic in terms of resource content [12, 57]. Such approaches are increasingly used to support symptom management is used to evaluate the patient's status after discharge from the hospital, and it depends on the available telemonitoring systems. Second, enhancing physical activity is based on local guidelines. Third, the mental health and wellbeing support targeting the anxiety and depression which are commonly associated with COPD. Delivering these types of content via digital health solutions requires a robust mechanism associated with the contents to explain how digital health solutions support feasibility and accessibility to improve health outcomes in people with COPD. [21, 30] Despite the variety in the content delivered using digital health information transfer for people with COPD, current approaches use almost exclusively text or video format. Text format could be delivered in many different modes like instruction books, written guidelines, websites and online resources, and SMS messages [49, 67, 74], while video format could be used to coach or teach the users a specific exercise and/or provide recorded education and instructions [26, 28, 75].

Mode of Delivery

Modes of delivery for digital health solutions in COPD care have been defined in the literature as the way the content is delivered to users [76]. Since technology is a fast-growing field, it is obvious that care can be delivered using many different styles and generations. In the literature, we found a variety of descriptions of modes of delivery for digital health support [77], but in this chapter, we consider ICT as a crucial factor contributing to the delivery of the content and, from that perspective, digital health support has been summarised as one of the three modes.

The first delivery mode used asynchronous digital health support [78], where the patient's data was stored on a secure modem. Then, COPD management was provided later by healthcare professionals through digital health. The second delivery mode used synchronised digital health support, where digital systems recognised data changes to alert the healthcare centre or healthcare team, but the system did not provide 24/7 communication (i.e., online chat, email) [78]. Both asynchronous and synchronous modes are considered as slow response digital health support [78]. The third mode used immediate and live analytics, support and decision-making from the monitoring centre and is available 24/7 for the users (i.e., predesigned algorithms and machine learning), and this mode is considered real-time digital health support [78]. Nowadays, advanced synchronised digital health support via machine learning (ML) and artificial intelligence (AI) are growing and getting more attention. It involves using existing data to develop and train statistical models to support the clinical judgment. The simple version of this method is described as reviewing the patterns in the data to reach an informed conclusion. It can be used to diagnose or treat people with COPD. Establishing these methods in COPD management requires a lot of data and is still under review by experts [79].

Strategies of Delivering COPD Management via Digital Health Support

Individual Strategy

The best example to describe this strategy is mobile health apps [7, 37, 75]. In terms of interaction, the users are required to access the mobile app to get feedback from the healthcare provider regarding their conditions and/or get feedback from a predesigned algorithm [80, 81]. In terms of technology, it also required advanced technology devices with internet access (i.e., smart cell phone or tablet) to visualise, send, or receive information. This mode has partial interaction between the users and the healthcare provider, but it has full interaction between the user and the technology device. For example, it could be delivered to the patient using well-known platforms such as "Living well with COPD" [82] and "my COPD" [83]. These platforms allow the patient to have access to the education programme, and it can be seen any time the patient pleases [37, 82-84]. Another proposed approach for individual strategy included using a designed platform based on the local guidelines. It required the patient to access the platform to do self-monitoring and receive education, support, and feedback from the healthcare provider [75]. This strategy mostly enhances personalised care for COPD patients [85].

Group Strategy

The best example of this strategy is providing services in regular meetings, also known as community-based health support [49, 67, 74, 86]. In terms of interaction, this digital health strategy engages interaction between consumers and healthcare professionals. It does not require advanced communication technology but it needs more effort from the patient and healthcare provider to complete the session or meet competencies [87]. For the healthcare provided, it required qualified healthcare professionals to deliver it. It might require the patient to attend the clinical or community centre to receive support [86]. The best example to explain this strategy is providing community-based pulmonary telerehabilitation for COPD [86, 87].

Intensity

Duration and Frequency

Treatment or management sessions for COPD via digital health solutions are presented at different intervals and durations. For example, some studies provide COPD management sessions for 10 to 20 minutes per day, which mostly consist of pulmonary rehabilitation and breathing exercises [28, 41, 88, 89]. Others provided the same session length per week [26, 46, 90, 91]. It seems that specific aspects of management via digital health (i.e., breathing exercise and pursed-lip breathing) take less time than comprehensive disease management (i.e., exercise coaching, energy conservation, medication follow-up, nutrition, stress management). Regarding the frequency of sessions, daily or weekly frequencies for a short time duration are seen more frequently in the literature [12, 92]. That frequency supports the ultimate goal of using digital health tools in disease management and assisting clinical decisions to improve patient health outcomes [12]. Technical aspects could play an important role here. For example, digital health solutions that used mobile devices were provided daily and follow-up and support were more frequent [28, 41, 75, 88], while the studies that used sedentary devices were less frequent [26, 46, 90, 91].

Outcomes

Health Outcomes

Digital health solutions that support COPD management have a variety of outcomes. That variety might come from the inconsistency in terms of using a theoretical model when the researchers designed a telehealth tool [93]. For example, if a researcher plans to design a study to understand the acceptance of digital health solutions for COPD, then the outcome measures for the study must be related to the constructs in that technology acceptance model, such as perceived ease of use and perceived usefulness [94]. Telehealth studies in the literature targeted various outcomes, including clinical outcomes, treatment costs or treatment adherence, and changes in patient behaviour [95-97]. Also, clinical outcomes such as time to exacerbation, emergency department (ED) visits, hospitalisation due to respiratory exacerbation [98], need for non-invasive mechanical ventilation [99], length of stay (LOS) [100], physical activity [101], health status, and health-related quality of life [102] were mostly measured as primary or secondary outcomes [97].

A study by Clave et al. found digital health solutions in COPD management are safe, useful tools to reduce healthcare utilisation [90]. However, evidence found no significant changes in these outcomes. Another example, a trial by Shay et al. evaluated ED visits, hospitalisation, and length of stay as clinical outcomes. The evidence showed that digital health solutions that support COPD management have no impact on ED visits [43].

Results were variable and controversial regarding the impact of digital health solutions on physical activity outcomes. For example, digital health applications could be promising in improving physical activity in COPD, either during the time of the exercise or the adherence to the exercise [28, 40]. However, studies show that physical activity could deteriorate with digital health applications [39, 103].

Looking at health status and health-related quality of life (HRQoL) outcomes, we found that studies used either specific or generic instruments to measure these outcomes. For example, HRQoL outcomes were measured using specific questionnaires such as the Saint George Respiratory Questionnaire (SGRQ) [104], the Chronic Respiratory Disease Questionnaire (CRQ) [46], and the Clinical COPD Questionnaire (CCQ) [105] and the studies found digital health solutions effective to improve HRQoL, while generic instruments such as the 36-item short-form survey (SF-36) [106] and the 12-item short-form survey (SF-12) [107] showed negative results or no change in the quality of life.

Additionally, the trend is to measure the cost-effectiveness of reducing healthcare utilisation in COPD management. Cost-effectiveness evaluations in the literature were presented according to the variation in the healthcare systems. However, evidence shows lower costs associated with digital health solutions in COPD management [108-110]. For example, it was found effective in saving healthcare resources (i.e., general practitioner visits, specialist visits) compared to traditional healthcare [111]. The same positive results regarding costs were found in a study by Koff et al., where digital health solutions minimised the cost of care by >20% per person [104].

Determinants of Digital Health Solutions

Before implementing digital health solutions for COPD management, stakeholders and policymakers must think about the factors that influence adaption and adherence (Figure 2). Providing individuals with easy access to basic and advanced communication technologies and digital health platforms is an important determinant. Other factors are the presence of well-trained healthcare experts to manage and administer the platform and a technical support team available 24 hours a day, seven days a week to resolve any technical issues. Third, data transformations on the envisaged digital health platforms must be safe. Fourth, platform users' needs must be taken into account, such as hearing and vision limitations in the elderly. [112].

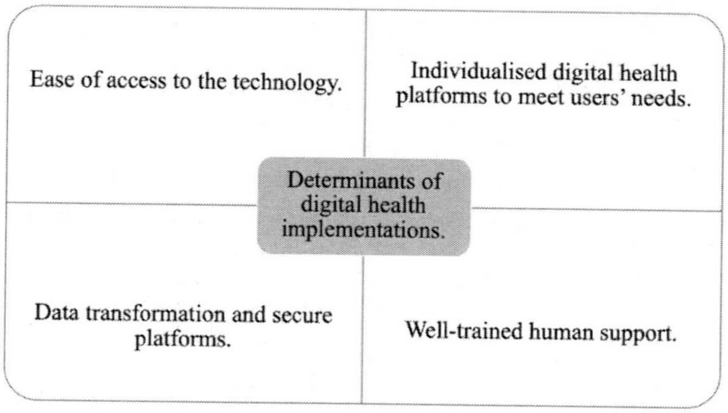

Figure 2. Determinants of digital health solutions.

Other Promising Applications for Digital Health in COPD Management

The use of digital health in giving medical education and training (tele-education) is evident, especially following a disruption in direct management, training sessions, seminars, and medical education. Even in intensive care units (ICUs), tele-education and/or remote training via Zoom (San Jose, California), Skype (Luxembourg), or Microsoft Teams (Redmond, Washington, United State) has supplanted traditional techniques in teaching and training programmes [113]. In the COPD management, this experience has positive influence [114, 115].

The use of virtual ICUs in management has risen rapidly to address a dearth of healthcare workers and to facilitate family visits to critically sick patients [116]. The use of virtual ICU had positive results in terms of reducing physiological stress and anxiety and enhancing staff morale, according to cross-sectional data [117]. In addition, virtual ICU is an excellent opportunity for family members to share their joy and relief [116].

Virtual reality (VR) has played a significant role in the treatment of COPD patients. One of the most important applications of VR is in pain management for COPD patients with back pain. Experts have proved that using VR to provide care to those people is a feasible and powerful tool in healthcare delivery. In addition, VR can be a fun tool to stimulate physical activity among persons in pulmonary rehabilitation programmes [118]. VR is extremely beneficial since it allows these patients to continue their treatment at home, avoiding the need to visit community centres and hospitals. As a result, VR plays a critical role, particularly for those who are highly fragile [119].

AI is considered one of the innovative new forms of technology that has helped in COPD diagnosis [120]. Kaplen et al. evaluated the ability of AI to detect COPD diagnosis, and the results showed that AI can distinguish between COPD and asthma [120]. AI can therefore provide rapid information for making medical decisions [121].

Conclusion

Digital health solutions in COPD management can be different in content, mechanism, and outcome, all of which have contributed to their efficiency and effectiveness. Current evidence suggested that using digital health solutions in COPD management can provide benefits such as detecting early exacerbations, enhancing physical activity, and managing symptoms. Implementing effective digital health solutions for COPD must consider determinants such as ease of use of the technology and the presence of well-trained healthcare professionals for support. Future research must focus on developing more smart interactive digital health solutions for people diagnosed with COPD.

Key Points

- Digital health for COPD management is a broad concept that covering different applications in planning, monitoring, assessment, diagnosis, education, and treatment.
- Digital health application for COPD management could range from simple additional components such as pedometers, to complex interventions such as telerehabilitation.
- Digital health solutions in COPD management can provide benefits such as detecting early exacerbations, enhancing physical activity, and managing symptoms.
- In order to implement digital health solutions for COPD management, stakeholders and policymakers must consider the determinants that influence adoption and adherence.
- Various advances in digital technology, such as artificial intelligence and machine learning, are being discussed and clarified in support of medical decisions.

References

[1] Venkatesan P. GOLD report: 2022 update. *The Lancet Respiratory Medicine*. 2022;10(2):e20.

[2] Criner GJ, Bourbeau J, Diekemper RL, Ouellette DR, Goodridge D, Hernandez P, Curren, K, Balter, MS, Bhutani, M, Camp, PG, Celli, BR, Dechman, G, Dransfield, MT, Fiel, SB, Foreman, MG, Hanania, NA, Ireland, BK, Marchetti, N, Marciniuk, DD, Mularski, RA, Ornelas, J, Road, JD, Sticklad, MKPrevention of acute exacerbations of COPD: American college of chest physicians and Canadian thoracic society guideline. *Chest Journal*. 2015;147(4):894-942.

[3] Jakobsen, AS, Laursen, LC, Rydahl-Hansen, S, Østergaard, B, Gerds, TA, Emme, C, Schou, L, & Phanareth, K. Home-based telehealth hospitalization for exacerbation of chronic obstructive pulmonary disease: findings from "the virtual hospital" trial. *Telemedicine Journal and E-health: The Official Journal of the American Telemedicine Association*. 2015;21(5):364-73.

[4] Effing, TW, Vercoulen, JH, Bourbeau, J, Trappenburg, J, Lenferink, A, Cafarella, P, Coultas, D, Meek, P, van der Valk, P, Bischoff, EWMA, Bucknall, C, Dewan, NA, Early, F, Fan, V, Frith, P, Janssen, DJA, Mitchell, K, Morgan, M, Nici, L, … van der Palen, J. Definition of a COPD self-management intervention: International Expert Group consensus. *European Respiratory Journal*. 2016:ERJ-00025-2016.

[5] Zwerink M, Brusse-Keizer M, van der Valk PD, Zielhuis GA, Monninkhof EM, van der Palen J, Frith, PA, & Effing, T. Self management for patients with chronic obstructive pulmonary disease. *The Cochrane Library*. 2014.

[6] Darkins A, Darkins AW, Cary MA, Cary M. *Telemedicine And Telehealth: Principles, Policies, Performances and Pitfalls:* Springer Publishing Company; 2000.

[7] Antoniades NC, Rochford PD, Pretto JJ, Pierce RJ, Gogler J, Steinkrug J, Sharpe, K, & McDonald, CF. Pilot study of remote telemonitoring in COPD. *Telemedicine Journal & E-Health*. 2012;18(8):634-40.

[8] Ding H, Fatehi F, Maiorana A, Bashi N, Hu W, Edwards I. Digital health for COPD care: the current state of play. *Journal of Thoracic Disease*. 2019;11(Suppl 17):S2210.

[9] Singh D, Agusti A, Anzueto A, Barnes PJ, Bourbeau J, Celli BR, Criner, GJ, Frith, P, Halpin, DMG, Han, M, Lopez Varela, MV, Martinez, F, Monta de Oca, M, Papi, A, Pavord, ID, Roche, N, Sin, DD, Stockley, R, Vestbo, J, Wedzicha, JA, Vogelmeier, C. Global strategy for the diagnosis, management, and prevention of chronic obstructive lung disease: the GOLD science committee report 2019. *European Respiratory Journal*. 2019;53(5).

[10] Brownsell S. Measuring the 'success' of telehealth interventions. *Journal of Assistive Technologies*. 2009.

[11] Currell R, Urquhart C, Wainwright P, Lewis R. Telemedicine versus face to face patient care: effects on professional practice and health care outcomes. *Cochrane Database of Systematic Reviews*. 2000(2).

[12] Alghamdi SM, Rajah AMA, Aldabayan YS, Aldhahir AM, Alqahtani JS, Alzahrani AA. Chronic Obstructive Pulmonary Disease Patients' Acceptance in E-Health Clinical Trials. *International Journal of Environmental Research and Public Health*. 2021;18(10):5230.

[13] Shaw DK, Heggestad-Hereford JR, Southard DR, Sparks KE. American Association of Cardiovascular and Pulmonary Rehabilitation telemedicine position statement. *Journal of Cardiopulmonary Rehabilitation and Prevention*. 2001;21(5):261-2.

[14] Alghamdi SM, Alsulayyim AS, Alqahtani JS, Aldhahir AM, editors. Digital Health Platforms in Saudi Arabia: Determinants from the COVID-19 Pandemic Experience. *Healthcare*; 2021: Multidisciplinary Digital Publishing Institute.

[15] Joseph V, West RM, Shickle D, Keen J, Clamp S. Key challenges in the development and implementation of telehealth projects. *Journal of Telemedicine andT*. 2011;17(2):71-7.

[16] Inskip J, Lauscher HN, Li L, Dumont G, Garde A, Ho K, Hoens, AM, Road, JD, Ryerson, CJ, & Camp, PG. Patient and health care professional perspectives on using telehealth to deliver pulmonary rehabilitation. *Chronic Respiratory Disease*. 2018;15(1):71-80.

[17] Nguyen HQ, Gill DP, Wolpin S, Steele BG, Benditt JO. Pilot study of a cell phone-based exercise persistence intervention post-rehabilitation for COPD. *International Journal of Chronic Obstructive Pulmonary Disease*. 2009;4:301.

[18] Calvo GS, Gómez-Suárez C, Soriano J, Zamora E, Gónzalez-Gamarra A, González-Béjar M, Jordán, A, Tadeo, E, Sebastián, A, Fernández, G, & Ancochea, J. A home telehealth program for patients with severe COPD: the PROMETE study. *Respiratory medicine*. 2014;108(3):453-62.

[19] Barlow J. *Managing Innovation in Healthcare*. World Scientific Publishing Company, 2016.

[20] Jonkman, NH, Westland, H, Trappenburg, JCA, Groenwold, RHH, Bischoff, EWMA., Bourbeau, J, Bucknall, CE, Coultas, D, Effing, TW, Epton, M, Gallefoss, F, Garcia-Aymerich, J, Lloyd, SM, Monninkhof, EM, Nguyen, HQ, van der Palen, J, Rice, KL, Sedeno, M, Taylor, SJC, … Schuurmans, MJ. Characteristics of effective self-management interventions in patients with COPD: individual patient data meta-analysis. *European Respiratory Journal*. 2016:ERJ-01860-2015.

[21] Newham JJ, Presseau J, Heslop-Marshall K, Russell S, Ogunbayo OJ, Netts P, Hanratty, B, Kaner, E. Features of self-management interventions for people with COPD associated with improved health-related quality of life and reduced emergency department visits: a systematic review and meta-analysis. *International Journal of Chronic Obstructive Pulmonary Disease*. 2017;12:1705.

[22] Alghamdi S, Alqahtani J, Aldhahir A, Alrajeh A, Aldabayan Y. Effectiveness of telehealth-based interventions with chronic obstructive pulmonary disease: A systematic review and meta-analysis. *B103 Treatment of Obstructive Lung Disease*. 2020:A4308-A.

[23] Alghamdi SM, Al Rajeh A. Top Ten Behavioral Change Techniques Used in Telehealth Intervention With COPD: A Systematic Review. *Respiratory Care*; 2019.

[24] Zhang X-Y, Zhang P. Telemedicine in clinical setting. *Experimental and Therapeutic Medicine*. 2016;12(4):2405-7.

[25] Velardo C, Shah SA, Gibson O, Clifford G, Heneghan C, Rutter H, Farmer, A, & Tarassenko, L. Digital health system for personalised COPD long-term management. *BMC Medical Informatics and Decision Making*. 2017;17(1):1-13.

[26] Nield M, Hoo GW. Real-time telehealth for COPD self-management using SkypeTM. *Copd: Journal of Chronic Obstructive Pulmonary Disease*. 2012;9(6):611-9.

[27] Nield M, Hoo GWS. Real-time telehealth for COPD self-management using Skype™. *COPD: Journal of Chronic Obstructive Pulmonary Disease*. 2012;9(6):611-9.

[28] Tsai LL, McNamara RJ, Moddel C, Alison JA, McKenzie DK, McKeough ZJ. Home-based telerehabilitation via real-time videoconferencing improves endurance exercise capacity in patients with COPD: The randomized controlled TeleR Study. *Respirology*. 2017;22(4):699-707.

[29] Trappenburg JC, Niesink A, de Weert-van Oene GH, van der Zeijden H, van Snippenburg R, Peters A, Lammers, JWJ, & Schrijvers, AJP. Effects of telemonitoring in patients with chronic obstructive pulmonary disease. *Telemedicine and e-Health*. 2008;14(2):138-46.

[30] Jonkman NH, Westland H, Trappenburg JC, Groenwold RH, Bischoff EW, Bourbeau J, Bucknall, CE, Coultas, D, Effing, TW, Epton, M, Gallefoss, F, Garcia-Aymerich, J, Lloyd, SM, Monninkhof, EM, Nguyen, HQ, van der Palen, J, Rice, KL, Sedeno, M, Taylor, SJC, … Schuurmans, MJ. Characteristics of effective self-management interventions in patients with COPD: individual patient data meta-analysis. *European Respiratory Journal*. 2016;48(1):55-68.

[31] Fromer L. Implementing chronic care for COPD: planned visits, care coordination, and patient empowerment for improved outcomes. *International Journal of Chronic Obstructive Pulmonary Disease*. 2011;6:605.

[32] Slevin P. *Human-centred recommendations to maximise the potential for digital health in the management of chronic obstructive pulmonary disease*. Doctoral Thesis, University College Dublin. 2020.

[33] Sorknaes AD, Bech M, Madsen H, Titlestad IL, Hounsgaard L, Hansen-Nord M, Jest, P, Olesen, F, Lauridsen, J, & Østergaard, B. The effect of real-time teleconsultations between hospital-based nurses and patients with severe COPD discharged after an exacerbation. *Journal of Telemedicine and Telecare*. 2013;19(8):466-74.

[34] Alqahtani JS, Oyelade T, Aldhahir AM, Mendes RG, Alghamdi SM, Miravitlles M, Mandal, S, & Hurst, JR. Reduction in hospitalised COPD exacerbations during COVID-19: A systematic review and meta-analysis. *PLoS One*. 2021;16(8):e0255659.

[35] Paré G, Sicotte C, St.-Jules D, Gauthier R. Cost-minimization analysis of a telehomecare program for patients with chronic obstructive pulmonary disease. *Telemedicine Journal & e-Health*. 2006; 12(2):114-21.

[36] Eysenbach G, Group C-E. CONSORT-EHEALTH: improving and standardizing evaluation reports of Web-based and mobile health interventions. *Journal of Medical Internet Research*. 2011;13(4).

[37] Marquis N, Larivee P, Saey D, Dubois MF, Tousignant M. In-Home Pulmonary Telerehabilitation for Patients with Chronic Obstructive Pulmonary Disease: A Pre-experimental Study on Effectiveness, Satisfaction, and Adherence. *Telemedicine Journal & E-Health*. 2015;21(11):870-9.

[38] Foundation BL. *COPD* (chronic obstructive pulmonary disease). 2022. https://www.blf.org.uk/support-for-you/copd.

[39] Cameron-Tucker HL, Wood-Baker R, Joseph L, Walters JA, Schuz N, Walters EH. A randomized controlled trial of telephone-mentoring with home-based walking preceding rehabilitation in COPD. *International Journal of Copd*. 2016;11:1991-2000.

[40] Franke KJ, Domanski U, Schroeder M, Jansen V, Artmann F, Weber U, Ettler, R, Nilius, G. Telemonitoring of home exercise cycle training in patients with COPD. *International Journal of COPD*. 2016;11(1):2821-9.

[41] Halpin DMG, Laing-Morton T, Spedding S, Levy ML, Coyle P, Lewis J, Newbold, P, & Marno, P. A randomised controlled trial of the effect of automated interactive calling combined with a health risk forecast on frequency and severity of exacerbations of COPD assessed clinically and using EXACT PRO. *Primary Care Respiratory Journal*. 2011;20(3):324-31.

[42] Rosenbek Minet L, Hansen LW, Pedersen CD, Titlestad IL, Christensen JK, Kidholm K, Rayce, K, Bowes, A, & Møllegård, L. Early telemedicine training and counselling after hospitalization in patients with severe chronic obstructive pulmonary disease: a feasibility study. *BMC Medical Informatics & Decision Making*. 2015;15(1):124-.

[43] Shany T, Hession M, Pryce D, Roberts M, Basilakis J, Redmond S, Lovell, N, & Schreier, G. A small-scale randomised controlled trial of home telemonitoring in patients with severe chronic obstructive pulmonary disease. *Journal of Telemedicine & Telecare*. 2017;23(7):650-6.

[44] Lundell S, Toots A, Sönnerfors P, Halvarsson A, Wadell K. Participatory methods in a digital setting: experiences from the co-creation of an eHealth tool for people with chronic obstructive pulmonary disease. *BMC Medical Informatics and Decision Making*. 2022;22(1):1-14.

[45] GOLD GIfCOLD. Diagnosis of Disease of Chronic Airflow Limitation: Asthma, COPD and Asthma-COPD Overlap Syndrome (ACOS). *Global Initiative for Chronic Obstructive Lung Disease GOLD, Disease GIFCOL*; 2017 2015.

[46] Chau JPC, Lee DTF, Yu DSF, Chow AYM, Yu WC, Chair SY, Lai, ASF, & Chick, YL. A feasibility study to investigate the acceptability and potential effectiveness of a telecare service for older people with chronic obstructive pulmonary disease. *International Journal of Medical Informatics*. 2012;81 (10):674-82.

[47] McDowell JE, McClean S, FitzGibbon F, Tate S. A randomised clinical trial of the effectiveness of home-based health care with telemonitoring in patients with COPD. *Journal of Telemedicine & Telecare*. 2015;21(2):80-7.

[48] Pearce G, Parke HL, Pinnock H, Epiphaniou E, Bourne CL, Sheikh A, Taylor, SJ. The PRISMS taxonomy of self-management support: derivation of a novel taxonomy and initial testing of its utility. *Journal of Health Services Research & Policy*. 2016;21(2):73-82.

[49] Berkhof FF, Van Den Berg JWK, Uil SM, Kerstjens HAM. Telemedicine, the effect of nurse-initiated telephone follow up, on health status and health-care utilization in COPD patients: A randomized trial. *Respirology*. 2015;20(2):279-85.

[50] Dale J, Connor S, Tolley K. An evaluation of the west Surrey telemedicine monitoring project. *Journal of Telemedicine & Telecare*. 2003;9 Suppl 1:S39-41.

[51] Schou L, Østergaard B, Rydahl-Hansen S, Rasmussen LS, Emme C, Svarre Jakobsen A, Phanareth, K. A randomised trial of telemedicine-based treatment versus conventional hospitalisation in patients with severe COPD and exacerbation - effect on self-reported outcome. *Journal of Telemedicine & Telecare*. 2013;19(3):160-5.

[52] Effing TW, Vercoulen JH, Bourbeau J, Trappenburg J, Lenferink A, Cafarella P, Coultas, D, Meek, P, van der Valk, P, Bischoff, EWMA, Bucknall, C, Dewan, NA, Early, F, Fan, V, Frith, P, Janssen, DJA, Mitchell, K, Morgan, M, Nici, L., … van der Palen, J. Definition of a COPD self-management intervention: International Expert Group consensus. *European Respiratory Journal*. 2016;48(1):46-54.

[53] Barlow J, Wright C, Sheasby J, Turner A, Hainsworth J. Self-management approaches for people with chronic conditions: a review. *Patient Education and Counseling*. 2002;48(2):177-87.

[54] Bourbeau J. Disease-specific self-management programs in patients with advanced chronic obstructive pulmonary disease. *Disease Management & Health Outcomes*. 2003;11(5):311-9.

[55] Baldwin JL, Singh H, Sittig DF, Giardina TD, editors. Patient portals and health apps: Pitfalls, promises, and what one might learn from the other. *Healthcare*; 2017: Elsevier.

[56] Johnston SK, Nguyen HQ, Wolpin S. Designing and Testing a Web-based Interface for Self-Monitoring of Exercise and Symptoms for Older Adults with COPD. *Computers, Informatics, Nursing: CIN*. 2009;27(3):166.

[57] Barbosa MT, Sousa CS, Morais-Almeida M, Simões MJ, Mendes P. Telemedicine in COPD: an overview by topics. *COPD: Journal of Chronic Obstructive Pulmonary Disease*. 2020;17(5):601-17.

[58] Wagner FM, Weber A, Park JW, Schiemanck S, Tugtekin SM, Gulielmos V, Schüler, S. New telemetric system for daily pulmonary function surveillance of lung transplant recipients. *The Annals of Thoracic Surgery*. 1999;68(6):2033-8.

[59] Tsai LLY, McNamara RJ, Moddel C, Alison JA, McKenzie DK, McKeough ZJ. Home-based telerehabilitation via real-time videoconferencing improves endurance exercise capacity in patients with COPD: the randomized controlled TeleR Study. *Respirology*. 2017;22(4):699-707.

[60] Velickovski F, Ceccaroni L, Roca J, Burgos F, Galdiz JB, Marina N, Lluch-Ariet, M. Clinical Decision Support Systems (CDSS) for preventive management of COPD patients. *Journal of Translational Medicine*. 2014;12(2):1-10.

[61] Shaw G, Whelan M, Armitage L, Roberts N, Farmer A. Are COPD self-management mobile applications effective? A systematic review and meta-analysis. *NPJ Primary Care Respiratory Medicine*. 2020;30(1):1-10.

[62] Jódar-Sánchez F, Ortega F, Parra C, Gómez-Suárez C, Jordán A, Pérez P, Bonachela, P, Leal, S, & Barrot, E. Implementation of a telehealth programme for patients with severe chronic obstructive pulmonary disease treated with long-term oxygen therapy. *Journal of Telemedicine and Telecare*. 2013;19(1):11-7.

[63] Stewart JI, Moyle S, Criner GJ, Wilson C, Tanner R, Bowler RP, Crapo, JD., Zeldin, RK, Make, BJ, Regan, EA, & for the COPDGene Investigators Automated telecommunication to obtain longitudinal follow-up in a multicenter cross-sectional COPD study. *COPD: Journal of Chronic Obstructive Pulmonary Disease*. 2012;9(5):466-72.

[64] Antoniades NC, Rochford PD, Pretto JJ, Pierce RJ, Gogler J, Steinkrug J, Sharpe, K, & McDonald, CF. Pilot study of remote telemonitoring in COPD. *Telemedicine and e-Health*. 2012;18(8):634-40.

[65] Berkhof FF, van den Berg JW, Uil SM, Kerstjens HA. Telemedicine, the effect of nurse-initiated telephone follow up, on health status and health-care utilization in COPD patients: A randomized trial. *Respirology*. 2015;20(2):279-85.

[66] Shany T, Hession M, Pryce D, Roberts M, Basilakis J, Redmond S, Lovell, N, & Schreier, G. A small-scale randomised controlled trial of home telemonitoring in patients with severe chronic obstructive pulmonary disease. *Journal of Telemedicine and Telecare*. 2017;23(7):650-6.

[67] Dinesen B, Haesum LK, Soerensen N, Nielsen C, Grann O, Hejlesen O, Toft, E, & Ehlers, L. Using preventive home monitoring to reduce hospital admission rates and reduce costs: A case study of telehealth among chronic obstructive pulmonary disease patients. *Journal of Telemedicine and Telecare*. 2012;18(4):221-5.

[68] Franke K-J, Domanski U, Schroeder M, Jansen V, Artmann F, Weber U, Ettler, R, Nilius, G.Telemonitoring of home exercise cycle training in patients with COPD. *International Journal of Chronic Obstructive Pulmonary Disease*. 2016;11:2821.

[69] Ringbæk T, Green A, Laursen LC, Frausing E, Brøndum E, Ulrik CS. Effect of tele health care on exacerbations and hospital admissions in patients with chronic obstructive pulmonary disease: a randomized clinical trial. *International Journal of Chronic Obstructive Pulmonary Disease*. 2015; 10:1801.

[70] Koff P, Jones RH, Cashman JM, Voelkel NF, Vandivier R. Proactive integrated care improves quality of life in patients with COPD. *European Respiratory Journal*. 2009;33(5):1031-8.

[71] McDowell JE, McClean S, FitzGibbon F, Tate S. A randomised clinical trial of the effectiveness of home-based health care with telemonitoring in patients with COPD. *Journal of Telemedicine and Telecare*. 2015;21(2):80-7.

[72] Pinnock H, Hanley J, McCloughan L, Todd A, Krishan A, Lewis S, Stoddart, A, van der Pol, M, MacNee, W, Sheikh, A, Pagliari, C, & McKinstry, B. Effectiveness of telemonitoring integrated into existing clinical services on hospital admission for exacerbation of chronic obstructive pulmonary disease: researcher blind, multicentre, randomised controlled trial. *Bmj*. 2013;347.

[73] Sicotte C, Pare G, Morin S, Potvin J, Moreault M-P. Effects of home telemonitoring to support improved care for chronic obstructive pulmonary diseases. *Telemedicine and e-Health*. 2011;17(2):95-103.

[74] Stickland MK, Jourdain T, Wong EYL, Rodgers WM, Jendzjowsky NG, MacDonald GF. Using Telehealth technology to deliver pulmonary rehabilitation to patients with chronic obstructive pulmonary disease. *Canadian Respiratory Journal*. 2011;18(4):216-20.

[75] Farmer A, Williams V, Velardo C, Shah SA, Yu LM, Rutter H, Jones, L, Williams, N, Heneghan, C, Price, J, Hardinge, M, & Tarassenko, L. Self-Management Support Using a Digital Health System Compared With Usual Care for Chronic Obstructive Pulmonary Disease: Randomized Controlled Trial. *Journal of Medical Internet Research*. 2017;19(5):e144.

[76] Vassilev I, Rowsell A, Pope C, Kennedy A, O'Cathain A, Salisbury C, Rogers, A. Assessing the implementability of telehealth interventions for self-management support: a realist review. *Implementation Science*. 2015;10(1):1-25.

[77] Webb T, Joseph J, Yardley L, Michie S. Using the internet to promote health behavior change: a systematic review and meta-analysis of the impact of theoretical basis, use of behavior change techniques, and mode of delivery on efficacy. *Journal of Medical Internet Research*. 2010;12(1):e1376.

[78] Scalvini S, Baratti D, Assoni G, Zanardini M, Comini L, Bernocchi P. *Information and communication Technology in Chronic Diseases: A Patient's Opportunity*. Springer; 2014. p. 91-5.

[79] Mekov E, Miravitlles M, Petkov R. Artificial intelligence and machine learning in respiratory medicine. *Expert Review of Respiratory Medicine*. 2020;14(6):559-64.

[80] Sobnath DD, Philip N, Kayyali R, Nabhani-Gebara S, Pierscionek B, Vaes AW, Spruit, MA, & Kaimakamis, E. Features of a mobile support app for patients with chronic obstructive pulmonary disease: literature review and current applications. *JMIR mHealth and uHealth*. 2017;5(2):e4951.

[81] Yang F, Wang Y, Yang C, Hu H, Xiong Z. Mobile health applications in self-management of patients with chronic obstructive pulmonary disease: a systematic review and meta-analysis of their efficacy. *BMC Pulmonary Medicine*. 2018;18(1):1-9.

[82] Boer L, Bischoff E, van der Heijden M, Lucas P, Akkermans R, Vercoulen J, Heijdra, Y, Assendelft, W, & Schermer, T. A smart mobile health tool versus a paper action plan to support self-management of chronic obstructive pulmonary disease exacerbations: randomized controlled trial. *JMIR mHealth and uHealth*. 2019;7(10):e14408.

[83] Cooper R, Giangreco A, Duffy M, Finlayson E, Hamilton S, Swanson M, Colligan, J, Gilliatt, J, McIvor, M, & Sage, EK. Evaluation of myCOPD Digital Self-management Technology in a Remote and Rural Population: Real-world Feasibility Study. *JMIR mHealth and uHealth*. 2022;10(2):e30782.

[84] Steurer-Stey C, Dalla Lana K, Braun J, Ter Riet G, Puhan MA. Effects of the "Living well with COPD" intervention in primary care: a comparative study. *European Respiratory Journal*. 2018;51(1).

[85] Bohingamu Mudiyanselage S, Stevens J, Watts JJ, Toscano J, Kotowicz MA, Steinfort CL, Bell, J, Byrnes, J, Bruce, S, Carter, S, Hunter, C, Barrand, C, & Hayles, R. Personalised telehealth intervention for chronic disease management: a pilot randomised controlled trial. *Journal of Telemedicine and Telecare*. 2019;25(6):343-52.

[86] Alwakeel AJ, Sicondolfo A, Robitaille C, Bourbeau J, Saad N. The accessibility, feasibility, and safety of a standardized community-based tele-pulmonary rehab program for chronic obstructive pulmonary disease: a 3-year real-world prospective study. *Annals of the American Thoracic Society*. 2022;19(1): 39-47.

[87] Tanguay P, Marquis N, Gaboury I, Kairy D, Touchette M, Tousignant M, Décary, S. Telerehabilitation for post-hospitalized COVID-19 patients: a proof-of-concept study during a pandemic. *International Journal of Telerehabilitation*. 2021;13(1).

[88] Lewis KE, Annandale JA, Warm DL, Rees SE, Hurlin C, Blyth H, Syed, Y, & Lewis, L. Does home telemonitoring after pulmonary rehabilitation reduce healthcare use in optimized COPD? A pilot randomized trial. *Copd: Journal of Chronic Obstructive Pulmonary Disease*. 2010;7(1):44-50.

[89] Marquis N, Larivee P, Dubois MF, Tousignant M. Are improvements maintained after in-home pulmonary telerehabilitation for patients with chronic obstructive pulmonary disease? *International Journal of Telerehabilitation*. 2014;6(2):21-30.

[90] Calvo GS, Gomez-Suarez C, Soriano JB, Zamora E, Gonzalez-Gamarra A, Gonzalez-Bejar M, Jordán, A, Tadeo, E, Sebastián, A, Fernández, G, & Ancochea, J. A home telehealth program for patients with severe COPD: The PROMETE study. *Respiratory Medicine*. 2014;108(3):453-62.

[91] Pedone C, Chiurco D, Scarlata S, Incalzi RA. Efficacy of multiparametric telemonitoring on respiratory outcomes in elderly people with COPD: a randomized controlled trial. *BMC Health Services Research*. 2013;13(1):82-.

[92] Tarigan AP, Pandia P, Tarigan AH, Eyanoer PC. Effectiveness of upper limb exercises and breathing exercises in COPD stable patients during COVID-19 pandemic era. *Advances in Respiratory Medicine*. 2022.

[93] Wade V, Gray L, Carati C. Theoretical frameworks in telemedicine research. *Journal of Telemedicine and Telecare*. 2017;23(1):181-7.

[94] Davis FD. Perceived usefulness, perceived ease of use, and user acceptance of information technology. *MIS Quarterly*. 1989:319-40.

[95] Baker E, Fatoye F. Clinical and cost effectiveness of nurse-led self-management interventions for patients with copd in primary care: A systematic review. *International Journal of Nursing Studies*. 2017;71:125-38.

[96] Chmiel FP, Burns DK, Pickering JB, Blythin A, Wilkinson TM, Boniface MJ. Prediction of Chronic Obstructive Pulmonary Disease Exacerbation Events by Using Patient Self-reported Data in a Digital Health App: Statistical Evaluation and Machine Learning Approach. *JMIR Medical Informatics*. 2022;10(3):e26499.

[97] Slevin P, Kessie T, Cullen J, Butler MW, Donnelly SC, Caulfield B. Exploring the potential benefits of digital health technology for the management of COPD: a qualitative study of patient perceptions. *ERJ Open Research*. 2019;5(2).

[98] Ancochea J, García-Río F, Vázquez-Espinosa E, Hernando-Sanz A, López-Yepes L, Galera-Martínez R, Peces-Barba, G, Pérez-Warnisher, MT, Segrelles-Calvo, G, Zamarro, C, González-Ponce, P, Ramos, MI, Conforto, JI, Jafri, S, & Soriano, JB. Efficacy and costs of telehealth for the management of COPD: the PROMETE II trial. *European Respiratory Journal*. 2018;51(5).

[99] Leonard R, Forte M, Mehta D, Mujahid H, Stansbury R. The impact of a telemedicine intervention on home non-invasive ventilation in a rural population with advanced COPD. *The Clinical Respiratory Journal*. 2021;15(7):728-34.

[100] Bhatt SP, Patel SB, Anderson EM, Baugh D, Givens T, Schumann C, Sanders, JG, Windham, ST, Cutter, GR, & Dransfield, MT. Video telehealth pulmonary rehabilitation intervention in chronic obstructive pulmonary disease reduces 30-day readmissions. *American Journal of Respiratory and Critical Care Medicine*. 2019;200(4):511-3.

[101] Guerra-Paiva S, Dias F, Costaa D, Santos V, Santos C. DPO2 Project: Telehealth to enhance the social role of physical activity in people living with COPD. *Procedia Computer Science*. 2021;181:869-75.

[102] Gregersen TL, Green A, Frausing E, Ringbaek T, Brøndum E, Ulrik CS. Do telemedical interventions improve quality of life in patients with COPD? A systematic review. *International Journal of Chronic Obstructive Pulmonary Disease*. 2016;11:809.

[103] Ringbaek TJ, Lavesen M, Lange P. Tablet computers to support outpatient pulmonary rehabilitation in patients with COPD. *European Clinical Respiratory Journal*. 2016;3:31016.

[104] Koff PB, Jones RH, Cashman JM, Voelkel NF, Vandivier RW. Proactive integrated care improves quality of life in patients with COPD. *European Respiratory Journal*. 2009;33(5):1031-8.

[105] Trappenburg JCA, Niesink A, De Weert-Van Oene GH, Van Der Zeijden H, Van Snippenburg R, Peters A, Lammers, JWJ, & Schrijvers, AJP. Effects of telemonitoring in patients with chronic obstructive pulmonary disease. *Telemedicine and e-Health*. 2008;14(2):138-46.

[106] Lilholt PH, Witt Udsen F, Ehlers L, Hejlesen OK. Telehealthcare for patients suffering from chronic obstructive pulmonary disease: effects on health-related quality of life: results from the Danish 'TeleCare North' cluster-randomised trial. *BMJ Open*. 2017;7(5):e014587.

[107] Sicotte C, Pare G, Morin S, Potvin J, Moreault MP. Effects of home telemonitoring to support improved care for chronic obstructive pulmonary diseases. *Telemedicine Journal & E-Health*. 2011;17(2):95-103.

[108] Haesum LK, Soerensen N, Dinesen B, Nielsen C, Grann O, Hejlesen O, Toft, E, & Ehlers, L. Cost-utility analysis of a telerehabilitation program: a case study of COPD patients. *Telemedicine and e-Health*. 2012;18(9):688-92.

[109] Paré G, Poba-Nzaou P, Sicotte C, Beaupré A, Lefrançois É, Nault D, Saint-Jules, D. Comparing the costs of home telemonitoring and usual care of chronic obstructive pulmonary disease patients: a randomized controlled trial. *European Research in Telemedicine*. 2013;2(2):35-47.

[110] Udsen FW, Lilholt PH, Hejlesen O, Ehlers L. Cost-effectiveness of telehealthcare to patients with chronic obstructive pulmonary disease: results from the Danish 'TeleCare North'cluster-randomised trial. *Bmj Open*. 2017;7(5):e014616.

[111] De San Miguel K, Smith J, Lewin G. Telehealth remote monitoring for community-dwelling older adults with chronic obstructive pulmonary disease. *Telemedicine Journal & E-Health*. 2013;19(9):652-7.

[112] Mihalj M, Carrel T, Gregoric ID, Andereggen L, Zinn PO, Doll D, Stueber, F, Gabriel, RA, Urman, RD, & Luedi, MM. Telemedicine for preoperative assessment during a COVID-19 pandemic: Recommendations for clinical care. *Best Practice & Research Clinical Anaesthesiology*. 2020;34(2): 345-51.

[113] Sharma D, Bhaskar S. Addressing the Covid-19 burden on medical education and training: the role of telemedicine and tele-education during and beyond the pandemic. *Frontiers in Public Health*. 2020: 838.

[114] Amorim P, Brito D, Castelo-Branco M, Fàbrega C, Gomes da Costa F, Martins H, Gonçalves, L, Gonçalves, LM, Martin, V, Milner, J, Nêveda, R, Ferreira, AN, Pardo, R, Peralta-Santos, A, Pessoa, T, Silva, J, & Salvador Vergès, À. Telehealth opportunities in the COVID-19 pandemic early days: what happened, did not happen, should have happened, and must happen in the near future? *Telemedicine and e-Health*. 2021;27(10):1194-9.

[115] Kim J, Kim S, Kim H, Kim K, Lee CT, Yang S, Kong, HJ, Shin, Y, & Lee, K. Acceptability of the consumer-centric u-health services for patients with chronic obstructive pulmonary disease. *Telemedicine and e-Health*. 2012;18(5):329-38.

[116] Dhala A, Sasangohar F, Kash B, Ahmadi N, Masud F. Rapid implementation and innovative applications of a virtual intensive care unit during the COVID-19 pandemic: case study. *Journal of Medical Internet Research*. 2020;22(9):e20143.

[117] Rose L, Yu L, Casey J, Cook A, Metaxa V, Pattison N, Rafferty, AM, Ramsay, P, Saha, S, Xyrichis, A, & Meyer, J. Communication and virtual visiting for families of patients in intensive care during the COVID-19 pandemic: a UK national survey. *Annals of the American Thoracic Society*. 2021;18(10): 1685-92.

[118] Rutkowski S, Rutkowska A, Kiper P, Jastrzebski D, Racheniuk H, Turolla A, Szczegielniak, J, Casaburi, R. Virtual reality rehabilitation in patients with chronic obstructive pulmonary disease: a randomized controlled trial. *International Journal of Chronic Obstructive Pulmonary Disease*. 2020;15:117.

[119] Colombo V, Aliverti A, Sacco M. Virtual reality for COPD rehabilitation: A technological perspective. *Pulmonology*. 2020.

[120] Kaplan A, Cao H, FitzGerald JM, Iannotti N, Yang E, Kocks JW, Kostikas, K, Price, D, Reddel, HK, Tsiligianni, I, Vogelmeier, CF, Pfister, P, & Mastoridis, P. Artificial intelligence/machine learning in respiratory medicine and potential role in asthma and COPD diagnosis. *The Journal of Allergy and Clinical Immunology: In Practice*. 2021;9(6):2255-61.

[121] Feng Y, Wang Y, Zeng C, Mao H. Artificial Intelligence and Machine Learning in Chronic Airway Diseases: Focus on Asthma and Chronic Obstructive Pulmonary Disease. *International Journal of Medical Sciences*. 2021;18(13):2871.

Chapter 27

COPD and COVID-19: Epidemiology at a Glance

Abdallah Y Naser*, Sami Qadus and Eman Zmaily Dahmash
[1]Department of Applied Pharmaceutical Sciences and Clinical Pharmacy, Faculty of Pharmacy, Isra University, Amman, Jordan

Abstract

Patients with asthma and chronic obstructive pulmonary disease (COPD) have been recognised as populations vulnerable to COVID-19 incidence and death. Because most COPD patients are old and have other comorbidities, those diagnosed with COVID-19 suffer worse outcomes, such as a greater rate of hospitalisation, admission to intensive care unit (ICU), and mortality. The COPD prevalence among COVID-19 patients varies by country, ranging from 0% to 14% worldwide, while data from ICUs range from 4% to 38%. Adults with COPD and asthma have greater rates of anxiety and depression symptoms, and they are more likely to seek medical treatment, putting them at risk for COVID-19 morbidity. It has been suggested to provide educational interventions for people with chronic respiratory diseases to aid them in symptom tracking, early diagnosis of COVID-19, and improved mental health support during the pandemic.

Keywords: COPD, coronavirus, COVID-19, epidemiology

Introduction

The COVID-19 pandemic has created numerous challenges in the diagnosis and management of patients with chronic obstructive pulmonary disease (COPD), as well as the management and prognosis of COPD patients who develop COVID-19. The patients themselves are fearful of contracting COVID-19, being denied treatment, coping with the symptoms, and dying [1]. The committee for the Global Initiative for the Management of Chronic Obstructive Lung Disease (GOLD) released their COPD management report for 2021 in November 2020 [2], which included important updates to the recommendations on COPD diagnosis, evaluation, and management [2]. The most significant change is the addition of a COPD and COVID-19 chapter reviewing current evidence and making recommendations based on current knowledge [3].

* Corresponding Author's Email: abdallah.naser@iu.edu.jo.

In: Chronic Obstructive Pulmonary Disease
Editor: Jaber S. Alqahtani
ISBN: 979-8-88697-333-4

COPD patients do not appear to be at higher risk of SARS-CoV-2 infection, which could be due to preventive mechanisms, at least in part. The majority of previous studies have not found COPD to be an independent risk factor for testing positive for COVID-19 [4, 5]. COPD patients have a slightly higher risk of COVID-19 hospitalisation, but data on the risk of developing severe disease and death are mixed: COPD has been linked to an increased risk of severe disease or death in certain studies [6], but not all [7]. Overall, the severity of the consequences appears to be smaller than anticipated [8].

According to GOLD's standards, patients with COPD should follow basic infection control measures and, if possible, wear masks. Although wearing a surgical mask does not appear to impair ventilation, even in patients with severe airflow limitation, a loose face covering or even a face shield is comfortable and successful in most cases [9], [4]. During the epidemic, many health systems curtailed face-to-face visits and implemented remote consultations via the web, phone, and video links.

Spirometry should only be used in an emergency or life-threatening conditions, such as before surgery. When standard spirometry is unavailable, home measurements of peak expiratory flow (PEF), paired with validated patient questionnaires, can be used to confirm or deny a COPD diagnosis. A PEF, on the other hand, does not correlate well with spirometry data, has low specificity, and cannot distinguish obstructive and restrictive lung function problems [10].

COVID-19 Epidemiology among COPD Patients

In the publications that have evaluated the epidemiology, there is significant diversity in the clinical settings, the type of data collected, the clinical characteristics, and the clinical outcomes of COVID-19 [6]. According to the results, the prevalence of mortality among patients with COVID-19 in a hospital setting is very high and ranges from 1 to 52% of the hospital admissions, while the prevalence of mortality among intensive care patients with COVID-19 is very high and ranges from 6% to 86% in admitted patients [11].

COPD is correlated with higher susceptibility to infections, including respiratory viral infections leading to acute exacerbations of COPD (AECOPD) [12]. Most COPD patients are old, with several comorbidities, making those diagnosed with COVID-19 exhibit significant outcomes including a higher incidence of hospitalisation, admission to intensive care units (ICUs), and mortality [13, 14]. Furthermore, a study by Lacedonia and coworkers (2021) reported that COVID-19 patients suffering from COPD were significantly older than COVID-19 patients without COPD (78.15 ±13.54 and 65.66 ± 16.85 respectively, $p < 0.001$) [15].

The prevalence of COPD among COVID-19 patients varies in different countries and ranges from 0 to 14% worldwide [16-19], while data from ICU are only cohorts, but are more variable in different countries, ranging from 4% in an Italian study to 38% in a Spanish one [20]. In a series of 257 critically ill patients admitted to the ICU with COVID-19 in New York, Cummings MJ et al. (2020) reported a 9% prevalence rate of COPD and a 33% prevalence rate of current or former smokers among those patients [21]. Also, in a meta-analysis including 15 studies with a total of 2473 confirmed COVID-19 patients, Alqahtani et al. (2020) reported that the pooled prevalence rates of COPD patients and smokers in COVID-19 cases were 2% and 9%, respectively [22]. Furthermore, the study reported that COPD patients were at a higher risk of more severe disease, with a risk of severity reaching 63%, compared to patients without COPD (risk severity of 33.4%). This was correlated with a higher mortality rate among the COPD group, reaching up to 60%. Figure 1 illustrates the comparison of the probability of survival in hospitalised COVID-19 patients with and without COPD. A significant difference and reduction in survival were observed in the COPD group [15]. Furthermore, the trend in hospitalisation among COVID-19 patients with COPD was higher than without COPD (48.2% vs. 26.5%) 22 [15].

Despite variability in prevalence, patients with COPD did not demonstrate a high risk of contracting COVID-19 but tended to develop severe clinical outcomes once infected. A possible explanation could be the chronic use of inhaled steroids, beta-agonists, or anticholinergics in COPD patients. This could be counteracted by lowering the COVID-19 receptor expression and modulating the inflammation induced by respiratory infection, therefore reducing the susceptibility to infection [23-25].

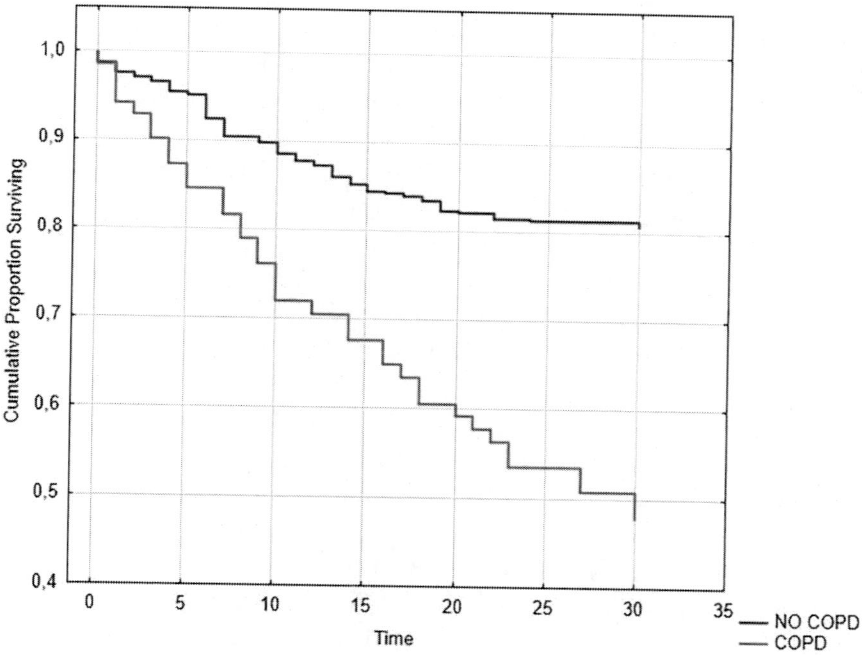

Figure 1. Kaplan–Meier plot of the probability of survival in COVID-19 patients hospitalized in four intermediate Respiratory Intensive Care Units according to the presence of COPD (with permission from Lacedonia et al. 2021).

Clinical Manifestations of COVID-19 in COPD Patients

The clinical presentation of COVID-19 in patients with COPD usually includes low grade fever (22.9% in COPD vs. 21% in non-COPD patients, $p < 0.001$), dyspnoea (72.3% vs. 56.2%, $p < 0.001$), and cough with expectoration (26.9% vs. 15.1%, $p < 0.001$), with less non-respiratory symptoms than in non-COPD COVID-19 patients. Upon clinical examination, COVID-19 COPD patients were more likely to have hypoxemia (38.8% vs. 20.6% in non-COPD patients,

$p < 0.001$), tachypnea (47.9% vs. 29.9%, $p < 0.001$), and confusional symptoms (17.3% vs. 11.5%, $p < 0.001$), with wheezing (17.3% vs. 5.3%, $p < 0.001$) on pulmonary auscultation [25].

In patients who died from COVID-19-associated respiratory failure, the histologic analysis of pulmonary vessels showed widespread thrombosis with microangiopathy compared to patients who died from influenza-associated respiratory failure. Also, their lungs showed distinctive vascular features and alveolar capillary microthrombi nine times as prevalent in patients with COVID-19 as in patients with influenza [26]. The severity of COVID-19 ranges from asymptomatic infections to mild self-limiting upper respiratory tract illness, severe pneumonia with respiratory failure, or death [27].

COPD patients were also more susceptible to vascular damage and thrombosis and coagulopathies during the SARS-CoV-2 infection [28-30], which may predispose them to an increased risk of worse outcomes from COVID-19. Breathlessness in patients with COPD during an acute exacerbation, apart from microbial infections, could also occur because of pulmonary thrombosis, which seems to be common in COVID-19 patients with severe diseases [31]. One observational study showed a cumulative incidence of venous and arterial thrombotic complications of 31% during the ICU admission of patients with COVID-19 pneumonia, pulmonary embolism being the most common thrombotic complication [32].

Acute exacerbations of COPD (AECOPD) are crucial events that occur in the natural course of COPD, and respiratory viral infections are an important cause of COPD exacerbations [33]. COPD exacerbations are often associated with an increased risk of myocardial infarction, stroke, all-cause mortality, and cardiovascular mortality, especially among those with associated pneumonia [34, 35]. Coronaviruses are recognised seasonal causes of acute exacerbations of COPD (AECOPD) [36]. However, imaging and postmortem studies have shown that the pathology of acute exacerbations of COPD is very different from COVID-19-associated viral pneumonia [26].

COPD patients were at a higher risk of more severe diseases compared to patients without COPD, and this was associated with a higher mortality rate of 60%. In a South Korean study, Lee SC et al. (2021) reported that in COVID-19 patients COPD was a significant independent risk factor for all-cause mortality, and a relatively greater proportion of COVID-19 patients with COPD received mechanical ventilation and intensive critical care than their counterparts without COPD [37]. Other studies reported that COPD patients had the highest hazard ratio for admission to the ICU, invasive ventilation, or death among COVID-19 patients with various types of underlying chronic diseases [15, 19]. This relationship between COPD and COVID-19 has been explained by the poor underlying lung reserve and the increased expression of angiotensin-converting enzyme 2 (ACE2) receptors in the small airways of COVID-19 patients with COPD [20]. A gene profile research reported that ACE2 expression is significantly higher on bronchial epithelial cells in COPD patients when compared to control patients, which might contribute to exacerbated progression (Leung et al. 2020). Furthermore, COPD can lead to systemic hypoxia sensitive to the induction of cytokine storms (Guo et al. 2017).

Evidence from COVID-19 convalescent patients without a pulmonary disease has shown a considerable reduction in lung function and computed tomography abnormalities after discharge [38]. Zhao YS et al. (2020) reported that radiological and physiological abnormalities were still found in a considerable proportion of COVID-19 survivors without critical cases 3 months after discharge [39]. In a cohort of fifty-seven COVID-19 patients, 40 were non-severe cases and 17 were severe cases; abnormal CT findings were noted in 54.3% of the patients and 75.4% had abnormal pulmonary function tests [38]. COPD patients demonstrate abnormal remodelling processes following lung injury, so one can expect significantly abnormal tissue remodelling following SARS-CoV-2 infection [29].

Risk Factors and Prevention

The COVID-19 pandemic is caused by severe acute respiratory syndrome coronavirus 2 (SARS-CoV-2). Clinical outcomes, including mortality, are worse in males, older individuals, and patients with comorbidities such as diabetes, cardiovascular diseases, and obesity [40].

COPD is a disease that occurs in later life and is associated with an increased risk of hospitalisation, multiple comorbidities, and a trend for increased mortality [28]. COPD covers many clinical subtypes with persistent airflow limitation in common [41]. Patients with COPD have increased general susceptibility to viral infections [42] and are more likely to progress to severe disease, leading to a higher mortality rate than those without COPD [43]. Similarly, patients with COPD have a significantly increased risk of severe respiratory failure [44]. Therefore, COPD patients are included in shielding strategies due to their susceptibility to exacerbations induced by viruses, compromised pulmonary function, and high prevalence of associated comorbidities [6]. The early shielding of older and high-risk populations, including patients with COPD, may account for the low prevalence of COPD observed in some populations [45].

Patients with COPD have a high risk for COVID-19 infection [20] and COVID-19 infection is associated with substantial severity and mortality rates in COPD patients [22]. Li et al. (2020) report that patients with severe COVID-19 are likely to develop acute respiratory distress syndrome (ARDS) and die of respiratory failure [46]. Based on data from over 20 000 patients hospitalised with COVID-19 infection, the International Severe Acute Respiratory and Emerging Infection Consortium (ISARIC) demonstrated that non-asthma chronic pulmonary diseases were associated with an increased risk of death [47]. Lee et al. (2021) reported that comorbidities like COPD, besides other factors such as old age, male sex, and a higher Charlson Comorbidity Index (CCI) score, were significant risk factors for respiratory failure and all-cause mortality [43].

Cigarette smoking appears to be an important risk factor in COVID-19 patients with COPD. Several studies reported that the expression level of ACE2 was significantly higher in COPD patients than in controls and in current smokers than in former or never smokers [48, 49]. Meta-analysis results showed also that 22% of current smokers and 46% of ex-smokers had severe complications, and that current smokers were 1.5 times more likely to have severe complications compared to former and never smokers [22]. The British Thoracic Society (BTS) (2020) reiterated the importance of smoking cessation [50]. Patients with COPD who were still smoking were strongly encouraged to stop in order to reduce the risk of poor outcomes from COVID-19 and their risk of acute exacerbations [51].

Preliminary evidence suggests that obesity may play a role in COPD patients as well [52]. In a cohort of 37 patients who were divided based on their Body Mass Index (BMI) into overweight and normal weight, Higham A and Singh D. (2020) have shown increased gene expression of ACE2 in the bronchial epithelium of COPD patients who were overweight compared to those who were not overweight, which indicates that comorbidities or even diet may regulate expression of ACE2 in the lungs [53].

Preventive Measures

COVID-19 may have many detrimental consequences on patients' well-being, and patients with COVID-19 and COPD have a worse clinical outcome compared with patients with other comorbidities [13, 22]. Coronaviruses are recognised seasonal causes of acute exacerbations of COPD (AECOPD) [36]. Ackermann M et al. (2020) reported that the pathology of a typical AECOPD is very different from viral pneumonia typical of COVID-19. However, physicians must take the underlying COPD into consideration when treating COVID-19 in COPD patients [26]. Also, diagnosing COVID-19 in a patient with COPD needs to take into consideration the treatment of concomitant acute exacerbations of COPD as well. Specific to treating patients with COPD is the necessity for bronchodilators, the beneficial effects of non-invasive ventilation (NIV), and the frequent need for antibiotics. Concerns have been raised as to whether to provide, and how, these therapies to patients with COPD during the pandemic [36].

The general preventive measures that need to be considered to help minimise the spread of COVID-19 include wearing masks that cover the mouth and nose in public; observing proper social distancing; washing hands often with soap for at least 15 to 20 seconds, or using a hand sanitiser that contains at least 60% alcohol if soap is not available; avoiding close contact with someone who is ill; staying at home if sick; using a tissue to cover mouth and nose in case of coughing or sneezing; frequently disinfecting surfaces and objects being touched; and avoiding touching eyes, nose, and mouth with unwashed hands. Patients with COPD should take extra appropriate preventive measures, as they are at a higher risk of developing a more severe COVID-19 than others [22]. These extra preventive measures include the following: smoking cessation; continuing their medications and current treatment plan as per physician advice; storing enough food to minimise trips to the grocery store; avoiding crowded areas and non-essential travel; staying at home as much as possible; seeking prompt medical attention if they or anyone in their family show symptoms of COVID-19 [2].

The strict isolation imposed on COVID-19 patients may amplify feelings of solitude and hopelessness [36]. Social isolation and loneliness are risk factors for poorer physical and mental health and increased mortality. They impact dietary behaviour and physical activity, which play a role in precipitating and maintaining obesity. Obesity is a very high risk for worsening the course of COVID-19, hospitalisation, and death [54]. This population may also be significantly impacted by the dietary and physical activity consequences resulting from lockdowns, social distancing, and isolation. Zeigler Z. identified the following as risk factors for weight gain during COVID-19 self-quarantines: increased sedentary behaviour, decreased physical activity, increased snacking frequency (particularly after dinner), increased alcohol intake, decreased water intake, emotional eating, decreased sleep quality, and being overweight/obese [54]. Simon et al. (2020) report that unintentional weight loss occurs in COVID-19 patients due to loss of taste and appetite in addition to difficulty in doing regular exercise, which could be in the initial hospitalised isolation phase [36]. However, the post-discharge self-quarantine period goes in favour of weight gain [54]. Hospital treatment should therefore include dietary as well as emotional and spiritual support in their management protocols of COVID-19 patients [36].

Early mobilisation is encouraged in recent COVID-19-specific physiotherapy guidelines, while airway clearance techniques should be provided cautiously as they carry the risk of aerosol spread. After discharge, smooth transfer from hospital to home care must be assured to ensure reducing the risk of readmission [2]. Although pulmonary rehabilitation (PR) is recommended for people with COPD, rehabilitation in general should be offered to all patients with COVID-19, and certainly after ICU admission because a prolonged ICU stay has a significant impact on the physical and emotional well-being of patients [55].

Social distancing and concerns about residual viral transmission may limit possibilities for centre-based PR and physiotherapy. Home-based, unsupervised PR might be a solution in these times of social distancing [2]. However, as soon as centre-based PR is possible, patients should change to such supervised programmes for optimal benefit [36].

Management of COPD with Co-Existing COVID-19

Diagnosing and treating the acute exacerbation of COPD (AECOPD) effectively in COVID-19 patients with COPD is important since patients with COPD are at an increased risk of poor outcomes [36]. Bronchodilators, NIV, and the use of antibiotics are central to treating patients with COPD [2]. Rawson TM et al. (2020) analyzed eighteen full texts for bacterial or fungal coinfection with COVID-19 and reported that only 8% of the patients were reported as experiencing bacterial or fungal coinfection with COVID-19 during hospital admission [56].

Bronchodilators are central medication for treating exacerbations of COPD all over the world [57]. Bronchodilators are frequently given via nebulizer in hospitalised patients with COPD. Despite the claim of Tran K et al. 2012 that some procedures are potentially capable of generating aerosols and have been associated with an increased risk of transmission of a severe acute respiratory syndrome (SARS-CoV) to health workers (HCWs) [58], the BTS's 2020 guidelines on treating patients with COPD and COVID-19 supported the use of nebulizers, claiming there is no evidence supporting an increased risk of viral transmission. The defence of the BTS is based on the notion that the aerosols surrounding the nebulizer come from the nebulizer, not from patients [50]. In treating acute exacerbations of COPD (AECOPD), the pressurized metered dose inhalers (pMDs) were not inferior to nebulizers [57]. Simons S et al. (2020) advocated the use of pressurized metered dose inhalers (pMDI) with a spacer, and that nebulized treatment should be reserved for those situations in which pMDI with a spacer is not possible, such as patients with severe, life-threatening diseases or those unable to use a pMDI [36].

Corticosteroids are beneficial to patients with severe acute exacerbations of COPD (AECOPD), especially in patients requiring ventilatory support, in whom steroids reduce ventilation days, and in case of non-invasive ventilation (NIV) failure [36]. In a cohort study involving 201 patients with confirmed COVID-19 pneumonia, Wu et al. (2020) reported that treatment with methylprednisolone may be beneficial to patients who develop acute respiratory distress syndrome (ARDS), which suggests that steroids might improve clinical outcomes in patients with COVID-19 [59]. The RECOVERY Collaborative Group (2020) reported that dexamethasone improved mortality in patients with COVID-19 requiring respiratory support [60]. Systemic glucocorticoids for treating acute exacerbations in hospitalised patients, or during emergency department visits, have been shown to reduce the rate of treatment failure and of relapse, and to improve lung function and breathlessness. Conversely, there are limited prospective studies on the long-term effects of oral glucocorticoids in stable COPD. Therefore, while oral glucocorticoids play a role in the acute management of exacerbations, they have no role in the chronic daily treatment of COPD because of a lack of benefit balanced against a high rate of systemic complications [2]. The World Health Organization (WHO) made a strong recommendation for systemic (i.e., intravenous or oral) corticosteroid therapy (e.g., 6 mg daily of dexamethasone orally or intravenously, or 50 mg of hydrocortisone intravenously, every 8 hours) for 7 to 10 days in patients with severe and critical COVID-19 [61].

The relationship between the use of inhaled corticosteroids (ICS) and SARS-CoV-2 infection is not absolutely clear. Higham et al. (2020) reported that with regard to SARS-CoV-2 infection the use of ICS in COPD patients may be a double-edged sword, benefitting some patients but harming others [29].

While there may be some benefits in reducing the ability of SARS-CoV-2 to proliferate [62], it is known that ICS can inhibit important antiviral mechanisms [63]. It is well known also that corticosteroids suppress pro-inflammatory cytokine production from various cell types, which confers protection against COPD exacerbations [63]. Bafadhel et al. (2018) also reported that ICS use in COPD patients prevented exacerbations in patients with higher blood eosinophils [64]. This is contrary to Choi et al. (2020) who reported that prior ICS use was not significantly associated with COVID-19 in patients with COPD or asthma, nor with the clinical outcomes among patients with COVID-19 [65]. The view of Choi et al. was supported by Schultze et al. (2020), who have also shown that regular use of ICS in patients with asthma or COPD did not show any beneficial role in protecting against COVID-19-related death [66].

COPD management guidelines provide recommendations as to the clinical situations where it is appropriate to withdraw ICS therapy [67]. Chalmers et al. (2020) reported that appropriate ICS withdrawal should continue to be considered in the absence of conclusive data showing a protective effect of using ICS against COVID-19 in COPD patients [67].

The impact of isolation on COPD progression is unclear; it may lead to reduced viral infections in the short term but may cause undesirable effects on the general physical and psychosocial health of the patients in the long term. The decrease in physical activities and exercise resulting from isolation may deprive patients of the beneficial effects that include improved quality of life, decreased symptoms burden, and risk of exacerbations and mortality [6, 68].

In general, viral infections may facilitate subsequent bacterial infections or increase the number of bacteria already present in the lower airways [69]. Bacterial co-infections appear infrequently in COVID-19 [56]; however, the risk of co-infections increases with the severity of COVID-19, and bacterial co-infections have been detected in up to 46% of COVID-19 patients admitted to an ICU [70]. When a COPD patient develops a new or increased productive cough or breathlessness, it should be evaluated and treated as an acute COPD exacerbation. Treatment can be initiated with short-acting inhaled beta$_2$-agonists with or without short-acting anticholinergics. Blanket antibiotic treatment is not started in all patients. If the patient has any signs of super-added infections, pyrexia, X-ray infiltrates, and/or an increase in inflammatory markers, antibiotics can be initiated considering the risks versus benefits [31]. Current WHO guidelines recommend broad-spectrum antibiotics in severe COVID-19 patients and in milder COVID-19 infections when there is clinical suspicion of bacterial infection [61]. Antibiotics should be used in COPD exacerbations, as indicated, whether or not there is evidence of COVID-19 infection [2]. Since it may be difficult to distinguish COVID-19 infections from bacterial pneumonia, and because patients with COPD are at risk for bacterial infections, Simons et al. (2020) suggest treating hospitalised patients with COPD and COVID-19 with broad-spectrum antibiotics [36], in line with the current WHO treatment guideline for severe

COVID-19 [61]. Microbiological analysis, such as sputum culture, should be performed on admission and, in the absence of a coinfection, the antibiotics can be stopped [36].

Mental Health Burden of COVID-19 on COPD Patients

Patients with asthma and COPD have been identified as sensitive populations for COVID-19 incidence and mortality by the Centers for Disease Control and Prevention (CDC) [71]. In addition to the physical effects of COVID-19 exposure, the COVID-19 pandemic has resulted in an increase in mental-health-related disorders as a result of advised preventive actions such as social distance and quarantining [72-78].

Adults with COPD and asthma have higher rates of anxiety and depressive symptoms, according to previous research conducted before the pandemic. Patients with these comorbid diseases have more symptom load and are more likely to seek medical help, which could place them at higher risk for COVID-19 morbidity [79]. Quantifying mental distress among COVID-19-vulnerable groups could help researchers create tailored therapies to improve their physical and mental health while also lowering their risk of acquiring COVID-19.

All sectors of society have been under different sources of financial, social, and psychological pressure as a result of the preventive measures taken by all governments around the world, including quarantine and lockdown, which have impacted their psychological well-being, leading to the development of social isolation, mental distress, anxiety, and depression [72-74, 76-78, 80, 81]. Previous research has found that the incidence of these psychological effects is not low, and that it is higher among university students than among healthcare professionals or the general population. Patients with comorbidities are also at a higher risk of being mentally ill during the pandemic. Individuals with chronic respiratory problems are more likely to report mental health symptoms during the COVID-19 pandemic than adults without chronic respiratory illnesses, according to a study in the United States [82]. These findings are similar to other published research showing an increase in mental health symptoms among people with other chronic health disorders during the COVID-19 pandemic [83]. People with respiratory conditions may be concerned because early public health reports indicated that adults with chronic conditions had a higher COVID-19 burden [82]. A previous study in the United States has recommended providing educational interventions via telehealth or mHealth tools to target individuals with chronic respiratory conditions to assist them with symptom tracking, early detection of COVID-19, and increased mental health support during the pandemic period [82].

Conclusion

When compared to individuals with other comorbidities, patients with COVID-19 and COPD have a worse clinical outcome. COPD patients should take extra precautions to help prevent the spread of COVID-19 since they have a higher chance of acquiring a more severe case of COVID-19 than others. Early detection and treatment of AECOPD are critical for lowering the risk of poor outcomes in COVID-19 patients with COPD. Adults with COPD and asthma have greater rates of anxiety and depression symptoms, and they are more likely to seek medical treatment, putting them at risk for COVID-19 morbidity. It is recommended to provide educational interventions for people with chronic respiratory diseases to help with symptom tracking, early diagnosis of COVID-19, and greater mental health support during the pandemic.

Key Points

- COPD patients are at higher risk of getting infected with COVID-19.
- COPD patients should take extra precautions to help prevent the spread of COVID-19.
- Early detection and treatment are important for lowering the risk of poor outcomes.
- Mental health and support should not be neglected in patients with COPD and COVID-19.
- For patients with COPD and COVID-19, educational interventions are critical for early identification and prevention.

References

[1] Philip, K., Lonergan, B., Cumella, A., Farrington-Douglas, J., Laffan, M., and Hopkinson, N. S. (2020). COVID-19 related concerns of people with long-term respiratory conditions: a qualitative study. *BMC Pulmonary Medicine*, 20(1), p. 1-10.

[2] Global Initiative for Chronic Obstructive Lung Disease (GOLD). *Global Strategy for the Diagnosis, Management, and Prevention of Chronic Obstructive Pulmonary Disease*. 2021 April 28, 2022], Available from: http://www.goldcopd.org/.

[3] Halpin, D., Criner, G. J., Papi, A., Singh, D., Anzueto, A., Martinez, F. J., Agusti, A. A., and Vogelmeier, C. F. (2021). Global Initiative for the Diagnosis, Management, and Prevention of Chronic Obstructive Lung Disease. The 2020 GOLD Science Committee Report on COVID-19 and Chronic Obstructive Pulmonary Disease. *American Journal of Respiratory and Critical Care Medicine*, 203(1), p. 24-36.

[4] Samannan, R., Holt, G., Calderon-Candelario, R., Mirsaeidi, M., and Campos, M. (2021). Effect of Face Masks on Gas Exchange in Healthy Persons and Patients with Chronic Obstructive Pulmonary Disease. *Annals of the American Thoracic Society*, 18(3), p. 541-544.

[5] Aggarwal, A.N., Gupta, D., and Jindal, S. K. (2006). The relationship between FEV1 and peak expiratory flow in patients with airways obstruction is poor. *Chest*, 130(5): p. 1454-61.

[6] Higham, A., Mathioudakis, A., Vestbo, J., and Singh, D. (2020). COVID-19 and COPD: a narrative review of the basic science and clinical outcomes. *European Respiratory Review: An Official Journal of the European Respiratory Society*, 29(158), p. 1-13.

[7] Pothirat, C., Chaiwong, W., Phetsuk, N., Liwsrisakun, C., Bumroongkit, C., Deesomchok, A., Theerakittikul, T., and Limsukon, A. (2015). Peak expiratory flow rate as a surrogate for forced expiratory volume in 1 second in COPD severity classification in Thailand. *International Journal of Chronic Obstructive Pulmonary Disease*, 10, p. 1213-8.

[8] Halpin, D., Faner, R., Sibila, O., Badia, J. R., and Agusti, A. (2020). Do chronic respiratory diseases or their treatment affect the risk of SARS-CoV-2 infection? *The Lancet: Respiratory Medicine*, 8(5), p. 436-8.

[9] Perencevich, E. N., Diekema, D. J., and Edmond, M. B. (2020). Moving Personal Protective Equipment Into the Community: Face Shields and Containment of COVID-19. *JAMA*, 323(22), p. 2252-2253.

[10] Jackson, H., and Hubbard, R. (2003). Detecting chronic obstructive pulmonary disease using peak flow rate: cross sectional survey. *BMJ (Clinical research ed.)*, 327(7416): p. 653-4.

[11] Mekonen, S., et al., (2020). *Prevalence and Risk Factors of Mortality among Hospitalized Patients with COVID-19: A Systematic Review and Meta-analysis.*

[12] Polverino, F., and Kheradmand, F. (2021). COVID-19, COPD, and AECOPD: Immunological, Epidemiological, and Clinical Aspects. *Frontiers in Medicine*, 7, p. 1-8.

[13] Lippi, G., and Henry, B. M. (2020). Chronic obstructive pulmonary disease is associated with severe coronavirus disease 2019 (COVID-19). *Respiratory Medicine*, 167(105941), p. 1-2.

[14] Wu, Z., and McGoogan, J. M. (2020). Characteristics of and Important Lessons From the Coronavirus Disease 2019 (COVID-19) Outbreak in China: Summary of a Report of 72 314 Cases From the Chinese Center for Disease Control and Prevention. *JAMA*, 323(13), p. 1239-42.

[15] Lacedonia, D., Scioscia, G., Santomasi, C., Fuso, P., Carpagnano, G. E., Portacci, A., Mastroianni, F., Larizza, G., Sabato, E., Profilo, E., Resta, E., Foschino Barbaro, M. P., and Resta, O. (2021). Impact of smoking, COPD and comorbidities on the mortality of COVID-19 patients. *Scientific Reports*, 11(1), p. 1-9.

[16] Guan, W. J., Liang, W. H., Zhao, Y., Liang, H. R., Chen, Z. S., Li, Y. M., Liu, X. Q., Chen, R. C., Tang, C. L., Wang, T., Ou, C. Q., Li, L., Chen, P. Y., Sang, L., Wang, W., Li, J. F., Li, C. C., Ou, L. M., Cheng, B., Xiong, S., … (2020). China Medical Treatment Expert Group for COVID-19, Comorbidity and its impact on 1590 patients with COVID-19 in China: a nationwide analysis. *The European Respiratory Journal*, 55(5), p. 1-14.

[17] Lagi, F., Piccica, M., Graziani, L., Vellere, I., Botta, A., Tilli, M., Ottino, L., Borchi, B., Pozzi, M., Bartalesi, F., Mencarini, J., Spinicci, M., Zammarchi, L., Pieralli, F., Zagli, G., Nozzoli, C., Romagnoli, S., Bartoloni, A., and COCORA working group members not listed as individual author. (2020). Early experience of an infectious and tropical diseases unit during the coronavirus disease (COVID-19) pandemic, Florence, Italy, February to March 2020. *European Communicable Disease Bulletin*, 25(17), p. 1-6.

[18] Richardson, S., Hirsch, J. S., Narasimhan, M., Crawford, J. M., McGinn, T., Davidson, K. W., the Northwell COVID-19 Research Consortium, Barnaby, D. P., Becker, L. B., Chelico, J. D., Cohen, S. L., Cookingham, J., Coppa, K., Diefenbach, M. A., Dominello, A. J., Duer-Hefele, J., Falzon, L., Gitlin, J., Hajizadeh, N., Harvin, T. G., … Zanos, T. P. (2020). Presenting Characteristics, Comorbidities, and Outcomes Among 5700 Patients Hospitalized With COVID-19 in the New York City Area. *JAMA*, 323(20), p. 2052-9.

[19] Tomlins, J., Hamilton, F., Gunning, S., Sheehy, C., Moran, E., and MacGowan, A. (2020). Clinical features of 95 sequential hospitalised patients with novel coronavirus 2019 disease (COVID-19), the first UK cohort. *The Journal of Infection*, 81(12), p. e59-61.

[20] Leung, J. M., Niikura, M., Yang, C., and Sin, D. D. (2020). COVID-19 and COPD. *The European Respiratory Journal*, 56(2).

[21] Cummings, M. J., Baldwin, M. R., Abrams, D., Jacobson, S. D., Meyer, B. J., Balough, E. M., Aaron, J. G., Claassen, J., Rabbani, L. E., Hastie, J., Hochman, B. R., Salazar-Schicchi, J., Yip, N. H., Brodie, D., and O'Donnell, M. R. (2020). Epidemiology, clinical course, and outcomes of critically ill adults with COVID-19 in New York City: a prospective cohort study. *Lancet* (London, England), 395(10239), p. 1763–1770.

[22] Alqahtani, J. S., Oyelade, T., Aldhahir, A. M., Alghamdi, S. M., Almehmadi, M., Alqahtani, A. S., Quaderi, S., Mandal, S., and Hurst, J. R. (2020). Prevalence, Severity and Mortality associated with COPD and Smoking in patients with COVID-19: A Rapid Systematic Review and Meta-Analysis. *PloS One*, 15(5).

[23] Yamaya, M., Nishimura, H., Deng, X., Sugawara, M., Watanabe, O., Nomura, K., Shimotai, Y., Momma, H., Ichinose, M., and Kawase, T. (2020). Inhibitory effects of glycopyrronium, formoterol, and budesonide on coronavirus HCoV-229E replication and cytokine production by primary cultures of human nasal and tracheal epithelial cells. *Respiratory Investigation*, 58(3), p. 155-68.

[24] Yin, T., Li, Y., Ying, Y., and Luo, Z. (2021). Prevalence of comorbidity in Chinese patients with COVID-19: systematic review and meta-analysis of risk factors. *BMC Infectious Diseases*, 21(1), p. 1-13.

[25] Gómez Antúnez, M., Muiño Míguez, A., Bendala Estrada, A. D., Maestro de la Calle, G., Monge Monge, D., Boixeda, R., Ena, J., Mella Pérez, C., Anton Santos, J. M., Lumbreras Bermejo, C., and SEMI-COVID-19 Network. (2021). Clinical Characteristics and Prognosis of COPD Patients

Hospitalized with SARS-CoV-2. *International Journal of Chronic Obstructive Pulmonary Disease*, 15, p. 3433-45.

[26] Ackermann, M., Verleden, S. E., Kuehnel, M., Haverich, A., Welte, T., Laenger, F., Vanstapel, A., Werlein, C., Stark, H., Tzankov, A., Li, W. W., Li, V. W., Mentzer, S. J., and Jonigk, D. (2020). Pulmonary Vascular Endothelialitis, Thrombosis, and Angiogenesis in Covid-19. *The New England Journal of Medicine*, 383(2), p. 120-8.

[27] Noh, J., Chang, H. H., Jeong, I. K., and Yoon, K. H. (2020). Coronavirus Disease 2019 and Diabetes: The Epidemic and the Korean Diabetes Association Perspective. *Diabetes & Metabolism Journal*, 44(3), p. 372-81.

[28] Aleva, F. E., Voets, L., Simons, S. O., de Mast, Q., van der Ven, A., and Heijdra, Y. F. (2017). Prevalence and Localization of Pulmonary Embolism in Unexplained Acute Exacerbations of COPD: A Systematic Review and Meta-analysis. *Chest*, 151(3), p. 544-54.

[29] Higham, A., Karur, P., Jackson, N., Cunoosamy, D. M., Jansson, P., and Singh, D. (2018). Differential anti-inflammatory effects of budesonide and a p38 MAPK inhibitor AZD7624 on COPD pulmonary cells. *International Journal of Chronic Obstructive Pulmonary Disease*, 13, p. 1279-88.

[30] Vaidyula, V. R., Criner, G. J., Grabianowski, C., and Rao, A. K. (2009). Circulating tissue factor procoagulant activity is elevated in stable moderate to severe chronic obstructive pulmonary disease. *Thrombosis Research*, 124(3), p. 259-61.

[31] Salvi, S. S., Dhar, R., Mahesh, P. A., Udwadia, Z. F., and Behra, D. (2021). COPD Management during the COVID-19 pandemic. *Lung India: Official Organ of Indian Chest Society*, 38, p. S80-5.

[32] Klok, F. A., Kruip, M., van der Meer, N., Arbous, M. S., Gommers, D., Kant, K. M., Kaptein, F., van Paassen, J., Stals, M., Huisman, M. V., and Endeman, H. (2020). Incidence of thrombotic complications in critically ill ICU patients with COVID-19. *Thrombosis Research*, 191, p. 145-7.

[33] Wedzicha, J. A. (2004). Role of viruses in exacerbations of chronic obstructive pulmonary disease. *Proceedings of the American Thoracic Society*, 1(2), p. 115-20.

[34] Shin, B., Kim, S. H., Yong, S. J., Lee, W. Y., Park, S., Lee, S. J., Lee, S. J., and Lee, M. K. (2019). Early readmission and mortality in acute exacerbation of chronic obstructive pulmonary disease with community-acquired pneumonia. *Chronic Respiratory Disease*, 16, p. 1-12.

[35] Wu, C., Chen, X., Cai, Y., Xia, J., Zhou, X., Xu, S., Huang, H., Zhang, L., Zhou, X., Du, C., Zhang, Y., Song, J., Wang, S., Chao, Y., Yang, Z., Xu, J., Zhou, X., Chen, D., Xiong, W., Xu, L., … Song, Y. (2020). Risk Factors Associated With Acute Respiratory Distress Syndrome and Death in Patients With Coronavirus Disease 2019 Pneumonia in Wuhan, China. *JAMA Internal Medicine*, 180(7), p. 934-43.

[36] Simons, S. O., Hurst, J. R., Miravitlles, M., Franssen, F., Janssen, D., Papi, A., Duiverman, M. L., and Kerstjens, H. (2020). Caring for patients with COPD and COVID-19: a viewpoint to spark discussion. *Thorax*, 75(12), p. 1035-9.

[37] Lee, S. C., Son, K. J., Han, C. H., Park, S. C., and Jung, J. Y. (2021). Impact of COPD on COVID-19 prognosis: A nationwide population-based study in South Korea. *Scientific Reports*, 11(1), p. 1-8.

[38] Huang, Y., Tan, C., Wu, J., Chen, M., Wang, Z., Luo, L., Zhou, X., Liu, X., Huang, X., Yuan, S., Chen, C., Gao, F., Huang, J., Shan, H., and Liu, J. (2020). Impact of coronavirus disease 2019 on pulmonary function in early convalescence phase. *Respiratory Research*, 21(1).

[39] Zhao, Y. M., Shang, Y. M., Song, W. B., Li, Q. Q., Xie, H., Xu, Q. F., Jia, J. L., Li, L. M., Mao, H. L., Zhou, X. M., Luo, H., Gao, Y. F., and Xu, A. G. (2020). Follow-up study of the pulmonary function and related physiological characteristics of COVID-19 survivors three months after recovery. *EClinicalMedicine*, 25(100463), p. 1-9.

[40] Wang, B., Li, R., Lu, Z., and Huang, Y. (2020). Does comorbidity increase the risk of patients with COVID-19: evidence from meta-analysis. *Aging*, 12(7), p. 6049-57.

[41] Vanfleteren, L., Spruit, M. A., Wouters, E., and Franssen, F. (2016). Management of chronic obstructive pulmonary disease beyond the lungs. *The Lancet. Respiratory Medicine*. 4(11), p. 911-24.

[42] Hsu, A. C., Parsons, K., Moheimani, F., Knight, D. A., Hansbro, P. M., Fujita, T., and Wark, P. A. (2016). Impaired Antiviral Stress Granule and IFN-β Enhanceosome Formation Enhances Susceptibility to Influenza Infection in Chronic Obstructive Pulmonary Disease Epithelium. *American Journal of Respiratory Cell and Molecular Biology*, 55(1), p. 117-27.

[43] Lee, S. C., Son, K. J., Han, C. H., Jung, J. Y., and Park, S. C. (2020). Impact of comorbid asthma on severity of coronavirus disease (COVID-19). *Scientific Reports*, 10(1), p. 1-9.

[44] Bartoletti, M., Giannella, M., Scudeller, L., Tedeschi, S., Rinaldi, M., Bussini, L., Fornaro, G., Pascale, R., Pancaldi, L., Pasquini, Z., Trapani, F., Badia, L., Campoli, C., Tadolini, M., Attard, L., Puoti, M., Merli, M., Mussini, C., Menozzi, M., Meschiari, M., … PREDICO study group. (2020). Development and validation of a prediction model for severe respiratory failure in hospitalized patients with SARS-CoV-2 infection: a multicentre cohort study (PREDI-CO study). *Clinical Microbiology and Infection: The Official Publication of the European Society of Clinical Microbiology and Infectious Diseases*, 26(11), p. 1545-53.

[45] Chu, D. K., Akl, E. A., Duda, S., Solo, K., Yaacoub, S., Schünemann, H. J., & COVID-19 Systematic Urgent Review Group Effort (SURGE) study authors. (2020). Physical distancing, face masks, and eye protection to prevent person-to-person transmission of SARS-CoV-2 and COVID-19: a systematic review and meta-analysis. *Lancet (London, England)*, 395(10242), p. 1973–1987.

[46] Li, X., Xu, S., Yu, M., Wang, K., Tao, Y., Zhou, Y., Shi, J., Zhou, M., Wu, B., Yang, Z., Zhang, C., Yue, J., Zhang, Z., Renz, H., Liu, X., Xie, J., Xie, M., and Zhao, J. (2020). Risk factors for severity and mortality in adult COVID-19 inpatients in Wuhan. *The Journal of Allergy and Clinical Immunology*, 146(1), p. 110-8.

[47] Docherty, A. B., Harrison, E. M., Green, C. A., Hardwick, H. E., Pius, R., Norman, L., Holden, K. A., Read, J. M., Dondelinger, F., Carson, G., Merson, L., Lee, J., Plotkin, D., Sigfrid, L., Halpin, S., Jackson, C., Gamble, C., Horby, P. W., Nguyen-Van-Tam, J. S., Ho, A., … (2020). ISARIC4C investigators, Features of 20 133 UK patients in hospital with covid-19 using the ISARIC WHO Clinical Characterisation Protocol: prospective observational cohort study. *BMJ (Clinical research ed.)*, 369(m1985), p. 1-12.

[48] Cai, G., Bossé, Y., Xiao, F., Kheradmand, F., and Amos, C. I. (2020). Tobacco Smoking Increases the Lung Gene Expression of ACE2, the Receptor of SARS-CoV-2. *American Journal of Respiratory and Critical Care Medicine*, 201(12), p. 1557-9.

[49] Smith, J. C., Sausville, E. L., Girish, V., Yuan, M. L., Vasudevan, A., John, K. M., and Sheltzer, J. M. (2020). Cigarette Smoke Exposure and Inflammatory Signaling Increase the Expression of the SARS-CoV-2 Receptor ACE2 in the Respiratory Tract. *Developmental Cell*, 53(5), p. 514-29.

[50] British Thoracic Society. *COPD and COVID-19 for Healthcare Professionals*. 2020 April 30, 2022]; Available from: https://www.brit-thoracic.org.uk/about-us/covid-19-information-for-the-respiratory-community.

[51] National Institute for Health and Care Excellence (NICE). (2020). *COVID-19 Rapid Guideline: Community-Based Care of Patients with Chronic Obstructive Pulmonary Disease (COPD).*

[52] Tamara, A., and Tahapary, D. L. (2020). Obesity as a predictor for a poor prognosis of COVID-19: A systematic review. *Diabetes & Metabolic Syndrome*, 14(4), p. 655-9.

[53] Higham, A., and Singh, D. (2020). Increased ACE2 Expression in Bronchial Epithelium of COPD Patients who are Overweight. *Obesity (Silver Spring, Md)*, 28(9), p. 1586-9.

[54] Zeigler, Z. (2021). COVID-19 Self-quarantine and Weight Gain Risk Factors in Adults. *Current Obesity Reports*, 10(3), p. 423-33.

[55] Dijkstra-Kersten, S., Kok, L., Kerckhoffs, M. C., Cremer, O. L., de Lange, D. W., van Dijk, D., Needham, D. M., and Slooter, A. (2020). Neuropsychiatric outcome in subgroups of Intensive Care Unit survivors: Implications for after-care. *Journal of Critical Care*, 55, p. 171-6.

[56] Rawson, T. M., Moore, L., Zhu, N., Ranganathan, N., Skolimowska, K., Gilchrist, M., Satta, G., Cooke, G., and Holmes, A. (2020). Bacterial and Fungal Coinfection in Individuals With Coronavirus: A Rapid Review To Support COVID-19 Antimicrobial Prescribing. *Clinical Infectious Diseases : An Official Publication of the Infectious Diseases Society of America*, 71(9), p. 2459-68.

[57] van Geffen, W. H., Douma, W. R., Slebos, D. J., and Kerstjens, H. A. (2016). Bronchodilators delivered by nebuliser versus pMDI with spacer or DPI for exacerbations of COPD. *The Cochrane Database of Systematic Reviews*, 2016(8), p. CD011826.

[58] Tran, K., Cimon, K., Severn, M., Pessoa-Silva, C. L., and Conly, J. (2012). Aerosol Generating Procedures and Risk of Transmission of Acute Respiratory Infections to Healthcare Workers: A Systematic Review. *PloS one*, 7(4), p. 1-8.

[59] Wu, F., Zhou, Y., Wang, Z., Xie, M., Shi, Z., Tang, Z., Li, X., Li, X., Lei, C., Li, Y., Ni, Z., Hu, Y., Liu, X., Yin, W., Cheng, L., Ye, F., Peng, J., Huang, L., Tian, J., Zhang, L., … Medical Treatment Expert Group for COPD and COVID-19, Clinical characteristics of COVID-19 infection in chronic obstructive pulmonary disease: a multicenter, retrospective, observational study. *Journal of Thoracic Disease*, (2020). 12(5), p. 1811-23.

[60] RECOVERY Collaborative Group, H., P., Lim, W. S., Emberson, J. R., Mafham, M., Bell, J. L., Linsell, L., Staplin, N., Brightling, C., Ustianowski, A., Elmahi, E., Prudon, B., Green, C., Felton, T., Chadwick, D., Rege, K., Fegan, C., Chappell, L. C., Faust, S. N., Jaki, T., … Landray, M. J., Dexamethasone in Hospitalized Patients with Covid-19. *The New England Journal of Medicine*, (2021). 384(8), p. 693-704.

[61] World Health Organization. *Clinical management of COVID-19: interim guidance*. 2020 April 30, 2022]; Available from: https://www.who.int/publications/i/item/WHO-2019-nCoV-clinical-2021-1.

[62] Jeon, S., Ko, M., Lee, J., Choi, I., Byun, S. Y., Park, S., Shum, D., and Kim, S. (2020). Identification of Antiviral Drug Candidates against SARS-CoV-2 from FDA-Approved Drugs. *Antimicrobial Agents and Chemotherapy*, 64(7), p. e00819-20.

[63] Skevaki, C. L., Christodoulou, I., Spyridaki, I. S., Tiniakou, I., Georgiou, V., Xepapadaki, P., Kafetzis, D. A., and Papadopoulos, N. G. (2009). Budesonide and formoterol inhibit inflammatory mediator production by bronchial epithelial cells infected with rhinovirus. *Clinical and Experimental Allergy: Journal of the British Society for Allergy and Clinical Immunology*, 39(11), p. 1700-10.

[64] Bafadhel, M., Peterson, S., De Blas, M. A., Calverley, P. M., Rennard, S. I., Richter, K., and Fagerås. M. (2018). Predictors of exacerbation risk and response to budesonide in patients with chronic obstructive pulmonary disease: a post-hoc analysis of three randomised trials. *The Lancet: Respiratory Medicine*, 6(2), p. 117-26.

[65] Choi, J. C., Jung, S. Y., Yoon, U. A., You, S. H., Kim, M. S., Baek, M. S., Jung, J. W., and Kim, W. Y. (2020). Inhaled Corticosteroids and COVID-19 Risk and Mortality: A Nationwide Cohort Study. *Journal of Clinical Medicine*, 9(11), p. 1-13.

[66] Schultze, A., Walker, A. J., MacKenna, B., Morton, C. E., Bhaskaran, K., Brown, J. P., Rentsch, C. T., Williamson, E., Drysdale, H., Croker, R., Bacon, S., Hulme, W., Bates, C., Curtis, H. J., Mehrkar, A., Evans, D., Inglesby, P., Cockburn, J., McDonald, H. I., Tomlinson, L., … OpenSAFELY Collaborative, Risk of COVID-19-related death among patients with chronic obstructive pulmonary disease or asthma prescribed inhaled corticosteroids: an observational cohort study using the OpenSAFELY platform. *The Lancet: Respiratory Medicine*, (2020). 8(11), p. 1106-20.

[67] Chalmers, J. D., Laska, I. F., Franssen, F., Janssens, W., Pavord, I., Rigau, D., McDonnell, M. J., Roche, N., Sin, D. D., Stolz, D., Suissa, S., Wedzicha, J., and Miravitlles, M. (2020). Withdrawal of inhaled corticosteroids in COPD: a European Respiratory Society guideline. *The European Respiratory Journal*, 55(6), p. 1-12.

[68] Vogelmeier, C. F., Criner, G. J., Martinez, F. J., Anzueto, A., Barnes, P. J., Bourbeau, J., Celli, B. R., Chen, R., Decramer, M., Fabbri, L. M., Frith, P., Halpin, D. M., López Varela, M. V., Nishimura, M., Roche, N., Rodriguez-Roisin, R., Sin, D. D., Singh, D., Stockley, R., Vestbo, J., … Agustí, A. (2017). Global Strategy for the Diagnosis, Management, and Prevention of Chronic Obstructive Lung Disease 2017 Report. GOLD Executive Summary. *American Journal of Respiratory and Critical Care Medicine*, 195(5), p. 557-82.

[69] Wilkinson, T., Hurst, J. R., Perera, W. R., Wilks, M., Donaldson, G. C., and Wedzicha, J. A. (2006). Effect of interactions between lower airway bacterial and rhinoviral infection in exacerbations of COPD. *Chest*. 129(2), p. 317-24.

[70] Verroken, A., Scohy, A., Gérard, L., Wittebole, X., Collienne, C., and Laterre, P. F. (2020). Co-infections in COVID-19 critically ill and antibiotic management: a prospective cohort analysis. *Critical Care (London, England)*, 24(1), p. 1-3.

[71] Sanchez-Ramirez, D. C., and Mackey, D. (2020). Underlying respiratory diseases, specifically COPD, and smoking are associated with severe COVID-19 outcomes: A systematic review and meta-analysis. *Respiratory Medicine*, 171, p. 1-10.

[72] Alqahtani, J. S., et al. (2022). Sleep Quality, Insomnia, Anxiety, Fatigue, Stress, Memory and Active Coping during the COVID-19 Pandemic. *International Journal of Environmental Research and Public Health*, 19(9).

[73] Abuhamdah, S. M. A., et al. (2021). The Prevalence of Mental Distress and Social Support among University Students in Jordan: A Cross-Sectional Study. *Int J Environ Res Public Health*, 18(21).

[74] Alyami, H. S., et al. (2021). Depression and anxiety during the COVID-19 pandemic in Saudi Arabia: A cross-sectional study. *Int J Clin Pract*. 75(7), p. e14244.

[75] Varghese, A., et al. (2021). Decline in the mental health of nurses across the globe during COVID-19: A systematic review and meta-analysis. *J Glob Health*, 11, p. 05009.

[76] Alsairafi, Z., et al. (2021). Mental Health Status of Healthcare Professionals and Students of Health Sciences Faculties in Kuwait during the COVID-19 Pandemic. *Int J Environ Res Public Health*, 18(4).

[77] Naser, A. Y., et al. (2021). The effect of the 2019 coronavirus disease outbreak on social relationships: A cross-sectional study in Jordan. *Int J Soc Psychiatry*, 67(6), p. 664-671.

[78] Naser, A. Y., et al. (2020). Mental health status of the general population, healthcare professionals, and university students during 2019 coronavirus disease outbreak in Jordan: A cross-sectional study. *Brain Behav*., 10(8), p. e01730.

[79] Atlantis, E., Fahey, P., Cochrane, B., and Smith, S. (2013). Bidirectional associations between clinically relevant depression or anxiety and COPD: a systematic review and meta-analysis. *Chest*, 144(3), p. 766-77.

[80] Abukhalaf, A. H. I. and Cohen, S. (2021). *COVID-19's Negative Mental Health Impact Goes Well Beyond Standard At-Risk Populations: Action Needs to be Taken to Combat Long-term Nationwide Emotional Disruption*. Academia Letters.

[81] Abukhalaf, A. H. I. and Cohen, S. (2022). *The Growing Mental Health Crisis Among America's Children, Adolescents, and Young Adults*. Academia Letters.

[82] Wei, L., Islam, J. Y., Mascareno, E. A., Rivera, A., Vidot, D. C., and Camacho-Rivera, M. (2021). Physical and Mental Health Impacts of the COVID-19 Pandemic among US Adults with Chronic Respiratory Conditions. *Journal of Clinical Medicine*, 10(7), p. 1-12.

[83] Islam, J. Y., Vidot, D. C., and Camacho-Rivera, M. (2021). Evaluating Mental Health-Related Symptoms Among Cancer Survivors During the COVID-19 Pandemic: An Analysis of the COVID Impact Survey. *JCO Oncology Practice*, 17(9), p. e1258-69.

Chapter 28

COPD Management during the COVID-19 Pandemic

Victor Manuel Mendoza Romero[1,*], MD, Rogelio García Torrentera[2], MD, Eduardo Vázquez Alcocer[3], MD, Omar Durán Nava[3], MD and Amaury Hernán González Molina[3], MD

[1]Lung Transplant Unit,
National Institute of Respiratory Diseases, Mexico City, Mexico
[2] Respiratory Emergency Unit,
National Institute of Respiratory Diseases, Mexico City, Mexico
[3]National Institute of Respiratory Diseases, Mexico City, Mexico

Abstract

It is estimated that there are approximately 300 million cases of COPD worldwide, considering it a vulnerable population for the development, worsening of symptoms and greater complications in SARS-CoV-2 infection. The suspected diagnosis, approach, treatment and follow-up of the population diagnosed with COPD and the development of COVID-19 represents a challenge for healthcare personal.

There is limited evidence whether COPD is an independent risk factor for the worsening of COVID-19, or whether the various comorbidities of patients with COPD determine a poor response to the SARS-CoV-2 infection.

Below we present a brief summary of the main interventions carried out in the management of patients diagnosed with chronic obstructive pulmonary disease during the COVID-19 pandemic.

Introduction

The COVID-19 pandemic caused by the SARS-CoV-2 virus was identified in December 2019 in the city of Wuhan (China) and subsequently spread worldwide. COVID-19 disease largely affects the respiratory tract, causing lower respiratory tract infections in about 20% to 25% of cases, some of which progress further to develop severe acute respiratory syndrome. Mortality

* Corresponding Author's Email: dr.victormendoza.iner@gmail.com.

In: Chronic Obstructive Pulmonary Disease
Editor: Jaber S. Alqahtani
ISBN: 979-8-88697-333-4

ranges from 2% to 15% and is higher among the elderly and those with associated comorbidities, such as ischemic heart disease, hypertension, diabetes, and chronic obstructive pulmonary disease (COPD) [1].

There are an estimated 300 million cases of COPD in the community worldwide who are more vulnerable not only to contracting the infection but also to developing the more severe form of COVID-19 disease, predisposing them to major complications [1].

COPD patients should follow and maintain basic infection control measures, including social distancing, handwashing, and wearing a mask or face covering. Patients should be brought up to date on appropriate vaccinations, particularly annual influenza vaccination. Although data are limited, inhaled corticosteroids, long-acting bronchodilators, roflumilast, or chronic macrolides should continue to be used as indicated for stable treatment of COPD. Systemic steroids and antibiotics should be used in COPD exacerbations according to the usual indications [2].

Differentiating symptoms of COVID-19 infection from chronic underlying symptoms or an acute exacerbation of COPD is challenging. Medical staff should take a detailed clinical history and support the diagnosis with SARS-CoV-2 PCR test [2].

Risk of SARS-CoV-2 Infection

ACE2 receptors are expressed on the apical surfaces of polarized epithelial cells of the lower and upper airways, including primary bronchial epithelial cells. The ACE2 receptors increase their expression by nicotine-dependent activation of the α7 subtype of acetylcholine receptors of acetylcholine (α7-nAChR). The levels of CHRNA7 (the gene that encodes α7-nAChR) in the bronchial epithelium are higher in smokers.

The expression of ACE2 and TMPRSS2 modulate the susceptibility of the individual and the clinical course of SARS-Cov2 infection, the expression of ACE2 mRNA is increased in COPD, this, might explain why people diagnosed with COPD are more susceptible of contracting COVID-19, at least in theory [3, 14].

At the moment it is not known with certainty if the fact that living with COPD represents a greater risk of suffering from a SARS-Cov-2 infection [17]. This is due to the fact that there are few studies with acceptable methodological quality that have solid conclusions.

Various observational studies around the world that report the accompanying diseases of patients with COVID-19 in its different presentations do not mention COPD as a significant disease, at least in frequency [17]. There are even studies that mention chronic obstructive pulmonary disease as a rare disease in patients with COVID-19. On the other hand, there are case series that mention information completely different from that mentioned above and even mention COPD as an independent risk factor that increases the risk of serious illness and death [17].

Finally, based on the evidence that has been generated in the last two years since the start of the pandemic, it is not known whether having chronic obstructive pulmonary disease constitutes an increased risk of infection and whether, once acquired, infection is more severe.

SARS-CoV-2 Infection Tests

Spirometry and Pulmonary Function Tests

The decision to perform spirometry for diagnostic purposes should be made based on the rate of transmission and prevalence of the disease according to local statistics where the patient resides [17]. During periods of high transmission in the community, it is recommended to perform spirometry only in patients who require it in a strictly urgently manner in order to make a diagnosis of COPD, as well as for patients with COPD who will undergo surgical intervention in whom spirometry is an integral part of the pre-surgical assessment. According to the ATS/ERS recommendations, it is recommended to perform a real-time polymerase chain reaction (RT-PCR) test whenever possible prior to performing spirometry, based on the previous recommendation, in patients who present a positive RT-PCR test should have spirometry deferred until they present a negative RT-PCR test [17].

Spirometry is the diagnostic test per excellence for COPD and should be performed in all patients to confirm the diagnosis. However, due to the effort required by the patient when performing the test, it is an aerosol-generating procedure, entailing a substantially higher risk of spreading the infection to other patients and health personnel. The 2020 GINA guidelines for asthma have recommended avoiding spirometry in patients with suspected/confirmed COVID-19 [16]. It is also suggested that spirometry should be performed under protective conditions within healthcare facilities if there is an urgent need [1].

In the absence of routine spirometry, home peak expiratory flow (PEF) measurement, combined with validated patient questionnaires, could be used to support or refute a possible diagnosis of COPD [4, 5]. However, PEF does not correlate well with spirometry results, it has low specificity and it has been demonstrated that it's not useful to differentiate between obstructive pattern and one suggestive of restriction [2, 6, 7].

Bronchoscopy

There is a select group of patients with obstructive pulmonary disease who may require diagnostic and/or therapeutic bronchoscopy during the course of their disease.

Elective bronchoscopy should be delayed until patients have a negative PCR test. In urgent cases where COVID-19 infection status is unknown, all cases should be handled as if symptom positive. A disposable bronchoscope should be used if available, with all personal protection measures, and limiting the test to the smallest number of healthcare personal [2].

Radiology

Recommendations have been made on the use of CT as part of diagnostic tests and evaluation of the severity of COVID-19, without special considerations for COPD patients. The initial characteristics of COVID-19 on CT and its progression over time have been reviewed. COPD patients with COVID-19 have a higher prevalence of bilateral and diffuse areas of increased attenuation, ground-glass opacities, and interstitial abnormalities on CT compared to the non-COPD population [2].

In COPD exacerbations, the possible habitual triggers must be individualized, differentiating the symptoms of COVID-19 infection from the underlying chronic symptoms, which is a challenge [2].

Pharmacological Maintenance Treatment of COPD during the COVID-19 Pandemic

There is currently no convincing evidence that the use of inhaled medications commonly used in COPD has a positive or negative impact on the severity of SARS-CoV-2 infection. It is recommended to continue with the same maintenance and exacerbation management for patients with COPD according to the most recent international guidelines. Based on what is known so far, maintaining patients on optimized controller therapy is the best way to prevent viral exacerbations, including those caused by SARS-CoV-2 [18]. This includes patients using short-acting and long-acting bronchodilators, as well as patients using inhaled corticosteroids.

Oral corticosteroids impair induction of antiviral Type-I interferon responses to a range of respiratory viruses, effects that are likely to also occur in the context of COVID-19. The use of ICS and systemic medications has been controversial in the treatment and prevention of COPD during the COVID-19 pandemic. Some laboratory experiments show that ICS may increase the replication of viruses such as rhinoviruses and influenza viruses. In contrast, other laboratory data show that long-acting bronchodilators and corticosteroids can decrease the replication of coronaviruses, including SARS-CoV-2. However, these data are limited on the use of long-acting bronchodilators, LAMAs or LABAs, roflumilast, macrolides in COPD patients and clinical outcomes of SARS-CoV-2 infection; therefore, until sufficient evidence emerges, these patients should continue with the drugs that generate stability in their disease [1, 2, 3].

A critical point in pharmacological therapy is the correct selection of the device, since it has been shown that the maneuvers performed during its use can be associated with the generation of aerosols. SARS-CoV-2 has been shown to be viable in aerosols for up to 90 minutes, and transmission to healthcare workers exposed to a hospitalized COVID-19 patient receiving nebulized therapy has been reported. If possible, the use of pressurized metered-dose inhalers, soft-mist inhalers, and dry-powder inhalers for medication delivery is suggested instead of nebulizers. Measures should be taken to prevent nebulized therapy from spreading infection to others in patients' homes by preventing its use in the presence of others and by ensuring that the nebulizer is used near open windows or in areas of increased air circulation [2, 12].

Non-Pharmacological Treatment of COPD during the COVID-19 Pandemic

During the COVID-19 pandemic, COPD patients must continue their non-pharmacological therapy. Patients must receive their annual influenza vaccine; this creates a challenge due to the restrictions implemented by the different health systems such as social distancing. There is no reason to change palliative care approaches due to COVID-19. It is imperative that patients currently receiving long-term oxygen therapy should continue with it. The patient should be monitored with a pulse oximeter and kept in the range prescribed by the health care provider. In case of decreased SpO2 and worsening of dyspnea, the patient should be recommended for evaluation in a hospital unit [1, 2].

COPD Exacerbations

To date, MERS-CoV, SARS-CoV, and SARS-CoV-2 infections have not been reported in COPD exacerbations. However, COPD patients with SARS-CoV-2 infection who present with respiratory symptoms that require changes in their maintenance medications would meet the definition of an exacerbation. Distinguishing these symptoms from a typical exacerbation of COVID-19 infection is diagnostic challenge due to the overlap of several symptoms.

If COVID-19 infection is suspected, RTPCR testing should be performed. If COVID-19 infection is confirmed, treatment for COVID-19 infection should be performed regardless of the presence of COPD. Patients with AECOPD and COVID-19 are at elevated risk of cardiovascular events and mortality after the acute phase of the disease. It has been recommended that in this vulnerable period, patients be monitored with a management plan that that focuses on detection to timely recognition of cardiovascular complications, especially in the first month after resolution of the acute phase [1, 2].

Systemic Corticosteroids

Observational studies in patients with SARS and MERS did not find an association between the use of steroids and better survival, however, it was shown that the use of steroids can be associated with adverse effects such as ostonecrosis and prolonged viral shedding; Due to these findings, routine use of corticosteroids was not recommended. The WHO only recommended the use of steroids in 2 specific clinical contexts: adult patients with ARDS and patients with COPD exacerbation and COVID-19 infection [2].

One of the main concerns during the development of the pandemic has been the use of systemic corticosteroids as a treatment for COPD exacerbations. In the current context, patients can be divided into 2 groups: the first is the group of patients with COPD exacerbation caused by SARS-CoV-2 and the second is the group with COPD exacerbation caused by any other agent.

In patients in whom the cause of the exacerbation is other than SARS-CoV-2 infection, the use of systemic corticosteroids should continue as recommended by international guidelines [17]. This is because if exacerbations are not treated correctly (including the use of systemic steroids), patients could present progression and deterioration with the need to go to the emergency room and even require hospitalization. At the moment, there is no evidence to recommend suspending the use of systemic corticosteroids in acute exacerbations of COPD that are not caused by SARS-CoV-2 [17].

The group of patients presenting with an acute exacerbation of COPD in whom a SARS-CoV-2 infection has been identified as the cause represent an exceptional group of patients.

Over the last two years and with the evidence generated regarding the use of systemic corticosteroids in the different stages of COVID-19 disease, concern has arisen regarding the use of systemic corticosteroids in the first 10 days of SARS-CoV-2 infection on the grounds of prolonging viral replication and, consequently, inducing more severe disease. Currently, the use of systemic steroids in patients with acute exacerbation of COPD secondary to SARS-CoV-2 infection has not been specifically studied and, due to the lack of evidence, it is suggested to prioritize the standardized management of an acute exacerbation of COPD which should include the use of systemic steroids [17].

Antibiotics

Antibiotic treatment for a COPD exacerbation is indicated if patients have at least two of the three cardinal symptoms, including increased sputum as well as purulence, or if the patient requires mechanical ventilation. Bacterial coinfections have been reported infrequently in COVID-19, however, the risk of co-infections increases with the severity of COVID-19. Antibiotics should be prescribed in COPD exacerbations in relation to the usual indications, whether or not there is evidence of SARS-COV-2 infection [2].

Many studies reporting various comorbidities in hospitalized COVID-19 patients suggest a lower-than-expected COPD prevalence [4, 14]. These determinations are limited by small sample sizes and incomplete data on comorbidities [2].

To explain the observed lower-than-anticipated prevalence of COPD among COVID-19 patients, it is proposed that treatment or disease may reduce the risk of infection [3, 13, 15]. Neither of these hypotheses has been proven somewhat suggesting that underdiagnosis of COPD is a well-known problem that may contribute to these conclusions, or that complete information on comorbidities, including COPD, was not completed in the medical records. It is also likely that early protection of older, high-risk populations, including COPD patients, is the real reason for the low prevalence observed in many countries [3, 15].

Self-Management in COPD

Due to the limitations in hospital care due to the pandemic, strategies were formulated for the self-management of the patient, from the recognition of symptoms, education, pulmonary rehabilitation, psychosocial support, and remote surveillance [8].

During the pandemic, patient education and pulmonary rehabilitation programs in hospitals or in specialized clinics were reduced, as many of them closed their face-to-face activities, leaving many patients with a gap in care in the aforementioned areas. Therefore, telemedicine programs were started. Some studies have demonstrated that telemedicine programs have positive results in health-related quality of life and activity level outcomes [18].

Although many face-to-face pulmonary rehabilitation programs may have closed during the pandemic, this does not mean that the patient's physical activity cannot be encouraged during the different periods of COVID-19 transmissibility.

Because of the aforementioned problems, it is essential that every time there is contact with the patient, either in person or through telemedicine, all behaviors that can promote a better evolution of the disease are reinforced. Some of the activities that should be favored are exercise programs which should include aerobic exercise, strengthening and flexibility. These activities should be individualized for the patient's environment, including activities that can be performed in the patient's home.

Patient attachment and commitment to self-care programs can be influenced by psychological, social, structural and disease-related factors [9]. Some systematic reviews have studied the impact of self-care in COPD, focusing interventions on: smoking cessation, correct medication administration, timely detection of exacerbations as well as diet and exercise programs. Most of the patients involved in these programs reported that they had a positive experience of their medical care, especially when a multidisciplinary team was included [9, 10].

The Impact of COPD and Smoking History on the Severity of COVID-19

Efforts have been made to determine whether being an active smoker and presenting acute COVID-19 is related to a more severe disease, or even if it is related to the persistence of symptoms in the long run. A systematic review indicated that active smokers have a higher risk of serious disease as well as the need for invasive mechanical ventilation [19].

On the other side, some reports have suggested and attenuating effect associated with smoking in people with COVID-19, by decreasing the probability of cytokine storm as well as a decrease in the severe inflammatory response through cholinergic-mediated anti-inflammatory mechanism, nevertheless, this mitigating effect may be caused by the high concentration of energy deposited from alpha particles emitted by natural radionuclides such as Po-210 in cigarette tobacco. It has previously been reported that a lower number of COVID-19 cases among smokers could be due to the effects of nicotine, noting that nicotine down regulates the ACE2 receptor. The effects of smoking on the suppression of SARS-CoV-2 are not defined, it is considered that there are positive effects in the consumption of 1 to 39 cigarettes per week, this effect is attributed to the presence of polonium-210 and lead-210 radioactive in tobacco smoke and cigarettes, the alpha emission associated with these natural radionuclides leads to the exposure of alveolar cells that line the alveoli, this energy deposit can lead to anti-inflammatory and antithrombotic effects and eventually reduce the risk of hospitalization due to COVID-19 [20].

In various studies, no association has been found between active smoking and the severity of the disease, therefore the impact of COPD and the susceptibility of active smoking in patients, as well as the severity of SARS-CoV-2 infection, is uncertain and controversial [21, 22].

Use of Supplemental Oxygen

Patients who were previously using oxygen should continue its use based on the recommendations established for patients with chronic obstructive pulmonary disease. They should be instructed regarding the proper cleaning of the equipment as well as reinforcing the fact of giving preventive maintenance to the devices used (stationary oxygen concentrator, portable or oxygen tank). In case of problems with the use of oxygen therapy equipment, they should be encouraged to seek immediate care and not avoid seeking timely care in the event of any failure of their equipment.

Home supply of oxygen represents a challenge during the pandemic, as its use has increased due to cases of COVID-19 with home treatment. This is why it is recommended that the COPD patient have backup providers available if needed.

Remote Patient Monitoring and Telemedicine of COPD Patients due to COVID-19 Restrictions

During the current pandemic, there has been a need for remote follow-up and telemedicine for patients with COPD, in order to meet the needs of continuous evaluation of patients and at the same time be able to maintain the isolation measures already known for this particular group of patients.

Remote monitoring represents an important measure to minimize the risk of community transmission of SARS-CoV-2.

Identification of Candidate Patients for Remote Follow-Up and Telemedicine

It is important to distinguish between patients who may be candidates for remote follow-up and to be aware of patients who necessarily require face-to-face follow-up due to their clinical condition.

Candidate patients for remote follow-up and telemedicine:

- The patient and caregiver understand the process, benefits, and limitations of remote monitoring, and are also able to provide information clearly to healthcare personnel.
- This is a previously known patient with regular follow-up and of whom there is full knowledge of accompanying conditions and important comorbidities.
- Medical records and laboratory studies are accessible to healthcare staff to be consulted when necessary.
- The patient has access to medications and in the event of an emergency, the patient also has adequate access to healthcare services.
- Candidates for face-to-face evaluation
- Caregiver or patient has difficulty providing information regarding their current clinical status.
- The patient has a serious medical condition and requires urgent medical attention.
- Recent change in the patient's symptoms and that requires a specific approach to be able to perform a differential diagnosis, requires laboratory or imaging studies as a priority.
- The treatment required by the patient can only be administered by health staff.

Once the correct patient has been identified to be able to be evaluated remotely, a series of evaluations must be completed during the consultation allow the patient's problem to be properly identified, complications to be detected, adequate treatment to be given, and adequate follow-up to be scheduled. The following items are suggested to be fulfilled during a remote evaluation in order to complete the assessment as complete as possible.

1. The beginning of the call must include the introduction by the doctor, verification of who is being spoken to and whether, in addition to the patient and the caregiver, someone else is listening to the call.
2. The technical aspects must be corroborated to allow adequate communication and always confirm that the medical staff, the patient and the caregiver can hear the conversation clearly and fluently. Likewise, a plan must be in place in case the connection fails during the call-in order to reestablish communication through an alternative route.
3. Explain to the patient about the advantages and limitations of a remote assessment.
4. Make clear what are the points to discuss and assess during the remote appointment
5. Consider scheduling a home visit as part of the follow-up
6. At the end of the consultation, confirm that the patient has understood each of the points evaluated and ask him directly to summarize what was explained in the consultation. A date for the next assessment must be set, as well as an action plan in the event of any possible complication or eventuality [11].

As part of the follow-up and monitoring strategies in patients diagnosed with COPD, surveys and consensus were carried out among patients and medical staff of which the respondents highlighted five activities as immediate priorities to improve distance communication: develop online education or improve the way in which video consultations are provided (81%), provision or loan of pulse oximeters for home measurement (83%), establish direct telephone access for emergencies, questions (87%), expand the availability of video consultations for healthcare professionals and patients, including training and support (87%), develop standard guidelines for remote consultations (80%). It is feasible to recognize that remote care for COPD came about rapidly in response to the COVID-19 pandemic. Perceived benefits of remote approaches included the ability to safely provide some type of continuity of care, especially for patients who were insured. Activities that required special equipment limited the extent to which specialized care could be provided by phone or video call [11].

Conclusion

Based on current knowledge, COPD by itself does not represent a risk for adverse outcomes from COVID-19. However, the association of COPD with other diseases (for example: obesity, type II diabetes, arterial hypertension) can be associated with a poor evolution of the disease. Broadly, it is recommended that patients continue their treatment according to current international guidelines, including inhaled and systemic medications. All the preventive measures recommended for the general population also apply to the COPD patient. Finally, the necessary adjustments must be made in each health system to ensure adequate monitoring of the disease.

Key Points

1. The expression of ACE2 and TMPRSS2 are increased in patients diagnosed with COPD, modulating the susceptibility of the individual and the clinical course of SARS-CoV-2 infection, so far it has not been concluded whether having COPD constitutes a greater risk of infection.
2. It is recommended to have a negative RT-PCR to perform lung function tests and invasive procedures such as bronchoscopy. In the event of an emergency with negative test available, the procedures must be carried out with the appropriate personal protective equipment.
3. It is recommended that the COPD patient continue treatment of stable disease with the medication considered by the attending physician. This includes LABA/LAMA/CSI. If possible, it is recommended to choose devices in DPI, soft mist or MDI presentation. All recommended vaccines must also be administered to prevent exacerbations.
4. In acute exacerbation of COPD of a cause other than SARS-CoV-2 infection, the use of systemic steroids is recommended, as well as evaluating the start of antibiotic treatment in suspected bacterial etiology.
5. Follow-up and self-care by telemedicine may be effective and safe in the management of patients diagnosed with COPD, without the need to go to a hospital unit, reducing the probability of SARS-CoV-2 infection.

References

[1] Salvi, Sundeep Santosh, Raja Dhar, P. A. Mahesh, Zarir Farooq Udwadia, Digambar Behra. "COPD Management during the COVID-19 pandemic." *Lung India: Official Organ of Indian Chest Society* vol. 38, Supplement (2021): S80-S85. doi: https://doi.org/10.4103/lungindia.lungindia_685_20.

[2] Higham, Andrew, Alexander Mathioudakis, Jørgen Vestbo, Dave Singh. "COVID-19 and COPD: a narrative review of the basic science and clinical outcomes." *European Respiratory Review: An Official Journal of the European Respiratory Society* vol. 29, 158 200199. 5 Nov. 2020, https://doi.org/10.1183/16000617.0199-2020/.

[3] Leung, Janice M., Masahiro Niikura, Cheng Wei Tony Yang, Don D. Sin. "COVID-19 and COPD." *The European Respiratory Journal* vol. 56, 2 2002108. 13 Aug. 2020, https://doi.org/10.1183/13993003.02108-2020.

[4] Martinez, Fernando J., David Mannino, Nancy Kline Leidy, Karen G. Malley, Elizabeth D. Bacci, R. Graham Barr, Russ P Bowler, MeiLan K. Han, Julia F. Houfek, Barry Make, Catherine A. Meldrum, Stephen Rennard, Byron Thomashow, John Walsh, Barbara P. Yawn, High-Risk-COPD Screening Study Group. "A New Approach for Identifying Patients with Undiagnosed Chronic Obstructive Pulmonary Disease." *American Journal of Respiratory and Critical Care Medicine* vol. 195, 6 (2017): 748-756. doi: https://doi.org/10.1164/rccm.201603-0622OC.

[5] Perez-Padilla, R., W. M. Vollmer, J. C. Vázquez-García, P. L. Enright, A. M. B. Menezes, A. S. Buist, BOLD and PLATINO Study. "Can a normal peak expiratory flow exclude severe chronic obstructive pulmonary disease?" *The International Journal of Tuberculosis and Lung Disease: The Official Journal of the International Union against Tuberculosis and Lung Disease* vol. 13, 3 (2009): 387-93.

[6] Aggarwal, Ashutosh N., Dheeraj Gupta, Surinder K. Jindal. "The relationship between FEV1 and peak expiratory flow in patients with airways obstruction is poor." *Chest* vol. 130, 5 (2006): 1454-61. doi: https://doi.org/10.1378/chest.130.5.1454.

[7] Llewellin, Peter, Gillian Sawyer, Simon Lewis, Soo Cheng, Mark Weatherall, Penny Fitzharris, Richard Beasley. "The relationship between FEV1 and PEF in the assessment of the severity of airways obstruction." *Respirology* (Carlton, Vic.) vol. 7, 4 (2002): 333-7. https://doi.org/10.1046/j.1440-1843.2002.00417.

[8] *Management of COPD during COVID-19: Ontario.* Toronto: Centre for Effective Practice and Department of Family and Community Medicine, University of Toronto. (July 2021).

[9] Elbeddini, Ali, and Yasamin Tayefehchamani. "Amid COVID-19 pandemic: Challenges with access to care for COPD patients." Research in social & administrative pharmacy: *RSAP* vol. 17, 1 (2021): 1934-1937. doi: https://doi.org/10.1016/j.sapharm.2020.06.002.

[10] Russell, Siân, Oladapo J. Ogunbayo, James J. Newham, Karen Heslop-Marshall, Paul Netts, Barbara Hanratty, Fiona Beyer and Eileen Kaner. "Qualitative systematic review of barriers and facilitators to self-management of chronic obstructive pulmonary disease: views of patients and healthcare professionals." *NPJ Primary Care Respiratory Medicine* vol. 28, 1 2. 17 Jan. 2018, doi: https://doi.org/10.1038/s41533-017-0069-z.

[11] Wu, Frances, Jenni Burt, Teena Chowdhury, Raymond Fitzpatrick, Graham Martin, Jan W. van der Scheer and John R. Hurst. "Specialty COPD care during COVID-19: patient and clinician perspectives on remote delivery." *BMJ Open Respiratory Research* vol. 8, 1 (2021): e000817. https://doi.org/10.1136/bmjresp-2020-000817.

[12] Yamaya, Mutsuo, Hidekazu Nishimura, Xue Deng, Mitsuru Sugawara, Oshi Watanabe, Kazuhiro Nomura, Yoshitaka Shimotai, Haruki Momma, Masakazu Ichinose, Tetsuaki Kawase. "Inhibitory effects of glycopyrronium, formoterol, and budesonide on coronavirus HCoV-229E replication and cytokine production by primary cultures of human nasal and tracheal epithelial cells." *Respiratory Investigation* vol. 58, 3 (2020): 155-168. doi: https://doi.org/10.1016/j.resinv.2019.12.005.

[13] Halpin, David M. G., Rosa Faner, Oriol Sibila, Joan Ramon Badia, Alvar Agusti. "Do chronic respiratory diseases or their treatment affect the risk of SARS-CoV-2 infection?" *The Lancet. Respiratory Medicine* vol. 8, 5 (2020): 436-438. doi: https://doi.org/10.1016/S2213-2600(20)30167-3.

[14] Leung, Janice M., Chen Xi Yang, Don D. Sin. "COVID-19 and nicotine as a mediator of ACE2." *The European Respiratory Journal* vol. 55, 6 2001261. 4 Jun. 2020, https://doi.org/10.1183/13993003.01261-2020.

[15] Guan, Wei-Jie, Zheng-yi Ni, Yu Hu, Wen-hua Liang, Chun-quan Ou, Jian-xing He, Lei Liu, Hong Shan, Chun-liang Lei, David S. C. Hui, Bin Du, Lan-juan Li, Guang Zeng, Kwok-Yung Yuen, Ru-chong Chen, Chun-li Tang, Tao Wang, Ping-yan Chen, Jie Xiang, Shi-yue Li, Jin-lin Wang, Zi-jing Liang, Yi-xiang Peng, Li Wei, Yong Liu, Ya-hua Hu, Peng Peng, Jian-ming Wang, Ji-yang Liu, Zhong Chen, Gang Li, Zhi-jian Zheng, Shao-qin Qiu, Jie Luo, Chang-jiang Ye, Shao-yong Zhu, and Nan-shan Zhong, for the China Medical Treatment Expert Group for COVID-19. "Clinical Characteristics of Coronavirus Disease 2019 in China." *The New England Journal of Medicine* vol. 382, 18 (2020): 1708-1720. doi: https://doi.org/10.1056/NEJMoa2002032.

[16] *Global Initiative for Asthma Strategy Document;* 2020. https://ginasthma.org/wp-content/uploads/2020/04/GINA-2020-full-report_-final-_wms.pdf. [Last accessed on 2020 Apr 25].

[17] Global Initiative for Chronic Obstructive Lung Disease. *Global Strategy for the Diagnosis, Management, and Prevention of Chronic Obstructive Pulmonary Disease 2022 report.*

[18] Bhutani, Mohit. Paul Hernandez, Jean Bourbeau, Gail Dechman, Erika Penz, Raymond Aceron, Marla Beauchamp, Joshua Wald, Michael Stickland, Sharla-Rae Olsen, and Donna Goodridge. "Key Highlights of the Canadian Thoracic Society's Position Statement on the Optimization of COPD Management During the Coronavirus Disease 2019 Pandemic." *Chest* vol. 158, 3 (2020): 869-872.

[19] Vardavas, Constantine I., and Katerina Nikitara. "COVID-19 and smoking: A systematic review of the evidence." *Tobacco Induced Diseases* vol. 18 20. 20 Mar. 2020, https://doi.org/10.18332/tid/119324.

[20] Mortazavi, Seyed Alireza, Joseph J. Bevelacqua, Payman Rafiepour, Abdol Karim Ghadimi-Moghadam, Pooya Saraie, Najmeh Jooyan, Seyedeh Hanieh Mortazavi, Seyed Mohammad Javad Mortazavi and James S. Welsh. "Revisiting the smoking paradox: radioactivity in tobacco smoke or suppression of the SARS-CoV-2 receptor, angiotensin-converting enzyme 2, via aryl-hydrocarbon

receptor signaling?" *Dose-response: A Publication of the International Hormesis Society* vol. 20.1 15593258221075111. April 1, 2022, doi: https://doi.org/10.1177/15593258221075111.

[21] Usman, Muhammad Shariq, Tariq Jamal Siddiqi, Muhammad Shahzeb Khan, Urvish K. Patel, Izza Shahid, Jawad Ahmed, Ankur Kalra, Erin D. Michos. "Is there a smoker's paradox in COVID-19?" *BMJ Evidence-Based Medicine* vol. 26, 6 (2021): 279-284. doi: https://doi.org/10.1136/bmjebm-2020-111492.

[22] Lacedonia, Donato, Giulia Scioscia, Carla Santomasi, Paolo Fuso, Giovanna Elisiana Carpagnano, Andrea Portacci, Franco Mastroianni, Giovanni Larizza, Eugenio Sabato, Emanuela Profilo, Emanuela Resta, Maria Pia Foschino Barbaro and Onofrio Resta. "Impact of smoking, COPD and comorbidities on the mortality of COVID-19 patients." *Scientific Reports* vol. 11, 1 19251. 28 Sep. 2021, https://doi.org/10.1038/s41598-021-98749-4.

Editor's Contact Information

Dr. Jaber S. Alqahtani, PhD, ACCP, CRT, AFHEA

Assistant Professor and Senior Specialist,
Department of Respiratory Care,
Prince Sultan Military College of Health Sciences,
Dammam, Saudi Arabia
Alqahtani-Jaber@hotmail.com

Index

B

C

D

E

F

G

H

I

L

M

N

O

P

Q

R

S

T

U

V

W